On Call Pediatrics

JAMES J. NOCTON, MD

Associate Professor of Pediatrics
Section of Rheumatology
Director, Pediatric Residency Training Program
Department of Pediatrics
Medical College of Wisconsin and the
  Children's Hospital of Wisconsin
Milwaukee, Wisconsin

RAINER G. GEDEIT, MD

Associate Professor of Pediatrics
Section of Critical Care
Associate Director, Pediatric Residency
  Training Program
Department of Pediatrics
Medical College of Wisconsin and the
  Children's Hospital of Wisconsin
Milwaukee, Wisconsin

*and the Pediatric Residents of Children's
Hospital of Wisconsin*

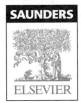

SAUNDERS

ELSEVIER

3rd edition

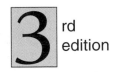

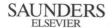

SAUNDERS
ELSEVIER

1600 John F. Kennedy Blvd.
Ste 1800
Philadelphia, PA 19103-2899

1004 966 700

ON CALL PEDIATRICS
Copyright © 2006 by Saunders, an imprint of Elsevier Inc.

ISBN-13: 978-1-4160-2393-7
ISBN-10: 1-4160-2393-3

Notice

Knowledge and best practice in this field are constantly changing. As new research and experience broaden our knowledge, changes in practice, treatment and drug therapy may become necessary or appropriate. Readers are advised to check the most current information provided (i) on procedures featured or (ii) by the manufacturer of each product to be administered, to verify the recommended dose or formula, the method and duration of administration, and contraindications. It is the responsibility of the practitioner, relying on their own experience and knowledge of the patient, to make diagnoses, to determine dosages and the best treatment for each individual patient, and to take all appropriate safety precautions. To the fullest extent of the law, neither the Publisher nor the Editors assume any liability for any injury and/or damage to persons or property arising out of or related to any use of the material contained in this book.

The Publisher

Previous editions copyrighted 2001, 1997.

Library of Congress Cataloging-in-Publication Data
On call: pediatrics / [edited by] James J. Nocton, Rainer G. Gedeit; and pediatric residents of Children's Hospital of Wisconsin. —3rd ed.
    p.;cm.
Includes index.
Rev. ed. of: On call : pediatrics / David A. Lewis, James J. Nocton. 2nd ed. ©2001.
ISBN 1-4160-2393-3
1. Pediatric emergencies—Handbooks, manuals, etc.
   [DNLM: 1. Pediatrics—Handbooks. 2. Child. 3. Emergencies—Handbooks. 4. Infant. WS 39 O58 2006] I. Title: Pediatrics. II. Nocton, James J. III. Gedeit, Rainer G. IV. Lewis, David, 1957—On call. V. Children's Hospital of Wisconsin.

RJ370.L49 2006
618.92—dc22

Acquisitions Editor: James Merritt
Developmental Editor: Nicole DiCicco
Publishing Services Manager: Linda Van Pelt
Project Manager: Linda Van Pelt
Cover Designer: Ellen Zanolle
Text Designer: Ellen Zanolle
Cover Art: Ellen Zanolle

Working together to grow
libraries in developing countries

www.elsevier.com | www.bookaid.org | www.sabre.org

ELSEVIER   BOOK AID International   Sabre Foundation

Printed in the United States of America

Last digit is the print number: 9 8 7 6 5 4 3 2 1

To all the children we care for, including our own—Amanda, Kay, Beth, and Claire Gedeit, and Jeff and Sara Nocton—who continue to be our greatest teachers; and to our wives, Margie Gedeit and Ellen Danto-Nocton, who have been consistently supportive of our endeavors to improve care for children.

T

Contributors

Elizabeth M. Galloway, MD

Senior Resident, Pediatrics
Children's Hospital of Wisconsin
Medical College of Wisconsin Affiliated Hospitals
Milwaukee, Wisconsin

Rainer G. Gedeit, MD

Associate Professor of Pediatrics
Section of Critical Care
Associate Director, Pediatric Residency Training Program
Department of Pediatrics
Medical College of Wisconsin and the Children's Hospital of Wisconsin
Milwaukee, Wisconsin

Wendy Z. Gavidia, MD

Senior Resident, Pediatrics
Children's Hospital of Wisconsin
Medical College of Wisconsin Affiliated Hospitals
Milwaukee, Wisconsin

Richard W. Hendershot, MD

Senior Resident, Pediatrics
Children's Hospital of Wisconsin
Medical College of Wisconsin Affiliated Hospitals
Milwaukee, Wisconsin

Tannaz G. Hild, MD

Senior Resident, Pediatrics
Children's Hospital of Wisconsin
Medical College of Wisconsin Affiliated Hospitals
Milwaukee, Wisconsin

Erica L. Kroncke, MD
Senior Resident, Pediatrics
Children's Hospital of Wisconsin
Medical College of Wisconsin Affiliated Hospitals
Milwaukee, Wisconsin

Rodney R. Mayhorn, MD
Senior Resident, Pediatrics
Children's Hospital of Wisconsin
Medical College of Wisconsin Affiliated Hospitals
Milwaukee, Wisconsin

David E. Melbye, MD
Senior Resident, Pediatrics
Children's Hospital of Wisconsin
Medical College of Wisconsin Affiliated Hospitals
Milwaukee, Wisconsin

David G. Meuler, MD
Senior Resident, Pediatrics
Children's Hospital of Wisconsin
Medical College of Wisconsin Affiliated Hospitals
Milwaukee, Wisconsin

Shenell Y. Miller, MD
Senior Resident, Pediatrics
Children's Hospital of Wisconsin
Medical College of Wisconsin Affiliated Hospitals
Milwaukee, Wisconsin

Thomas H. Nichols, MD
Senior Resident, Pediatrics
Children's Hospital of Wisconsin
Medical College of Wisconsin Affiliated Hospitals
Milwaukee, Wisconsin

James J. Nocton, MD
Associate Professor of Pediatrics
Section of Rheumatology
Director, Pediatric Residency Training Program
Department of Pediatrics
Medical College of Wisconsin and the Children's Hospital of
    Wisconsin
Milwaukee, Wisconsin

Erin C. Nunnold, MD

Senior Resident, Pediatrics
Children's Hospital of Wisconsin
Medical College of Wisconsin Affiliated Hospitals
Milwaukee, Wisconsin

Priya Pais, MD

Senior Resident, Pediatrics
Children's Hospital of Wisconsin
Medical College of Wisconsin Affiliated Hospitals
Milwaukee, Wisconsin

Ushma Patel, MD

Senior Resident, Pediatrics
Children's Hospital of Wisconsin
Medical College of Wisconsin Affiliated Hospitals
Milwaukee, Wisconsin

B. Joann Patterson, MD

Senior Resident, Pediatrics
Children's Hospital of Wisconsin
Medical College of Wisconsin Affiliated Hospitals
Milwaukee, Wisconsin

Marlene Peng, MD

Senior Resident, Pediatrics
Children's Hospital of Wisconsin
Medical College of Wisconsin Affiliated Hospitals
Milwaukee, Wisconsin

Lori A. Porter, DO

Senior Resident, Pediatrics
Children's Hospital of Wisconsin
Medical College of Wisconsin Affiliated Hospitals
Milwaukee, Wisconsin

Christopher J. Schwake, MD

Senior Resident, Pediatrics
Children's Hospital of Wisconsin
Medical College of Wisconsin Affiliated Hospitals
Milwaukee, Wisconsin

Rebecca S. Severe, MD
Senior Resident, Pediatrics
Children's Hospital of Wisconsin
Medical College of Wisconsin Affiliated Hospitals
Milwaukee, Wisconsin

Nosheen N. Shaikh, MD
Senior Resident, Pediatrics
Children's Hospital of Wisconsin
Medical College of Wisconsin Affiliated Hospitals
Milwaukee, Wisconsin

Caroline C. Shieh, MD
Senior Resident, Pediatrics
Children's Hospital of Wisconsin
Medical College of Wisconsin Affiliated Hospitals
Milwaukee, Wisconsin

Lacy E. Taylor, MD
Senior Resident, Pediatrics
Children's Hospital of Wisconsin
Medical College of Wisconsin Affiliated Hospitals
Milwaukee, Wisconsin

Heather L. Toth, MD
Senior Resident, Pediatrics
Children's Hospital of Wisconsin
Medical College of Wisconsin Affiliated Hospitals
Milwaukee, Wisconsin

Katrina R. Ubell, MD
Senior Resident, Pediatrics
Children's Hospital of Wisconsin
Medical College of Wisconsin Affiliated Hospitals
Milwaukee, Wisconsin

Teresa M. Uy, MD
Senior Resident, Pediatrics
Children's Hospital of Wisconsin
Medical College of Wisconsin Affiliated Hospitals
Milwaukee, Wisconsin

Kishore Vellody, MD
Senior Resident, Pediatrics
Children's Hospital of Wisconsin
Medical College of Wisconsin Affiliated Hospitals
Milwaukee, Wisconsin

Elizabeth A. Walenz, MD
Senior Resident, Pediatrics
Children's Hospital of Wisconsin
Medical College of Wisconsin Affiliated Hospitals
Milwaukee, Wisconsin

Keri A. Wheeler, MD
Senior Resident, Pediatrics
Children's Hospital of Wisconsin
Medical College of Wisconsin Affiliated Hospitals
Milwaukee, Wisconsin

Preface

We are pleased to have the opportunity to write this third edition of *On Call Pediatrics*. For this edition, we have changed the organization of some of the material and have included additional chapters that we believe will be helpful and will make the book a more comprehensive resource. A chapter on "Remembering Your ABCs" has been added, which we hope will help alleviate some of the fear that is experienced immediately after being summoned to care for a critically ill patient. A chapter on "Genitourinary Problems" has also been added to discuss some problems that had not been addressed in the previous editions. We have added a chapter on teaching while on call to address the needs of pediatric residents, who are often responsible for teaching students and other residents while attending to their own on-call responsibilities. Finally, the introductory chapters regarding communication have been revised and consolidated, and each of the problem-related chapters has been revised and updated.

The most significant change to this edition is that we have used the knowledge and practical expertise of the senior residents of the Children's Hospital of Wisconsin, who have contributed to the revisions of most of the chapters. There is no substitute for being on the "front lines," and we therefore believe that the contributions of the residents will make this book more practical and helpful, particularly to other pediatric residents.

Being on call is not just a necessary experience but is also a valuable educational undertaking for the resident or medical student. It is our intent that this book will be a helpful resource for those who are on call. We hope that by using this book, individuals who are on call will be able to provide the best care to their pediatric patients and will also learn in the process. The experience of being on call should not be one that simply has to be endured. It should be appreciated as an opportunity to help one's patients, an opportunity to improve one's skills and knowledge, and an opportunity to build one's confidence and independence. We hope that this book will contribute to these goals.

James J. Nocton, MD
Rainer G. Gedeit, MD

Acknowledgments

We are indebted to Robert M. Kliegman, MD, whose support and encouragement have made each edition of this book possible, and to Mr. Jim Merritt and Ms. Nicole DiCicco of Elsevier, whose patience and assistance were phenomenal during the preparation of this edition. We would also like to thank our colleagues at the Medical College of Wisconsin for their encouragement and understanding, and the residents of the Children's Hospital of Wisconsin, who continue to make teaching and writing worthwhile.

Structure of the Book

The book is divided into three main sections: I (introduction), II (patient-related problems), and III (laboratory-related problems).

Section I covers introductory material in five chapters: The Diagnosis and Management of On-Call Problems, Communicating with Colleagues and Families, Common Mistakes, Remembering Your ABCs, and Teaching (and Learning) While On Call.

Section II discusses the common calls associated with patient-related problems. Each problem is approached from its inception, beginning with the relevant questions that should be asked over the phone, the temporary orders that should be given, and the major life-threatening problems to be considered as one approaches the bedside. The setup of Section II is as follows.

PHONE CALL

Questions

Pertinent questions to assess the urgency of the situation.

Orders

Urgent orders to be carried out before the housestaff arrives at the bedside.

Inform RN

Nurse to be informed of the time the housestaff anticipates arrival at the bedside.

ELEVATOR THOUGHTS

The differential diagnosis to be considered by the housestaff while they are on their way to assess the patient (i.e., while they are in the elevator).

MAJOR THREAT TO LIFE

Identification of the major threat to life, which is essential in providing focus for the subsequent effective management of the patient.

BEDSIDE

Quick-Look Test

The quick-look test is a rapid visual assessment to place the patient into one of three categories: well, sick, or critical. This helps determine the necessity of immediate intervention.

Airway and Vital Signs

Selective History and Chart Review

Selective Physical Examination

MANAGEMENT

Section III contains the common calls associated with laboratory-related problems.

The Appendices consist of reference items that we have found useful in managing calls.

The On Call Formulary is a compendium of commonly used medications that are likely to be prescribed by the student or resident on call. The formulary serves as a quick, alphabetically arranged reference for indications, drug dosages, routes of administration, side effects, contraindications, and modes of action.

Commonly Used Abbreviations

ABCs	Airway, breathing, and circulation
ABD	Abdomen
ABG	Arterial blood gas
AC	Before meals
ACE	Angiotensin-converting enzyme
ACLS	Advanced cardiac life support
AIDS	Acquired immunodeficiency syndrome
ANA	Antinuclear antibody
A/P	Anteroposterior
aPTT	Activated partial thromboplastin time
ARDS	Adult respiratory distress syndrome
ASD	Atrial septal defect
ASO	Antistreptolysin O
AV	Atrioventricular
BID	Twice a day
BP	Blood pressure
BPD	Bronchopulmonary dysplasia
BPM	Beats per minute
BSA	Body surface area
CBC	Complete blood count
CF	Cystic fibrosis
CHF	Congestive heart failure

CMV	Cytomegalovirus
CNS	Central nervous system
CO	Cardiac output
CO_2	Carbon dioxide
CPK	Creatine phosphokinase
CSF	Cerebrospinal fluid
CT	Computed tomography
CVAT	Costovertebral angle tenderness
CVS	Cardiovascular system
CXR	Chest x-ray
DDAVP	Desmopressin
DIC	Disseminated intravascular coagulation
DKA	Diabetic ketoacidosis
D_5NS	5% dextrose in normal saline solution
DOE	Dyspnea on exertion
DVT	Deep venous thrombosis
D_5W	5% dextrose in water
$D_{25}W$	25% dextrose in water
ECG	Electrocardiogram
EEG	Electroencephalogram
ELISA	Enzyme-linked immunosorbent assay
ENT	Ears, nose, and throat
ESR	Erythrocyte sedimentation rate
EXT	Extremities
F_IO_2	Fraction of inspired oxygen
Fr	French (unit of measurement for catheters and tubes)
FUO	Fever of unknown origin
GI	Gastrointestinal
G-6-PD	Glucose-6-phosphate dehydrogenase
GU	Genitourinary
Hb	Hemoglobin
HCT	Hematocrit

HEENT	Head, eyes, ears, nose, and throat
HIV	Human immunodeficiency virus
HPI	History of present illness
Hr	Hour
HR	Heart rate
HS	At bedtime
HSV	Herpes simplex virus
HUS	Hemolytic-uremic syndrome
ICU	Intensive care unit
ICP	Intracranial pressure
IDDM	Insulin-dependent diabetes mellitus
IgG	Immunoglobulin G
IM	Intramuscular
INR	International normalized ratio
ITP	Idiopathic thrombocytopenic purpura
IV	Intravenous
IVIG	Intravenous immunoglobulin
JRA	Juvenile rheumatoid arthritis
LDH	Lactate dehydrogenase
LOC	Loss of consciousness
LP	Lumbar puncture
LV	Left ventricle
LVH	Left ventricular hypertrophy
MAO	Monoamine oxidase
MCV	Mean corpuscular volume
mm Hg	Millimeters of mercury
MRI	Magnetic resonance imaging
NEC	Necrotizing enterocolitis
NEURO	Neurologic system
NG	Nasogastric
NIDDM	Non–insulin-dependent diabetes mellitus
NPH	Neutral protamine Hagedorn (insulin)

NPO	Nothing by mouth
NS	Normal saline
NSAID	Nonsteroidal anti-inflammatory drug
O$_2$	Oxygen
Osm	Osmolality
P/A	Posteroanterior
PAC	Premature atrial contraction
PALS	Pediatric Advanced Life Support
PC	After meals
PCA	Patient-controlled analgesia
PCO$_2$	Partial pressure of carbon dioxide
PEEP	Positive end-expiratory pressure
PICU	Pediatric intensive care unit
PMI	Point of maximal intensity
PO	By mouth
PO$_2$	Partial pressure of oxygen
PPD	Purified protein derivative
PPHN	Persistent pulmonary hypertension of the newborn
PR	Per rectum
PRBCs	Packed red blood cells
PRN	As necessary
PT	Prothrombin time
PTH	Parathyroid hormone
PTT	Partial thromboplastin time
PVC	Premature ventricular contraction
Q	Each
QHS	Each night at bedtime
QID	Four times a day
RBC	Red blood cell
RESP	Respiratory system
RN	Registered nurse
RR	Respiratory rate

RSV	Respiratory syncytial virus
RTA	Renal tubular acidosis
RV	Right ventricle
RVH	Right ventricular hypertrophy
SBE	Subacute bacterial endocarditis
SC	Subcutaneous
Sec	Second
SI	International System of Units
SIADH	Syndrome of inappropriate antidiuretic hormone
SL	Sublingual
SLE	Systemic lupus erythematosus
SOB	Shortness of breath
STAT	Immediately
SVT	Supraventricular tachycardia
T_3	Triiodothyronine
T_4	Thyroxine
TB	Tuberculosis
TCA	Tricyclic antidepressants
TKVO	To keep vein open
TORCH	Toxoplasmosis, other infections, rubella, cytomegalovirus, herpes (congenital infections)
TPN	Total parenteral nutrition
TSH	Thyroid-stimulating hormone
TTP	Thrombotic thrombocytopenic purpura
UAC	Umbilical arterial catheter
URI	Upper respiratory infection
UTI	Urinary tract infection
UVC	Umbilical venous catheter
V/Q	Ventilation/perfusion
VSD	Ventricular septal defect
VT	Ventricular tachycardia
WBC	White blood cell
WPW	Wolff-Parkinson-White syndrome

Contents

Laboratory-Related Problems

Appendices

Introduction

1

The Diagnosis and Management of On-Call Problems

James J. Nocton, MD

The approach to the evaluation and management of problems that arise while on call is similar to that taken in other clinical situations. Initially, information about the patient and the specific problem must be collected. This information is acquired by obtaining a history, performing a physical examination, and reviewing pertinent laboratory data or imaging studies. While collecting information, the physician is considering possible diagnoses. Eventually, a diagnostic impression is formulated, and appropriate management is undertaken. Although this general scheme is identical to that used when admitting a new patient or evaluating a patient in the emergency department, the approach does need to be modified when one is informed about a problem that arises in a patient already in the hospital.

The primary distinction between the approach to an on-call problem and a problem in a "new" patient is that the goals are different. In most cases, patients who are in the hospital have already undergone a complete history and physical examination, a diagnostic impression has already been formulated regarding their problems at the time of admission, and management of these problems has begun. It is not the goal of the physician on call to repeat this process. Instead, the physician on call is expected to evaluate and manage acute problems that either are causing discomfort or have the potential to lead to deterioration in the patient's condition. It is appropriate to ask the question, "What might happen **today** that may be causing this problem and may adversely affect the patient?" When one is admitting multiple patients and is responsible for many others, time is always a factor. Some problems need to be given priority over others. Rarely does one have time to deliberate extensively about problems that are not going to lead to immediate harm to the patient. These problems can be addressed at a later time. In some cases, the cause of a problem may not be easily diagnosed, and specific management may therefore be deferred until the problem

3

"declares itself." This approach may be acceptable if one keeps in mind that the goals are to maintain the comfort of the patient and exclude (or empirically treat) potential causes of significant morbidity or mortality.

Because the goal of a physician on call is limited, the approach to a patient in whom a problem develops can be much more focused. One does not need to take a complete history or perform an exhaustive physical examination. Chart reviews may provide helpful information but should also be directed at answering specific questions. In many cases, historical information may have already been obtained during "sign-out." The sign-out process is the ideal time to enhance efficiency in managing on-call problems. Potential problems can often be anticipated by those who have been caring for a patient on a daily basis. Specific details about patients can be relayed to the on-call house officer, and management suggestions for anticipated problems can be discussed. Such a "sign-out" process can be extremely helpful, for example, when a recurrent problem develops and previously successful or unsuccessful management strategies have been used. The key to addressing on-call problems is **efficiency**. Being only as thorough as one needs to be and prioritizing appropriately allow one to be a successful physician on call.

The approach suggested in this book is designed to be efficient, yet thorough. For each problem, the sequence of thought processes that the physician should go through is discussed from the time that a problem is identified (usually with a phone call from a nurse) until the problem is managed. These thought processes are discussed in four separate parts for each chapter:

1. Phone call
2. Elevator thoughts
3. Major threat to life
4. Bedside

PHONE CALL

The phone call is usually how one first hears about a problem. The initial call should not simply be for notification but should also allow the physician to indirectly assess the severity of the problem, to begin developing a differential diagnosis, and when necessary, to begin management. In this section of each chapter, questions that should be asked **immediately**, before hanging up the phone, are listed. If the severity of the problem can be determined, the physician can then appropriately decide how to prioritize the call. If the severity cannot be determined, the patient needs to be seen fairly quickly. Orders that may enhance efficient evaluation or management are also suggested in this section, and other information important for the nurse to know is discussed, such as when the physician will arrive at the bedside.

Not every call requires that the physician evaluate the patient directly. For quick, minor problems that pose no immediate threat to the patient, taking a history from the nurse may be sufficient to allow one to determine appropriate management. In these instances, it is reasonable to ask the nurse, "Do you think I need to see the patient?" If there is any doubt in either the nurse's or the physician's mind, the patient should be seen.

ELEVATOR THOUGHTS

After the physician has finished discussing the problem with the nurse, some time is usually required to travel from another ward or call room to the patient's bedside. The time that it takes to walk or ride the elevator to see a patient can be used to reflect on the situation and to think about differential diagnoses. In this section of each chapter, the differential diagnosis for each problem is listed. The lists are not exhaustive but are intended to present the most common possibilities and those considered life threatening.

MAJOR THREAT TO LIFE

As part of the differential diagnosis, it is important for the physician on call to identify the possible diagnoses that are the most severe or potentially life threatening. One should ask, "What should I be considering that might be life threatening?" By asking this question, one ensures that even if definitive solutions are not found, the most serious possibilities have been considered and either excluded or empirically treated.

BEDSIDE

This section describes the approach that should be taken on arrival at the bedside. By this time, the chief complaint is known (the reason for the phone call from the nurse), possible diagnoses have been considered on the basis of the information available (elevator thoughts), and the major threat or threats to life have been identified (elevator thoughts). The steps to be taken at the bedside are presented in the following subsections in each chapter:

1. Quick-look test
2. Airway and vital signs
3. Selective history
4. Selective physical examination
5. Selective chart review
6. Management

The quick-look test and evaluation of the airway and vital signs should always be the first things done on arrival at the bedside, regardless of the complaint. The quick-look test involves an overall impression gained by observing the patient. The goal is to rapidly evaluate the patient's condition. The patient may appear comfortable and in no distress (e.g., sitting in bed having a conversation), mildly uncomfortable or distressed (e.g., crying, worried), or severely ill (e.g., comatose). Combined with evaluation of the airway and vital signs, the quick-look test enables the physician to determine the urgency of the situation and whether immediate intervention is necessary before obtaining a history and performing a physical examination. If the patient appears comfortable and has stable vital signs and an intact airway, the physician can proceed with less urgency. The sequence of the subsections describing the history, physical examination, chart review, and management varies among the chapters according to the problems presented. For some problems (e.g., hypotension and shock), some form of management probably needs to be undertaken before additional history is obtained or a selective chart review is performed. In other instances (e.g., constipation), the sequence is as expected, with management suggestions offered after suggestions regarding the history, physical examination, and chart review.

We believe that this approach to problems that may arise in a pediatric patient is helpful for the physician on call. As outlined here and presented in the individual chapters, this approach should provide an organized way for the physician to thoroughly and efficiently evaluate the common problems that arise in hospitalized pediatric patients.

Communicating with Colleagues and Families

James J. Nocton, MD

As with all other clinical situations, appropriate communication is an essential component of the evaluation and management of a patient while one is on call. The results of the evaluation and management of the problem, if any, must be effectively communicated to the patient, the family, the nurse, and others responsible for care of the patient. Communicating while on call occurs in two ways: (1) discussions in person or by telephone and (2) documentation in the patient's chart. When one is busy admitting patients and evaluating patients with problems, taking the time for appropriate communication and documentation may often seem less important than the actual process of caring for the patients. However, the time spent talking with families, discussing the patient with the nurse, writing a note, or making the extra phone call is much appreciated by everyone, including your colleagues who will resume responsibility for the patient in the morning.

Communicating with the child and usually the parents of the child will begin as soon as you arrive at the bedside and will continue until you have addressed the problem and answered the family's questions. The family of a child in the hospital is under great stress. Their child's illness is a tremendous source of worry and anguish and causes significant upheaval in their daily lives. When a problem arises on the weekend or at night, the family may feel lost without the usual physicians available to them and their child. They may feel as though no one knows what is happening with their child and may not trust that the physician on call will know what to do. It will be up to you to evaluate and manage the problem and to communicate to the family in a manner that is comforting, gains their trust, and reassures them that their child will receive excellent care, regardless of the day or the time.

Once you arrive to evaluate the child, you need to formally introduce yourself to the family and the child and address the family by name, not as "Mom" or "Dad." This takes very little time, but it may make a difference in how the family reacts to you. Explain who you are and why you have been called to see their child. Stating that you know why the child is in the hospital and what issues are being evaluated or treated during this hospitalization will reassure the family that you do know something about their child and will hopefully build their trust in you. Then proceed with your evaluation quickly and thoroughly.

After you have finished your selective examination, history, and chart review and have developed an assessment and plan of action, this should be communicated directly to the family. The family will want to know whether their child is becoming "sicker" or is in danger of becoming critically ill as a result of the problem for which you have been called. You will need to address these issues and inform the family if there appears to have been a change in the child's status. When the findings of your evaluation imply a serious change in the child's condition, the family needs to be informed in a clear, understandable, and honest manner. Bad news is always difficult to deliver. The physician must **never** delegate this duty to a student or nurse. If the family is not present, the on-call physician should contact the family by telephone promptly, introduce himself or herself clearly, and truthfully explain the situation to the family.

One decision that will need to be made when managing problems on call is when to notify a supervising resident or attending physician. This is a process that must be individualized. The status of the patient, the severity of the problem, and the experience and degree of comfort of the house officer are all factors that affect the decision to immediately notify others who are supervising care of the patient. Early in the first year of residency, nearly every problem is discussed immediately with a senior resident. As experience is gained, the physician on call is able to manage many of these problems independently, with discussion at a later time or at morning rounds. In some cases it is obvious that the senior resident must be notified, such as when a patient's condition changes significantly, transfer to an intensive care setting appears imminent, or diagnostic or therapeutic uncertainty exists. As a general rule, **if there is any doubt** regarding a problem that arises while one is on call, it is always best to discuss the problem with a senior resident. Knowing one's limitations is an extremely valuable asset that should not be forgotten while on call.

Deciding when to discuss problems immediately with attending physicians is often more difficult. One has a tendency to "not want to bother them" if they are not in the hospital. One may also fear appearing foolish or inadequate because one could not evaluate and manage the problem without calling them. These notions should be dismissed, and the same general rule described for senior residents should hold true for attending physicians as well: **if there is any doubt**, make the phone call. Responsible attending physicians always want to know immediately of changes in their patients' status and always want to be part of diagnostic and therapeutic decisions. The same is true for consulting physicians. If a subspecialty consultant's advice will help in the evaluation or management of a problem, the subspecialist should be called, regardless of the hour. By adopting this approach, physicians on call soon realize that they are not really alone. Senior residents, attending physicians, and consultants are only as far as the phone, a thought that can be very comforting in the middle of the night.

Discussing problems and their management with the nurse caring for the child is also essential. In many instances, the nurse knows the patient well, may have more experience with specific problems, and has seen how others have managed similar problems successfully. The nurse can be a great resource in these circumstances and may be able to offer very helpful suggestions. Listening to the nurse, involving the nurse in the decision-making process, and keeping the nurse informed of your plans will allow you to provide the best care to the patient and will keep everyone "on the same page," thereby minimizing the potential for errors.

Regardless of whether a particular problem requires immediate discussion or notification of others, documentation of the problem, the evaluation, and the action taken is mandatory. With the exception of minor problems that can be resolved over the phone without seeing the patient, all other problems require at least some documentation. It is extremely helpful for those caring for the patient on a daily basis to know what happened in the middle of the night and to have access to such information via the patient's chart. The written documentation of the evaluation and management of a problem that arises while one is on call can take several forms. Simple problems may require only a few sentences. For example,

> Called to see patient for sore throat. Patient afebrile, HR 84, RR 20, BP 120/75. Appeared comfortable. No complaints other than throat. Posterior pharynx slightly erythematous with patches of exudate on tonsils. Mild cervical adenopathy. Obtained throat culture. Will not administer antibiotics until results of culture known.

For other problems (e.g., new fever in an immunocompromised patient), a more extensive note may be required, and the **SOAP** format generally works well—listing the **s**ubjective complaint, **o**bjective findings, **a**ssessment, and **p**lan of management. One should be as concise as possible, describing only as much historical, subjective information as is essential and providing a brief summary of your assessment and management plan. It is necessary to perform and document only the pertinent parts of the physical examination. The goal is to notify those who will be seeing the patient the following day that a problem arose and that the problem was evaluated. As with all other types of documentation, notes should be dated **and** timed. All procedures should be described. If the problem was discussed with the family, attending physician, or consultants, this should be documented along with the time that the discussion took place. Finally, your name should be signed clearly or printed, followed by a phone or pager number. If someone has a question regarding what happened in the middle of the night, that person should be able to reach you easily.

Discussing problems with colleagues and families and documenting the evaluation and management of problems are tasks that are easy to ignore when one is on call and extremely busy. However, maintaining communication should be a priority. Communicating with the family promptly, honestly, and in person when possible is essential. Communicating with senior colleagues in all situations in which there is any doubt is in the patient's best interest. By documenting problems, you are helping your colleagues and others caring for the patient. Through verbal communication and documentation, you can also remind yourself that you are never alone when you are on call.

Common Mistakes

James J. Nocton, MD

Everyone makes mistakes. Although some mistakes are the result of fatigue and lack of sleep, the most common mistakes are made by physicians in a hurry. Therefore, many mistakes are preventable. This chapter briefly discusses a few of the most common and most preventable errors made in the care of hospitalized children, including

- Illegible signatures
- Poorly written orders
- Failure to communicate with the nurse
- Failure to communicate with the attending physician
- Failure to listen to the family
- Failure to document in the chart while on call

The issue of handwriting legibility is enormous and is one of the factors driving the move to electronic medical records. Illegible orders may lead to medication errors, patient morbidity, and unnecessary deaths. Illegible writing is inexcusable and indefensible and only makes more work for the physician on call. You will be forced to answer innumerable calls and pages from nurses, pharmacists, and other members of the health care team to clarify what they cannot read clearly. Illegibility wastes your time and erodes the confidence of others in your ability. It starts with your signature. Every time you sign your name, especially to orders, you should print your name and your pager number immediately below the signature so that there is no question about who has written the order or whom to call with a question. Not doing so is just being lazy. You have the time. As the saying goes, "Just do it!"

The way you write orders is also important. Calls requesting clarification of confusing or incomplete orders will plague you and eat away at your time if you do not take this issue seriously. Write every order so that any 10-year-old could accurately interpret what is requested. Be meticulous. **Write the weight of the patient on every order sheet**. Specify the preparation of any medication, the dose, the route of administration, and the dosing frequency clearly. Be extra careful about decimal points! Always precede a decimal point by a 0 when prescribing less than a milligram, for example, digoxin, **0.25** mg by mouth every day. Never follow the tenths or hundredths place with a 0; for example, captopril, **6.250** mg, could be misread easily

11

as 6,250 mg. Try to avoid abbreviations. Instead of writing "qd" or "bid," write "once a day" or "twice a day." When ordering a liquid preparation, write the concentration of the liquid as well as the amount to be given.

Another way to save yourself time and get things started for your patient is to communicate what you have ordered directly to the nurse. Having the nurse review the orders allows immediate clarification and prevents annoyingly time-consuming pages and clarification calls later. It also facilitates prompt and appropriate action on those orders by the nursing staff and other ancillary personnel.

As mentioned in Chapter 2, Communicating with Colleagues and Families, communication with the attending physician should never be delegated to the nurse or student in any emergency situation. Remember that notification of laboratory data or test results does not always require a telephone conversation. Do not hesitate to fax results and your analysis or plan of action to the office with a note to page you with any questions. Faxing information provides written notification but allows attending physicians to act at their convenience, and you will not have to wait on hold while they are interrupted during office hours. Remember, if you think that the attending physician **might** want to know, **make the call, send a fax, communicate!**

The same policy applies for the family. The more willing you are to communicate with the family, the more confident they will be having you care for their child. Families have many reasons for being present with their child in the hospital and equally many reasons why they sometimes cannot be with their child. Do not judge them. Involve them in their child's care and communicate freely, frequently, and honestly. No family has ever complained or filed a lawsuit because they were told **too much** or because people in the hospital communicated **too often** with them.

Finally, as discussed in Chapter 2, if you go to the effort of evaluating a patient when on call or if you spend time communicating with the attending physician or the family, **write a note!** It only takes a moment to write, "Asked to evaluate [*the patient's name*] for [*fever, chest pain, wheezing, etc.*]. Vital signs stable. Cardiorespiratory exam normal. No signs of sepsis, shock, or meningitis. Tylenol ordered for fever control. No studies at this time. Attending notified [*or will be notified in* AM]. Discussed with family." Always record the date **and time** in on-call documentation. Charting on-call encounters not only is for your protection but also serves a vital role in communicating with the team caring for the patient during the daytime. **It is too important to neglect**.

Each of these mistakes occurs when physicians become hasty, and none of these actions is so time consuming that you can afford to postpone or ignore them. Each is a fundamental part of conscientious care and ultimately improves your efficiency. Improved efficiency will give you the time to call home, grab dinner, shower before rounds, or even catch a little sleep.

Remembering Your ABCs

Rainer G. Gedeit, MD

Nothing strikes fear in a house officer more than the "code page." When the "code team" is activated, there is a flurry of activity not seen at any other time or place in the hospital. The "code team" responds, as does everyone else within earshot of the page. A frenzied group of doctors, nurses, medical students, respiratory therapists, chaplains, pharmacists, phlebotomists, security guards, and anyone else who is curious enough to see what the commotion is all about show up. The team awaits orders from the "team leader." As you view the chaotic scene of a cardiac arrest in the hospital, many people are busy doing things but may not truly be helping. When you arrive at the scene, you must not be one of these people. You need to be caring for the patient, not getting in the way. The most important thing to remember comes from the novel *House of God* by Samuel Shem, MD. "AT A CARDIAC ARREST, THE FIRST PROCEDURE IS TO TAKE YOUR OWN PULSE!" Stop, take a breath, assess the situation, determine what you should be doing, and do it. Your role in the "code" will depend on the situation. You may be the first person on the scene, the first MD on the scene, the fifth MD on the scene, or the team leader. Think about what you need to do and do it. If you are not needed, move away.

THE BASICS

When you walk into a code situation, the things you learned in kindergarten will come in handy. Go back and think about the ABCs. You will probably not know the patient in front of you or why that patient is dying; that is not what is important. The thing to do is to try to reverse that process. Whether the patient you were examining just stopped breathing or you have responded to the "code page," the same response is required.

A = Airway

See whether the patient responds to stimulation. Call the child's name or gently shake the child; if there is no response, open the airway. A jaw thrust or chin lift along with placing the patient supine is the first thing to do. Make sure that suction equipment is available in case the child vomits or has excessive airway secretions. If it is not within reach, direct someone to get the equipment needed.

B = Breathing

Is the patient breathing? Look, listen, and feel. Is the chest rising, can you feel air moving in and out, are there breath sounds? If yes, maintain the airway and assess for cardiac output. If the patient is not breathing, begin assisted breathing. Most hospital rooms will have some type of resuscitation device (know where these are in your institution), or the "code cart" that should have been brought to the bedside will have a self-inflating bag and mask. Get the correct size mask and begin respirations. If this is not available, begin mouth-to-mouth or mouth-to-mask rescue breathing. Two people are often needed to accomplish effective breathing: one to open the airway and hold the mask in place and the other to ventilate with the bag. Once intubation equipment arrives, an artificial airway should be placed. This is the best way to assist breathing and can be used as a portal to deliver drugs if intravenous (IV) access is absent. The size of endotracheal tube that should be used can be estimated by the formula (age in years/4) + 4. Make sure that all the equipment works before attempting intubation. Nothing is worse than placing a laryngoscope and having a dead light bulb.

C = Circulation

This is the most difficult part of the entire assessment. Feeling a weak pulse in an infant who is receiving artificial respirations is difficult, if not impossible. Your own adrenaline is rushing and your hand is shaking. Take time to feel multiple areas for a pulse (brachial, femoral, carotid). If there is no pulse, begin chest compressions. Use the appropriate rate and method for the patient's age and size.

Placement of an IV catheter is required for drug delivery. Using a large vein such as the antecubital should be attempted. If a catheter is already in place, flush it to ensure patency. Placing a second IV catheter is never wrong, in case the first one fails. Place the largest catheter possible. If an IV catheter cannot be placed within 15 to 30 seconds, place an intraosseous catheter.

As the basics are started, it is important to get an idea of what might have precipitated this event. Someone familiar with the patient (nurse, medical student, resident) must be available to consult with the team leader, and the chart must be brought to the bedside. Always show up if a patient you know is in trouble.

If you are the team leader, you must take control of the situation at the bedside. Your job is to ask for information and request that medications be given, as well as control flow in the room. The most difficult part of running the "code" is keeping control. Keep control of your own emotions; a panicked leader makes a panicked team. Make sure that everyone in the room is supposed to be there. Excuse extraneous persons. If there are persistent "pests," give these people a job to do to keep them out of the way. The best team leader I ever saw was a senior resident who looked the extraneous personnel in the eye and gave them each a job to do, outside the room (get ice for labs, get the chart, check on the family, get equipment for a blood draw). This left only the needed team members in the room. Make sure that those performing ventilation and chest compressions are doing an adequate job, and replace them every few minutes as they fatigue (performing cardiopulmonary resuscitation [CPR] is physically and emotionally draining).

As a team member, know your role (perform CPR, get information, place an IV line, ventilate the patient, communicate with the family). Do that job until you are told otherwise, or tell the leader that you cannot perform the assigned duty or are becoming fatigued (while performing CPR).

In some institutions, rapid-response extracorporeal support is possible. Know your institution's policies and procedures so that this resource can be activated. Know what the response time will be and what needs to be done to prepare the patient.

If the child is successfully resuscitated, transfer to a higher level of care is required. The pediatric intensive care unit (PICU) should be notified of the patient's condition and needs (ventilator, pressors, etc.). The team leader should accompany the patient to inform the accepting team in the PICU of the situation.

The outcome of resuscitation becomes less favorable as time goes on. At some point the team leader must "call the code." This is the worst time for any physician, and how to do this is important. Verify how long the code has been ongoing, what medications were given, and that there has been no response to resuscitation. Make sure all agree that the code is to be stopped. Thank everyone for their hard work. Stay with the patient and help clean up. If the doctors help when it is over, it makes it easier for everyone, including yourself.

When a code is over, whether the patient survived or not, those involved are shaken. Take time to decompress. Get a drink of water, coffee, or soda. Talk with those involved. At times a formal debriefing may be needed, and most institutions can accommodate this. Ask about a debriefing if you think it is needed.

Remember that the most common reason for a pediatric cardiac arrest is progression of respiratory disease and that it usually has a poor outcome. Prevention is the key.

Teaching (and Learning) While on Call

James J. Nocton, MD

Although the first priority for physicians on call is always to care for the patients, the hours spent on call are also of tremendous educational value. Every question, every call from a nurse, every discussion with a family, and every problem provide you with opportunities to learn something new and to share things you already know. The number of questions received from nurses and families, the number of patients who require evaluation, and the number of problems that you will need to manage will usually be far greater while you are on call than at other times. Although you will probably be very busy responding to these situations, your on-call experience will be much more rewarding and useful to you if you remember to make an effort to teach, as well as remember to learn, while you are taking care of patients.

Teaching while on call may initially seem to be an impossible task. You may ask yourself, "How will I possibly find time to teach when I will be taking care of so many patients, getting so many pages, admitting so many new patients, and evaluating the other problems that will invariably arise?" The answer to this question involves understanding something about adult learning and using some very effective methods of efficient teaching. Most of us think of teaching as the active process of sharing information and learning as the passive process of receiving information from the teacher. This is how we recall most of our formal education, with heavy emphasis on "the lecture." Needless to say, it will generally be impossible for you to plan on giving lectures while you are on call, and as it turns out, this is not a very effective way for adults to learn anyway. Adults learn best when they are invested in the learning process and take an active role in their own education. Therefore, the optimal way to teach is to allow your learners to be actively involved in everything you are doing. When evaluating a problem, evaluate it together with your student: inform the student of the problem as it was presented to you, and give the student an opportunity to think about it.

Most importantly, give students an opportunity to **commit** to a specific plan of action, whether it be diagnostic testing, treatment, or both. Whenever possible, do this before informing the student of your own plan of action. It is the **commitment** on the part of students that gets them actively invested in the learning process and permits you to teach more effectively. Once a student has thought the problem through independently, developed an assessment, and formulated a plan, you are then in a position to discuss that student's thought process and explain why or why not the assessment and plan are appropriate. You will be a better teacher, and your student will learn far more in this way than if you simply told the student what should be done.

Two specific types of teaching can be very effective when time is at a premium. The first is known as "priming." Priming involves setting a specific expectation for learners before engaging them actively in the learning process. For example, if you are called to see a child who has a sudden onset of abdominal pain, you might ask your student, "When we go in to examine this patient, how will we determine whether or not this may be appendicitis?" The student can then respond, hopefully with a reasonable answer, and you can comment on the answer and then proceed to examine the patient. This process should not take a great deal of time, it allows you to teach about a specific topic (the expected physical findings in someone with appendicitis), and it permits the learner to be invested in the learning process by making a commitment in responding to your question.

"Modeling" is an even more efficient method of teaching. Modeling is a more passive learning process than priming, but it can also be very effective; it involves preparing the student for a specific behavior or skill that you are about to demonstrate. For example, if you are called to a child's room by the nurse because the child has a high fever, you may say to the student, "I want you to watch how I discuss the significance of a fever with this child's parents." Modeling requires that you choose a specific teaching point and make sure that the student focuses on learning about this specific topic. In this case, the teaching point is the significance of fever and how to explain it to families. You will be discussing many other issues when you go into the room to see the patient, but your student will understand what you would like him or her to learn from this individual patient interaction. You have been able to teach, while not spending any more time than you would have had the student not been present.

When teaching an adult learner, particularly when using priming or modeling as a teaching method, it is important to keep two additional things in mind. First, teaching needs to occur at a suitable level for the learner. It may be appropriate to ask an average third-year medical student about the expected physical findings in someone with abdominal pain and appendicitis. It may not be appropriate, even for the most advanced third-year student, to ask about the expected physical findings, genetics, and treatment of familial Mediterranean fever. Of course, students will vary with regard to their knowledge and skill, and you will need to determine the individual level that is appropriate for each student. This can be accomplished by asking students questions and evaluating the appropriateness of their responses. Initially, the questions may be very basic or super-ficial ("What are the physical findings in appendicitis?"). If the student answers the initial questions easily, you can then determine the depth of the student's understanding by asking additional ques-tions ("What are the expected laboratory and radiographic findings in appendicitis? Which patients should be taken to surgery? What is the prognosis and long-term outcome of appendicitis?"). In this way, you should be able to roughly determine the appropriate level at which to teach.

The second principle to keep in mind is that teaching should involve general rules that will be relevant to all learners. Physical examination of the abdomen is a skill that nearly every physician will need. Teaching about the genetics of familial Mediterranean fever may be interesting, but it will not necessarily be relevant to most medical students. They will remember a general rule that they are able to apply repeatedly to the care of their future patients. They will forget the specific minutiae regarding a rare disease that they are unlikely to see very often.

As you are making efforts to teach while on call, you may not realize quite how much you have learned. When called regarding a problem that you have never been confronted with before, you may need to quickly review a textbook or an on-line database for information. You may need to call your supervising resident or attending physician. You may need to discuss the problem with a consultant. It is to your educational benefit to take advantage of as many of these resources as you can, as time permits. Sharing what you are learning from these resources with your student will sharpen your understanding of the problem. Reviewing published informa-tion and discussing the problem with those who have more experi-ence will also enable you to feel reassured regarding your evaluation and treatment of the patient.

Much of the learning that you will experience while on call will occur as you discuss problems with those supervising you, either while you are on call or at a later time, such as during morning rounds. Presenting your patients at rounds and discussing how you evaluated and managed problems will give you an opportunity to ask how others might have proceeded in certain situations. This will permit you to reflect on your own decisions and allow you to ask the question to yourself, "What could I have done differently?" By doing so, you will increase your knowledge, improve your decision-making, and improve the care you will provide to your patients the next time you are on call.

Teaching (and learning) can occur while you are on call. All that is required is some effort on the part of the teacher and willingness to invest in learning by the student. Hopefully, this chapter has explained how teaching can be very effective without taking a great deal of time away from patient care responsibilities. By making the effort to teach, the physician on call can make the on-call experience more educational, rewarding, and satisfying.

Patient-Related Problems

Abdominal Pain

Elizabeth A. Walenz, MD

Abdominal pain in a hospitalized pediatric patient should **always** be evaluated promptly. Although it is an extremely common and often benign complaint in all children, abdominal pain should never be dismissed as insignificant until a thorough evaluation has excluded potentially serious causes. In addition, abdominal pain should not be empirically treated with analgesics until a thorough evaluation has determined that the patient does not have a surgical or other life-threatening condition. In some instances, the cause of the abdominal pain may not be clear. After an initial evaluation, it may be necessary to adopt an expectant approach that involves performing serial examinations at regular intervals, prescribing analgesics when necessary for discomfort, and continuing to consider possible diagnoses until the cause becomes clear or the pain resolves.

PHONE CALL

Questions

1. How old is the patient?
2. Why is the patient in the hospital?
3. What are the patient's vital signs?
4. How does the patient rate the pain?
5. How long has it been present?
6. Is it localized?
7. Does the child have any nausea, vomiting, or diarrhea?
8. Has the child complained of abdominal pain previously during this admission?

The patient's vital signs, the degree of severity, and the duration of pain allow the physician to quickly determine the urgency of the situation. Stable vital signs with mild pain present for several hours do not imply an acute intra-abdominal process. The location of the pain, the age of the child, the underlying diagnosis, and any associated symptoms allow you to begin to consider a specific diagnosis. Previous complaints may signal that an evaluation has been performed before or that the cause of the pain is known.

Orders

1. **NPO.** The patient should have nothing by mouth (NPO) until further evaluated.
2. **Place IV.** If pain is severe and the vital signs indicate shock (tachycardia and hypotension), an intravenous (IV) line should be placed and a 20-mL/kg bolus of isotonic fluid (normal saline or lactated Ringer's solution) should be infused.

Inform RN

If the pain is severe or the vital signs make you concerned about an intra-abdominal emergency or shock, alert the RN that the patient will be evaluated immediately. If the pain is mild and vital signs are normal, the nurse should be informed of when you expect to see the patient.

ELEVATOR THOUGHTS

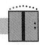

On your way to evaluate the patient, you can contemplate the many causes of abdominal pain. One useful way of remembering this long list is to think of the location of the organs within the abdomen, pelvis, and retroperitoneum and the potential pathologic processes that may affect each organ. There are two types of pain in relation to organs: pain at the site of the organ and referred pain. When abdominal pain is generalized or cannot be localized (e.g., in an infant or toddler), all causes are possible and should be considered. It is also important to think of not only the organs within the abdomen but also the vessels that supply the organs because interruption of the blood supply can lead to pain.

It should also be remembered that abdominal pain may result from systemic metabolic abnormalities (e.g., diabetic ketoacidosis, porphyria), as well as processes at distant anatomic sites (e.g., streptococcal pharyngitis, pneumonia):

Epigastric pain	Aortic dissection
	Carditis (pericarditis, myocarditis)
	Pancreatitis
	Peptic ulcer (perforation)
	Gastroesophageal reflux (heartburn)
	Gastritis
	Esophagitis
Left upper quadrant pain	Splenic rupture
	Splenic infarct
	Splenic abscess
	Subphrenic abscess
Right upper quadrant pain	Hepatitis
	Cholecystitis
	Biliary obstruction (gallstones)

Right upper quadrant pain—Cont'd	Liver abscess
	Subphrenic abscess
	Fitz-Hugh–Curtis syndrome (gonococcal perihepatitis)
Left lower quadrant pain	Ovarian torsion
	Mittelschmerz (ovulation)
	Psoas abscess
	Ectopic pregnancy
	Renal stone
	Colitis (infectious or inflammatory)
	Incarcerated hernia
	Typhlitis
Right lower quadrant pain	Appendicitis
	Ruptured appendix/abscess
	Mesenteric adenitis
	Ovarian torsion
	Psoas abscess
	Ectopic pregnancy
	Pelvic inflammatory disease
	Renal stone
	Incarcerated hernia
Hypogastric pain	Cystitis
	Bladder obstruction
	Ovarian torsion
	Pelvic inflammatory disease
	Testicular torsion
Generalized pain	Any of the preceding conditions
	Constipation
	Gastroenteritis
	Viral infection (e.g., mononucleosis)
	Inflammatory bowel disease
	Lactose intolerance
	Vasculitis (Henoch-Schönlein purpura, polyarteritis nodosa, systemic lupus erythematosus)
	Mesenteric thrombosis (resulting in ischemic bowel)
	Trauma (including child abuse)
	Lower lobe pneumonia
	Pharyngitis
	Diskitis
	Porphyria
	Bezoar
	Peritonitis
	Sterile peritonitis (systemic juvenile rheumatoid arthritis, familial Mediterranean fever, lupus)
	Hereditary angioedema

Generalized pain— Cont'd	Abdominal epilepsy
	Abdominal migraine
	Tumor
	Adrenal insufficiency
	Bowel obstruction (volvulus, malrotation)
	Superior mesenteric artery syndrome
	Sickle cell crisis
	Pregnancy
	Meckel's diverticulum (with secondary intussusception)
	Intussusception
	Behavioral (somatization)

MAJOR THREAT TO LIFE

- Perforated viscus
- Ischemic bowel (e.g., from volvulus, intussusception, or vasculitis)
- Infectious peritonitis (with or without a perforated viscus)
- Ectopic pregnancy
- Splenic rupture
- Pericardial tamponade or myocarditis
- Aortic dissection

The biggest concern is shock. Exsanguination and infection are the most worrisome immediate sequelae of the possible causes just listed because hypovolemic or septic shock may occur quickly. Cardiogenic shock may also occur if severe pericarditis or myocarditis is the cause of the abdominal pain.

BEDSIDE

How Does the Patient Look?

Does the patient appear comfortable, uncomfortable, or severely ill?

An uncomfortable or severely ill patient should be examined immediately to look for signs of peritonitis. If peritonitis is suspected, antibiotic treatment, IV fluids, and surgical evaluation may be needed as soon as possible. In general, patients with peritonitis appear uncomfortable and may prefer to lie motionless and avoid any movement of the peritoneum. A patient who has recently ruptured a viscus (e.g., a perforated appendix) may actually suddenly appear more comfortable because the painful pressure and obstruction have been relieved. The degree of discomfort may also be intermittent, as in the case of intussusception or renal colic, with episodic pain being punctuated by periods of relative comfort. An infant or a child who has been receiving narcotics or steroids may appear deceptively comfortable despite a significant intra-abdominal pathologic condition. It is important to obtain a medication history.

Airway and Vital Signs

Hypotension and tachycardia are signs that septic, hypovolemic, or cardiogenic shock may be present. Fever and abdominal pain should raise suspicion regarding infectious causes, which could be relatively mild (gastroenteritis) or life threatening (peritonitis). Tachypnea suggests pneumonia or an attempt to compensate for a metabolic acidosis associated with diabetes, shock, or ischemic bowel. If a patient has abdominal pain and is tachypneic with shallow respirations, the patient may be splinting secondary to the pain.

Selective History

When gathering information about pain in any location, including the abdomen, precise characterization of the pain is essential.

Duration: How long has the pain been present?
   If the pain has been ongoing for several days, most likely it is not an intra-abdominal emergency. Acute onset or sudden worsening of chronic pain is concerning and warrants immediate evaluation.

Location: Where is the pain? Does it radiate? Has it changed location?
   As noted earlier, the location of the pain may help narrow the diagnostic possibilities. Pain moving from the umbilicus to the right lower quadrant is strongly suggestive of appendicitis. Pain radiating to the shoulder suggests pericarditis or irritation of the diaphragm, as with a subphrenic abscess, perforated ulcer, or irritation of the capsule of the liver (Fitz-Hugh–Curtis syndrome). Pain radiating to the back may occur with aortic dissection or pancreatitis. Pain with radiation to the groin suggests ureteral irritation, as with renal stones. In young children, the response to "Where does it hurt?" invariably involves pointing directly to the umbilicus and therefore may be less reliable than in older patients.

Character: Is the pain aching, burning, crushing, or sharp? Is it constant or intermittent? Does it vary in intensity? What makes it feel better? Worse?
   Esophagitis, gastritis, or peptic ulcers may often be described as burning. Aching pain generally indicates a more diffuse or distant cause (e.g., pneumonia, porphyria), whereas sharp pain tends to be indicative of a more localized process. Biliary or renal colic and intussusception may cause severe but intermittent pain. If walking or moving seems to provide relief, peritonitis is much less likely.

Associated symptoms: Does the child have any related symptoms?
   If diarrhea is present, infectious causes need to be considered further. In children, vomiting may occur with any intra-abdominal process but should raise suspicion of infection or bowel obstruction. Bloody vomiting is strongly suggestive of gastritis, esophagitis, or an ulcer. Bilious or fecal vomiting implies bowel obstruction. Dark black stools are suggestive of bleeding in the upper

gastrointestinal (GI) tract. Grossly bloody stools indicate bleeding in the lower GI tract. Constipation may cause pain by itself, particularly in young children, or may also be a sign of bowel obstruction. Pharyngitis, coughing, rashes, headache, and other systemic symptoms may likewise help with the differential diagnosis. If the child has been eating normally and appears well, the likelihood of a significant problem is very small.

Selective Physical Examination

Vital signs	Hypotension may ensue rapidly; therefore, repeating blood pressure and other vital sign measurements is a good idea. Remember that in infants and young children, tachycardia alone may be indicative of shock. By increasing the heart rate, cardiac output can be enhanced enough to maintain "normal" blood pressure; hypotension may not occur until relatively late in the course of septic or hypovolemic shock.
HEENT	Scleral icterus (suggestive of hyperbilirubinemia and possible liver disease), pharyngeal erythema or exudate (streptococcal infection, infectious mononucleosis), periorbital edema (angioedema).
Neck	Adenopathy (streptococcal pharyngitis, mononucleosis), jugular venous distention (cardiac tamponade).
Chest	Rales, wheezes, decreased breath sounds (pneumonia, congestive heart failure [CHF] from myocarditis, pericarditis).
Heart	Muffled or distant heart sounds (pericardial effusion), friction rub (pericarditis).
Abdomen	1. *Observe.* Protuberance may be a sign of bowel obstruction, ascites, or an intra-abdominal mass (intussusception, hernia). 2. *Auscultate.* The purpose of auscultation is twofold. You can begin to listen to the abdomen but also lightly palpate simultaneously. The absence of bowel sounds is consistent with ileus (which may occur with any condition) or obstruction. 3. *Palpate.* Rigidity, rebound tenderness, and guarding all suggest peritonitis. Localized tenderness may be present even if the pain is described as generalized. A fluid wave may be palpable if ascites is present.

Abdomen—Cont'd	Cautiously palpate the liver and spleen because an enlarged spleen may be more easily ruptured.
	4. *Percuss.* Evaluate the size of the liver. Shifting dullness is indicative of ascites.
Rectal	Tenderness (appendicitis, pelvic inflammatory disease), impacted stool (constipation), positive occult blood test result (gastritis, bleeding peptic ulcer, ischemic bowel, Meckel's diverticulum, inflammatory bowel disease, intussusception, vasculitis). **Note: A patient with abdominal pain has not been fully evaluated without a rectal examination!**
Genitourinary	All adolescent girls should undergo a pelvic examination for any unexplained abdominal pain (pelvic inflammatory disease, ectopic pregnancy); prepubescent and pubescent boys should undergo testicular examination (torsion, edema associated with vasculitis).
Skin	Rashes (vasculitis, lupus, systemic juvenile rheumatoid arthritis, scarlet fever), Cullen's sign (purpuric discoloration of the skin of the abdomen seen in hemorrhagic pancreatitis), hyperpigmentation (adrenal insufficiency).
Extremities	Peripheral edema (CHF, renal disease, vasculitis), pulses and capillary refill (assess for potential shock).
Neurologic examination	Altered mental status (shock, toxin, porphyria, diabetic ketoacidosis).

Selective Chart Review

After the history and physical examination, the cause of the abdominal pain may still be unclear. Selectively reviewing the medical record may provide useful information.

What medications is the patient taking?

Some medications are notorious for causing abdominal symptoms, and abdominal pain is listed as a potential side effect of nearly all drugs. Attributing pain to a medication may be reasonable but should be considered a diagnosis of exclusion. Steroids and nonsteroidal anti-inflammatory medications may potentially cause gastritis, esophagitis, and peptic ulcer. The increasing use of ibuprofen, naproxen, and ketorolac as pain relievers and antipyretics may be placing more patients at risk. Narcotics and other medications may induce constipation and thereby result in abdominal pain. Pancreatitis and hepatitis are also side effects of several medications. Remember that *Clostridium difficile* infection, colitis, and subsequent abdominal pain may develop in any patient who has been receiving antibiotics. Conversely, both narcotics and steroids can mask abdominal pain.

If the child is an adolescent girl, when was the last menstrual period? Is she sexually active?

Missed menses is suggestive of pregnancy, ectopic or intrauterine. Known sexual activity confirms the possibility of pelvic inflammatory disease.

Has the child complained of this type of pain before?

If the same pain has prompted several previous calls, the problem is much less likely to be an acute one requiring extensive evaluation and emergency management in the middle of the night. However, acute changes in chronic pain need to be evaluated. The child may have a significant problem causing the pain (lactose intolerance, inflammatory bowel disease), but further evaluation may be able to be deferred after life-threatening possibilities are excluded.

Management

At this point, either a specific diagnosis is evident or you are able to shorten the list of potential causes. If the specific cause of the abdominal pain remains questionable, you should at least be able to determine whether the patient (1) is critically ill and requires immediate intervention, (2) is in discomfort but has no evidence of an immediately life-threatening process, or (3) is only mildly uncomfortable and life-threatening processes can be excluded. If the patient is critically ill, you need to pursue management and additional diagnostic studies simultaneously. A patient who is stable but uncomfortable may require further diagnostic studies before appropriate management is begun. A mildly uncomfortable patient may not require any specific diagnostic tests or management at the moment and may often be managed expectantly.

Critically Ill Patients

A critically ill patient with abdominal pain usually has hypovolemic shock, septic shock, or a combination of both as a result of perforation, peritonitis, or exsanguination. Immediate management of a critically ill patient with abdominal pain involves addressing the issues of shock and infection simultaneously and necessitates consultation with pediatric surgeons. Management should proceed as follows:

    1. Volume

        Immediate expansion of intravascular volume helps improve tissue perfusion. Normal saline or lactated Ringer's solution can be given as a 20-mL/kg IV bolus. Evaluate the response of the heart rate, capillary refill, and blood pressure and repeat if indicated. If cardiogenic shock is a possibility, volume expansion should still be a priority, but one should avoid exacerbating CHF with excess IV fluids. If the patient is known to be bleeding, whole blood can also be used to expand intravascular volume. If time does not permit cross-matching, O-negative blood should be used.

2. Oxygenation

   Oxygen should be administered and an arterial blood gas measurement obtained to assess the adequacy of oxygenation and tissue perfusion.

3. Laboratory studies

   Additional laboratory tests include a complete blood count with differential, prothrombin time, partial thromboplastin time, blood culture, urinalysis, urine culture, human chorionic gonadotropin-β (HCG-β) if female, amylase, lipase, lactate dehydrogenase, blood gas, and electrolyte determinations, as well as blood for typing and cross-matching. Optional tests at this time are dictated by your differential diagnosis. If concerned about a renal etiology, add blood urea nitrogen (BUN) and creatinine. If the liver or biliary tract is concerning, aspartate transaminase (AST), alanine transaminase (ALT), γ-glutamyl-transferase (GGT), and bilirubin would be appropriate.

4. Paracentesis

   If sepsis is suspected and the patient has ascites, diagnostic paracentesis should be performed and the fluid cultured to evaluate for bacterial peritonitis.

5. Antibiotics

   After cultures are obtained, broad-spectrum antibiotics should be started immediately to empirically treat gut anaerobes, as well as gram-positive and gram-negative pathogens (the combination of ampicillin, gentamicin, and clindamycin is one possible choice).

6. Radiography

   Radiographic studies need to be performed with a portable machine at the patient's bedside and should include antero-posterior (AP) views of the abdomen, supine and erect if possible. If the patient is an infant, a cross-table lateral view allows the detection of free air in the peritoneum. A patient who cannot stand should have a lateral decubitus view. An AP view of the chest should also be obtained to evaluate the lung fields (the potential exists for acute respiratory distress syndrome, pneumonia) and heart size (to exclude pericardial effusion, myocarditis, CHF) and to look for free air under the diaphragm. Air-fluid levels suggest bowel obstruction or ileus. A "sentinel" loop suggests pancreatitis. Lead may be seen as radiopaque "chips" throughout the bowel. Constipation should be fairly obvious, as should an intra-abdominal mass. A fecalith in the right lower quadrant is suggestive of appendicitis.

7. Consultation

Surgical consultation is mandatory if a perforated viscus, splenic rupture, intra-abdominal abscess, aortic dissection, appendicitis, intussusception, volvulus, malrotation, psoas abscess, incarcerated hernia, ischemic bowel, Meckel's diverticulum, tumor, or testicular torsion is suspected. Gynecologic consultation may be necessary if ovarian torsion, pelvic abscess, or ectopic pregnancy is suspected.

8. Vasopressors

If fluid resuscitation alone does not improve the signs of shock, vasopressors may be necessary (see Chapter 25, Hypotension and Shock).

Patients Who Are Uncomfortable but Do Not Have Cardiorespiratory Compromise

If the patient is not in shock, additional evaluation may proceed before any specific intervention is made. However, one should remain alert for the possibility that the patient may suddenly become critically ill (e.g., if ischemic bowel progresses to a perforated bowel or if intussusception progresses to ischemia and necrosis). Laboratory studies and radiographs as outlined for critically ill patients may be helpful diagnostically. If gastroenteritis is a consideration, stool may be tested for rotavirus, *Salmonella, Shigella, Yersinia, Escherichia coli,* and if the patient has been taking antibiotics, *C. difficile* toxin. If laboratory testing and initial radiographs do not lead to a diagnosis, consideration may be given to performing abdominal or pelvic ultrasound studies (to exclude an abscess, tumor, ovarian torsion, ectopic pregnancy, urolithiasis), a barium enema (if intussusception is suspected), computed tomography (CT) of the abdomen and pelvis (abscess, tumor, appendicitis), angiography (mesenteric thrombosis or vasculitis), or a Meckel scan. Whether these tests are performed immediately or the next day depends on clinical suspicion and the potential for morbidity if the diagnosis is delayed. If significant abdominal pain persists, the patient should remain NPO with IV hydration at a maintenance rate until the cause is found. Further management depends on the diagnosis.

Patients with Mild Discomfort

In some cases, a patient with mild discomfort may need additional studies immediately to exclude the possibility of bacterial infection or a surgical abdomen. Laboratory studies and radiographs as outlined earlier may provide additional evidence of infection (dramatic increase in the white blood cell count with a left shift) or a surgical abdomen (free air), or they may help exclude these possibilities. Not every patient, however, requires further study beyond a history and physical examination. If a potentially serious cause of the abdominal pain is unlikely, expectant management is reasonable, provided that the patient is observed carefully and frequently. If the patient wants to eat, maintenance of NPO status is usually unnecessary. Acetaminophen, 10 mg/kg every 4 to 6 hours, may be used to alleviate pain. In such circumstances you need to use your "gut" feeling about the patient to guide further evaluation and management. Serial examinations should be performed at frequent intervals until the pain resolves or a specific diagnosis is made.

Altered Mental Status

Kishore Vellody, MD

Altered mental status can be simply defined as an alteration in consciousness. Mental status can become "altered" in many different ways. In general, any pathologic process affecting the central nervous system (CNS) is capable of producing a wide spectrum of changes, including irritability, lethargy, syncope, seizures, and unresponsiveness. Defining the type of alteration is therefore often less important than recognizing that a change in mental status has occurred. Nevertheless, the specific details of how the patient's mental status has changed can help narrow the list of diagnostic possibilities and may change the initial approach to management. This chapter discusses the evaluation and management of children in whom irritability, lethargy, syncope, delirium, or coma develop while in the hospital. *Delirium* is defined as confusion and disorientation and is usually manifested as inappropriate speech or bizarre behavior. The term *lethargy* implies sleepiness and limited interest in any activity or conversation. If the lethargy is severe, the term *obtundation* is sometimes used. *Stupor* refers to a state characterized by lapses of consciousness, with the ability to be aroused. Finally, *coma* is a condition of profound unconsciousness. Irritability in an infant (see Chapter 12) and seizures (see Chapter 29) are discussed elsewhere.

PHONE CALL

Questions

1. How old is the patient?
2. Why is the patient in the hospital?
3. What are the patient's vital signs, including temperature?
4. How is the child breathing? Is the airway compromised?
5. How is the child behaving? Was there a brief period of unresponsiveness suggesting seizure or syncope?
6. Has this occurred in the past? What is the child's baseline mental status?

The child's vital signs, respiratory pattern, and current behavior help determine whether the change in mental status is associated with a critical ongoing process, such as increased intracranial pressure (ICP), or a self-limited event, such as a seizure or syncope. If the airway is compromised, plans should be made to intubate the child **immediately**. The responses to these questions also help differentiate between the various types of alterations in mental status. If the child's mental status changes appear to be resolving, an "event" may have occurred but does not require immediate treatment. On the other hand, if hypertension, bradycardia, and respiratory changes are present, increased ICP should be suspected and management begun immediately. The reason for hospitalization and determining whether such an episode has occurred before may help direct your initial thoughts regarding the cause of the change in mental status. Defining the child's baseline mental status and history of previous alterations in mental status helps clarify the potential significance of the current change.

Orders

1. A bedside blood glucose measurement should be requested. If hypoglycemia is present (<40 mg/dL), 2 mL/kg of 25% dextrose or 5 mL/kg of 10% dextrose should be given intravenously.
2. Pulse oximetry analysis should be ordered if the patient has abnormal respirations or a cardiac or respiratory illness.
3. If the vital signs indicate increased ICP or the airway appears to be compromised, preparation should be made for intubation.
4. If the history is suspicious for syncope, an electrocardiogram (ECG) should be performed at the bedside to evaluate for cardiac dysrhythmia.
5. An intravenous (IV) line should be placed in most patients with delirium, obtundation, stupor, or coma. If an IV line is to be placed, you may ask the nurse to draw off some blood in anticipation of the need for laboratory studies.

Inform RN

An acute alteration in mental status always requires immediate evaluation. It is critical that the cause be determined as soon as possible so that appropriate management can be initiated.

ELEVATOR THOUGHTS

Altered mental status may occur because of a primary intracranial process or a metabolic disturbance, or it may be due to a systemic illness or disorder. Almost any illness can lead to irritability or lethargy in a young child. Therefore, in these children it is important to also consider illnesses localized to organ systems other than the CNS. If consciousness is impaired, the process must be affecting both cerebral hemispheres or the brainstem.

Intracranial processes	Infection (meningitis, encephalitis, abscess)
	Hemorrhage (subarachnoid, subdural, epidural, parenchymal) secondary to aneurysm, trauma (including shaken baby syndrome), coagulopathy, or arteriovenous malformation
	Tumor
	Concussion secondary to head trauma
	Cerebral edema secondary to trauma
	Cerebral thrombosis
	Cerebral vasculitis
	Cerebritis
	Psychosis
	Hydrocephalus
	Seizure disorder
	Acute confusional migraine ("Alice in Wonderland" syndrome)
	Acute disseminated encephalomyelitis
Metabolic disturbances	Diabetic ketoacidosis
	Hyperammonemia (e.g., Reye's syndrome, urea cycle disorders, liver disease)
	Hypoglycemia
	Hyponatremia, hypernatremia
	Hypocalcemia, hypercalcemia
	Hypokalemia
	Hypoxemia (e.g., carbon monoxide poisoning, cardiac failure, respiratory failure)
	Drugs and toxins (e.g., narcotics, lead, barbiturates, alcohol, salicylates, acetaminophen)
	Mitochondrial encephalomyopathies (e.g., Leigh disease, Zellweger syndrome)
Systemic illnesses	Hypothyroidism, hyperthyroidism
	Uremia (e.g., hemolytic-uremic syndrome)
	Addison's disease
	Congestive heart failure
	Cardiac dysrhythmia
	Pulmonary failure
	Hypertension with encephalopathy
	Heat stroke
	Shock (septic, hypovolemic, cardiogenic, anaphylactic)
	Fever
	Human immunodeficiency virus (HIV) encephalopathy
	Systemic lupus erythematosus with cerebritis
	Malnutrition (with thiamine deficiency)

Systemic illnesses— Cont'd	Thrombotic thrombocytopenic purpura
	Burn encephalopathy
	"Hospital" or "intensive care unit" encephalopathy
	In children and adolescents who have had an episode of what appears to have been syncope, the following should also be considered:
	Vasovagal episode
	Cardiac conduction disturbance (heart block)
	Dysrhythmia (e.g., supraventricular tachycardia, long QT syndrome)
	Narcolepsy
	Cough syncope
	Severe anemia
	Breath holding
	Hyperventilation
	Cervical vertebral anomalies

MAJOR THREAT TO LIFE

- CNS infection
- Intracranial hemorrhage
- Increased ICP
- Metabolic disturbance
- Shock
- Dysrhythmia
- Organ failure (e.g., heart, lung, liver, or kidney)
- Status epilepticus
- Aspiration resulting from an inability to protect the airway

Infection, hemorrhage, and mass lesions leading to increased ICP and subsequent brain herniation are the most worrisome possibilities. Metabolic disturbances, shock, dysrhythmias, and organ failure may potentially have multiple systemic life-threatening consequences in addition to their effects on the CNS. Status epilepticus may also have substantial deleterious effects on the CNS. Regardless of the underlying cause, a stuporous, obtunded, or comatose patient may not be able to protect the airway and is therefore at greater risk for aspiration.

BEDSIDE

Quick-Look Test

Is the patient currently alert, comfortable, and oriented (suggesting an episodic event, e.g., a self-limited seizure or syncope), or is the patient actively seizing, unconscious, lethargic, irritable, combative, or sleepy (suggesting an ongoing process)?

The latter patient needs to be examined immediately with a focus on signs that would suggest infection, shock, increased ICP, brain herniation, or a combination of these conditions. If the patient is seizing, management to control the seizure should begin simultaneously with further examination (see Chapter 29, Seizures). Generally, irritability alone is less worrisome than confusion, disorientation, lethargy, or alterations in the level of consciousness. Isolated irritability is present in many hospitalized children and, if unaccompanied by other abnormal neurologic findings, is not necessarily an indicator of CNS pathology. Keep in mind, however, that mental status may change rapidly and a child who is irritable initially may progress to stupor, obtundation, or coma.

Airway and Vital Signs

Can the child protect his or her airway? (Are cough and gag reflexes present?)

If the answer is no, the child should be intubated as soon as possible.

The vital signs should be checked, with particular attention paid to signs of infection or increased ICP—two of the major threats to life. Fever should raise the suspicion of CNS infection or septic shock. Patients with brain abscesses are not necessarily febrile; consequently, the absence of fever makes infection less likely but does not exclude the possibility. Cushing's triad (bradycardia, hypertension, and irregular respirations) is an ominous finding that occurs in the presence of significantly increased ICP. It is considered a late finding; therefore, normal vital signs may be present in a patient in whom increased ICP is developing. Management should begin **immediately** if Cushing's triad is noted.

Hypertension may also be the cause (rather than the result) of an encephalopathy, usually associated with renal disease. Hypotension implies shock (septic, hypovolemic, cardiogenic, or anaphylactic) and also requires immediate management (see Chapter 25, Hypotension and Shock). Tachycardia may be present in a septic patient or one with hyperthyroidism, but an increase in heart rate is also a common finding in any ill child. Heart rates greater than 200 beats per minute are suggestive of supraventricular tachycardia. Tachypnea may reflect pulmonary disease with secondary hypoxemia or compensation for metabolic acidosis, as in diabetic ketoacidosis.

Selective Physical Examination I

After the quick-look test and a check of vital signs, an initial selective physical examination should be performed with the goal of determining the likelihood of increased ICP, impending brain herniation, or CNS infection (meningitis, encephalitis, or abscess) because immediate management is necessary if any of these conditions is suspected.

Head	Bruising over the mastoid (Battle's sign), "raccoon eyes," or depressions or deformity of the skull (all indicators of significant head trauma); bulging or sunken fontanelle
Eyes	Pupil size and reactivity to light. A single dilated, unreactive pupil may indicate herniation of the ipsilateral temporal lobe. Bilateral dilatation is associated with a postictal state and certain drugs (e.g., atropine, cocaine, mydriatic agents)
	Fundi. Retinal hemorrhage is associated with trauma. Papilledema suggests increased ICP (Fig. 7-1)
	Extraocular movements. Third nerve palsy (dilated pupil, lateral and inferior displacement of the eye, ptosis) may be associated with temporal lobe herniation.

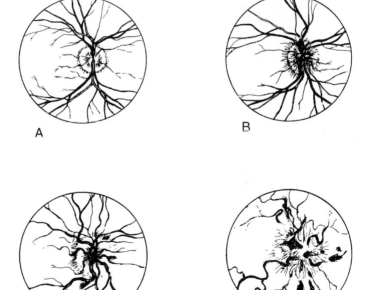

Figure 7–1 Disk changes seen in papilledema. **A,** Normal. **B,** Early papilledema. **C,** Moderate papilledema with early hemorrhage. **D,** Severe papilledema with extensive hemorrhage. (From Marshall SA, Ruedy J: On Call: Principles and Protocols, 4th ed. Philadelphia, Elsevier, 2004, p 123.)

TABLE 7–1 **Localization of Cerebral Dysfunction**

Level of Injury	Breathing Pattern	Pupils	Ocular Palsies	Posturing
Hemispheres, diencephalon	Cheyne-Stokes*	Normal or dilated	Upgaze difficulty	Decorticate
Midbrain	Central neurogenic hyperventilation[†]	Dilated	Cranial nerves III, IV	Decerebrate
Pons	Apneustic[‡]	Normal or miotic reflex	Loss of oculocephalic reflex[§]	Flaccid
Medulla	Ataxic or Biot[¶]	Midposition reflex	Loss of oculocephalic reflex[§]	Flaccid

*Cheyne-Stokes breathing refers to alternating hyperpnea and apnea.
[†]Central neurogenic hyperventilation refers to persistent tachypnea and hyperpnea.
[‡]Apneustic breathing is similar to Cheyne-Stokes breathing except that the periods of hyperpnea and apnea cycle at very short intervals.
[§]The oculocephalic reflex ("doll's eyes" maneuver) is elicited by passively turning the head to one side and noting that the eyes move in the opposite direction.
[¶]Ataxic or Biot breathing is irregularly irregular with respect to both the rate and depth of breathing.
Adapted from Graef JW, Cone TE (eds): Manual of Pediatric Therapeutics, 3rd ed. Boston, Children's Hospital, 1985.

Eyes—Cont'd	Sixth nerve palsy (absence of lateral movement) may be associated with increased ICP and may be unilateral or bilateral
Ears	Hemotympanum or blood in the external canal (head trauma)
Nose	Cerebrospinal fluid (CSF) rhinorrhea (trauma)
Neck	Nuchal rigidity (meningitis), Kernig's and Brudzinski's signs (meningitis)
Chest	Respiratory pattern (Table 7-1) (may indicate herniation)
Cardiac	Bradycardia (increased ICP), extreme tachycardia, or abnormal rhythm
Extremities	Posturing (Table 7-1) (may indicate herniation)
Neurologic	Level of consciousness, orientation, focality, Glasgow Coma Scale (GCS) score (asymmetry in muscle tone, strength, spontaneous movement, reflexes)

What is the Glasgow Coma Scale (GCS) (Table 7-2)?
A GCS score less than 8 is an indication that severe CNS abnormalities are present and the child is at risk for respiratory compromise. Intubation is indicated.

TABLE 7–2 **Modified Glasgow Coma Scale**

Score	Eyes Opening	
	>1 Year Old	<1 Year Old
4	Spontaneously	Spontaneously
3	To verbal command	To shout
2	To pain	To pain
1	No response	No response
Score	**Best Motor Response**	
6	Obeys	Spontaneous
5	Localizes pain	Localizes pain
4	Flexion: withdrawal	Flexion: withdrawal
3	Flexion: abnormal (decorticate rigidity)	Flexion: abnormal (decorticate rigidity)
2	Extension (decerebrate rigidity)	Extension (decerebrate rigidity)
1	No response	No response

Score	Best Verbal Response		
	>5 Years Old	2–5 Years Old	0–23 Months Old
5	Oriented, converses	Appropriate words and phrases	Smiles, coos appropriately
4	Disoriented, converses	Inappropriate words	Cries, consolable
3	Inappropriate words	Persistent cries	Persistent, inappropriate cries
2	Incomprehensible sounds	Grunts	Grunts, agitated or restless
1	No response	No response	No response

Management I

Increased Intracranial Pressure

If elevated ICP is suspected, treatment must be initiated in an attempt to reduce the volume of the intracranial contents (i.e., brain, CSF, and blood) and ensure adequate cerebral perfusion pressure. This is done by the following techniques:

1. *Positioning.* The head of the bed should be raised to 30 degrees.
2. *Hyperventilation.* Intubation plus mechanical ventilation adjusted to keep the arterial partial pressure of CO_2 at approximately 25 mm Hg reduces blood flow to the brain and is the fastest way to reduce ICP. However, prolonged hyperventilation may reduce cerebral blood flow enough to cause cerebral ischemia. Hyperventilation should be used only in acute situations.

3. *Osmotherapy.* Increasing serum osmolarity to 300 to 320 mOsm/L may establish a gradient that allows brain water to be drawn into the circulation. Three percent NaCl, 2 to 4 mL/kg, or mannitol, 0.25 to 1.0 g/kg, can be given every 2 to 4 hours. Serum osmolarity must be measured when using this therapy.

After these steps have been performed, computed tomography (CT) should be performed to help confirm the presence of a mass lesion, hemorrhage, or cerebral edema as a potential cause of the increased ICP. Neurosurgical consultation may be helpful because surgery and/or an ICP monitor may be necessary.

Infection

If meningitis, abscess, or encephalitis is suspected, further evaluation should be expedited and empiric treatment begun as quickly as possible. Ideally, the results of blood and CSF culture should be obtained before the administration of antibiotics. However, in a critically ill child, no more than a 15-minute delay in the administration of antibiotics for suspected meningitis should be allowed. If suspicion of increased ICP necessitates a CT scan before lumbar puncture, the antibiotics should be administered and the lumbar puncture performed after the CT scan. An opening pressure should be obtained during the lumbar puncture because high pressure is suggestive of bacterial meningitis. IV ceftriaxone (200 mg/kg/day divided every 6 hours) and vancomycin (40 mg/kg/day divided every 6 hours) are the empiric treatments of choice for suspected meningitis. Consideration should be given to administering dexamethasone (0.15 mg/kg) shortly before the antibiotics to help prevent complications related to bacterial lysis. In geographic areas that are endemic for Rocky Mountain spotted fever, the addition of IV doxycycline may be considered. The presence of focality on physical examination, hemorrhagic CSF, or associated focal seizures should raise suspicion of herpes encephalitis, and empiric treatment with acyclovir (10 mg/kg per dose every 8 hours) is then indicated.

Selective Physical Examination II

If the patient has no signs of significant cardiorespiratory compromise, the initial selective physical examination does not reveal evidence of increased ICP or CNS infection, and the patient is not believed to be actively seizing, a more detailed physical examination can be performed before further evaluation and management. The goal should be to locate findings that can help narrow the list of diagnostic possibilities.

| HEENT | Intracranial bruits (arteriovenous malformations), periorbital edema (anaphylaxis), or mastoid edema and erythema (cellulitis); perioral cyanosis (hypoxemia), fruity breath (diabetic ketoacidosis) |

Neck	Jugular venous pulsations (congestive heart failure), goiter (thyroid disease)
Chest	Rales, intercostal retractions, tachypnea (respiratory failure, pneumonitis)
Cardiac	Murmurs, muffled heart sounds, friction rub (pericarditis, pericardial effusion)
Abdomen	Hepatomegaly (liver disease, congestive heart failure), splenomegaly (portal hypertension)
Extremities	Paresis, paralysis, arthritis (systemic lupus erythematosus, vasculitis), edema (congestive heart failure)
Skin	Palpable purpura (vasculitis), petechiae, ecchymoses (hemolytic-uremic syndrome, thrombotic thrombocytopenic purpura, coagulopathy, child abuse), jaundice (liver disease)
Neurologic	Responsiveness (see Table 7-2, Modified Glasgow Coma Scale); cranial nerves; doll's eyes reflex; muscle bulk, tone, and strength; reflexes (to evaluate the extent of and potentially localize a nervous system lesion); if possible in an adolescent, assessment of mood, affect, and thought processes (psychosis)

Selective History and Chart Review

After the airway and vital signs have been stabilized, treatment of increased ICP or infection has been initiated if necessary, and the patient has been examined, further information should be obtained from the patient, family members, and the chart.

Has there been a history of trauma?

Keep in mind that a traumatic event may have occurred before hospitalization. Symptoms secondary to a subdural hematoma may occur well after the injury.

Are there any concerns for shaken baby syndrome?

Recall that infants may not have any external signs of injury.

Has the child been complaining of headaches? Nausea or vomiting? Visual disturbances?

Symptoms of increased ICP that have been present for some time suggest a mass lesion such as tumor or abscess.

Has the child had any recent infections?

A recent infection raises the suspicion of encephalitis, meningitis, or abscess.

Does the child have any underlying illnesses that may affect the CNS? Have there been any symptoms to suggest a systemic illness that might be affecting the CNS?

Diabetes, chronic pulmonary, cardiac, renal, or liver disease, HIV infection, and lupus are examples of underlying conditions that may affect the CNS. Approximately 25% of diabetic children are initially found to have ketoacidosis.

What medication is the child receiving? Do any of these medications have CNS effects? In an adolescent, is there a history of drug or alcohol use?

Accidental or intentional overdosing of numerous medications may alter mental status. In addition, secondary metabolic effects from medications, such as hypoglycemia or hypokalemia, may be contributing to the altered mental status.

Is there a family history of migraine or psychosis? Has the child been acting depressed or abnormally lately?

Acute confusional migraine or psychosis may begin suddenly but should be considered after the more life-threatening possibilities have been excluded. In addition, keep in mind that a psychotic or depressed child is at increased risk for toxic ingestion.

If the episode was thought to be syncopal, what was happening at the time of the event? Did the child feel anxious, flushed, nervous, or sweaty? Is there a family history of heart disease or premature death? Did the child feel palpitations?

Such symptoms suggest vasovagal syncope. A family history of early death raises the suspicion of long QT syndrome or cardiomyopathy. Palpitations also increase suspicion for a dysrhythmia.

Management II

Nearly all children and adolescents who have had an alteration in mental status require additional laboratory or radiographic evaluation. The exceptions to this generalization include young children who are irritable but consolable, have normal neurologic examination findings, and have been hospitalized for an illness that might be expected to cause some irritability. Such children may simply be observed as their illness is being treated, with the expectation that the irritability will resolve as soon as they are feeling better. However, if there is any suspicion of CNS pathology, additional evaluation is warranted.

The following tests should be performed in patients in whom syncope has been excluded and the cause of the altered mental status remains unclear:

1. Complete blood count and differential (infection, anemia, thrombocytopenia)
2. Electrolytes, glucose, calcium, ammonia
3. Blood and urine toxicology screen
4. Head CT or magnetic resonance imaging (mass lesion)
5. Lumbar puncture with an opening pressure, unless there are signs of increased ICP, focal neurologic findings, risk of cardiorespiratory compromise, or a skin/soft tissue infection overlying the site of the lumbar puncture

Additional blood and CSF should be collected and saved because further studies may be necessary if the diagnosis remains unclear.

The following tests may be helpful if some evidence suggests a specific illness:

1. Hepatic transaminases, blood urea nitrogen, creatinine, urinalysis (liver or renal disease)
2. Arterial blood gas (hypoxemia, hypercapnia)
3. Chest radiographs (cardiac or pulmonary failure)
4. Peripheral blood smear, prothrombin time, partial thromboplastin time (microangiopathy, coagulopathy)

If the alteration in mental status is thought to be consistent with syncope or if cardiac failure with decreased cerebral perfusion is suspected, an ECG should be obtained.

Additional diagnostic evaluation such as thyroid studies, cerebral angiograms, electroencephalograms, echocardiograms, antinuclear antibody studies, and other tests aimed at excluding specific diseases should be considered for individual patients. Similarly, further evaluation of a patient with syncope, such as electroencephalographic studies or tilt-table testing, may need to be scheduled the next day. In most cases, the cause of the altered mental status is apparent after the history, physical examination, and laboratory evaluation as outlined earlier. At a minimum, the major threats to life are considered, and if necessary, the child is receiving treatment aimed at reducing increased ICP or resolving a possible CNS infection. Definitive treatment depends on the cause of the altered mental status.

Infection

As outlined previously, suspected bacterial meningitis is treated with antibiotics, and IV ceftriaxone and vancomycin (with or without dexamethasone) is a good choice of initial empiric therapy beyond the neonatal period because it is effective against the most common pathogens: *Streptococcus pneumoniae* (*including penicillin- and cephalosporin-resistant strains*) and *Neisseria meningitidis*. Brain abscess may be caused by a large group of aerobic and anaerobic bacteria, and therefore empiric treatment with appropriate broad-spectrum IV antibiotics is necessary. In addition, neurosurgical consultation is helpful because most children require excision or drainage of the abscess. Encephalitis should be treated empirically with acyclovir if herpes infection is suspected.

Mass Lesion

Intracerebral hemorrhage or tumor requires surgical evacuation or resection, and a neurosurgeon should be consulted promptly. Any alteration in mental status associated with trauma is also an indication for neurosurgical consultation.

Metabolic Disturbance

Diabetic ketoacidosis should be managed with insulin, hydration, and correction of associated electrolyte abnormalities. Likewise, other electrolyte disturbances should be corrected by specific replacements. Inborn errors of metabolism (particularly partial/incomplete forms) can occur at any age and require prompt evaluation and possible consultation with a geneticist to ascertain the cause and begin emergency therapy (i.e., reducing the serum ammonia level in patients with urea cycle defects).

Drugs and Toxins

If overdose is suspected, treatment should be directed at decontamination and supportive therapy. Treatment of ingestions includes gastric lavage, which may require prior intubation in patients with altered mental status who cannot protect their airway. Charcoal, diuresis, and specific antidotes may all be used, depending on the substance ingested. Dialysis or exchange transfusion is reserved for the most severe cases.

Psychosis

A psychotic child should be managed in consultation with psychiatrists. Chlorpromazine, haloperidol, or diazepam may be considered in an extremely agitated or violent child.

Systemic illnesses such as liver or renal disease, thyroid disease, lupus, or vasculitis should be managed appropriately while keeping in mind that associated increased ICP may also need to be treated.

Analgesics and Antipyretics

Ushma Patel, MD

Analgesics and antipyretics are two classes of medications that are among the most commonly prescribed in hospitalized pediatric patients. Although writing orders for these medications can become very routine, it is important to remember that like all medications, these drugs are to be prescribed with careful thought and attention to detail. When asked to write an order for analgesics and/or antipyretics, it is important that you (1) determine the need for the medication, (2) understand why the child needs these medications, and (3) realize the potential consequences of using these medications in the individual patient, including adverse effects, as well as the effect that limiting pain and/or fever will have on your ability to accurately evaluate a patient's status.

ANALGESICS

PHONE CALL

Questions

1. Why is an analgesic being requested?
2. Where is the pain?
3. How severe is the pain?
4. Is this pain new?
5. What interventions have been tried thus far?
6. What is the child's admitting diagnosis?
7. How old is the child?
8. How much does the child weigh?
9. Does the child have any allergies?

The answers to these questions should allow you to understand the cause of the pain and the child's need for an analgesic, as well as the urgency of the situation.

In children it is sometimes difficult to know whether the problem is truly one of pain. Parents, nurses, and physicians may assume that pain is present because a young child is crying or screaming. Temper tantrums, night terrors, nightmares, and/or fear may be the problem rather than pain. Similarly, pain may be the result of behavioral issues, depression, anxiety, or other psychogenic and psychosocial factors, in which case analgesics may be ineffective. It is important to consider these possibilities before immediately ordering medication.

If the child's diagnosis is unclear or if masking the pain will make it difficult to evaluate the child's status (e.g., abdominal pain that may require surgery or joint pain that may be associated with rheumatic fever), you must carefully consider these factors before immediately prescribing an analgesic.

Orders

Table 8-1 lists selected analgesics and antipyretics. In most situations, acetaminophen is the best initial choice because it is well tolerated, it does not usually mask significant pain, and there are no concerns regarding dependency. Ibuprofen or another nonsteroidal anti-inflammatory drug (NSAID) is generally the next best choice if acetaminophen is insufficient. However, in children with abdominal pain or renal disease, one needs to be aware of the potential for gastritis or nephrotoxicity with these drugs. Because of their anti-inflammatory effect, NSAIDs also have greater potential to mask the symptoms and signs associated with progression of disease.

Narcotics should not be ordered unless the cause of the pain is clearly understood and not until the child has already failed a trial of acetaminophen and NSAIDs. Narcotics have greater potential for serious adverse events such as respiratory depression, they may alter mental status, their potency results in significant masking of signs and symptoms, and they may result in dependency. Narcotics also slow gastrointestinal motility and may therefore cause adynamic ileus and subsequent constipation.

Inform RN

"Will arrive at the bedside in … minutes."

ELEVATOR THOUGHTS

If there is any doubt regarding the origin or cause of the pain, if the pain is a new complaint, if the character of the pain has changed, or if the pain is severe, you must evaluate the child at the bedside before ordering an analgesic.

REMEMBER

1. It is easy to both overestimate and underestimate the severity of pain in pediatric patients. You need to make sure that you

TABLE 8–1 Commonly Used Analgesics and Antipyretics

Drug	Dose	Comments
Acetaminophen (Tylenol)	10-15 mg/kg PO q4-6h	Analgesia and antipyresis
Ibuprofen (Motrin, Advil)	10-15 mg/kg PO q6h	Analgesia and antipyresis
Naproxen (Aleve)	7.5-10 mg/kg PO bid	Generally used for analgesia and anti-inflammatory effect, but also for antipyretic effect
Codeine*	1 mg/kg PO q4-6h (maximum dose, 60 mg)	Analgesia only; often used in combination with acetaminophen: Tylenol No. 2 = 15 mg codeine + 300 mg acetaminophen Tylenol No. 3 = 30 mg codeine + 300 mg acetaminophen Tylenol No. 4 = 60 mg codeine + 300 mg acetaminophen
Morphine*	0.1-0.2 mg/kg IV, IM, SC q2-4h	Analgesia only; 10 mg morphine = 100 mg meperidine; naloxone is antidote
Meperidine (Demerol)*	1.0-1.5 mg/kg PO, IM, IV, SC q3-4h	Analgesia only; use with caution in renal failure; naloxone is antidote

*Narcotics are addictive and may cause respiratory depression; therefore, they should be used only for severe pain and when the cause of pain is understood.

understand the cause of the pain as clearly as possible while making the patient as comfortable as possible. Overprescribing narcotics and other analgesics, as well as withholding medication from a child in pain, should both be avoided. The severity of pain can be assessed and monitored over time with a simple 0 to 10 scale for older children or with the Bieri faces scale (see Fig. 21-1) for younger children.

2. Escalating the potency of the analgesic you order without re-evaluating the patient should also be avoided. After ordering acetaminophen or an NSAID for a patient, if the nurse calls you several hours later to tell you the child is still in pain, you must see that patient before simply ordering a more potent analgesic, such as a narcotic.

3. When the cause of pain is poorly understood, you should not order analgesics as "PRN pain." You must instead be notified if the patient remains in pain and how severe it is. In this situation, ask the nurse to call you back in several hours if the child remains in pain.

4. When the cause of pain is clearly understood and there is an anticipated need for multiple doses of intravenous (IV) narcotic medication, patient-controlled analgesia (PCA) should be considered. PCA should be ordered after consultation with an anesthesiologist or other pain specialist.

5. Narcotic overdosage can be reversed with naloxone (Narcan), 0.01 to 0.1 mg/kg per dose intramuscularly (IM), IV, or subcutaneously (SC) (maximum, 2 mg per dose). This dose can be repeated every 3 to 5 minutes as needed. Reversal may induce nausea and vomiting. Therefore, be prepared to protect the airway because the child is at risk for aspiration.

ANTIPYRETICS

PHONE CALL

Questions

1. How old is the child?
2. How high is the fever?
3. What is the child's admitting diagnosis?
4. How much does the child weigh?
5. Is the fever a new finding?

Orders

See Table 8-1 for dosing of antipyretics.

Inform RN

"Will arrive at the bedside in ... minutes."

Any child with a new fever must be evaluated (see Chapter 18, Fever) before ordering antipyretics.

REMEMBER

1. Although you are ordering these medications for fever, they also have an analgesic effect, and therefore you need to consider this potential effect on your ability to evaluate the patient as described earlier under "Analgesics."
2. There is no longer any need to use aspirin as an antipyretic. Acetaminophen and ibuprofen are alternatives that in general are better tolerated and entail less risk.
3. There are fewer concerns with the use of antipyretics in a patient in whom the diagnosis remains unclear. Decreasing the fever rarely results in difficulty arriving at a diagnosis, and it allows the child to be much more comfortable.
4. When fever is persistently high and unresponsive to acetaminophen alone, acetaminophen and ibuprofen may be ordered together (acetaminophen every 4 to 6 hours and ibuprofen every 6 hours).

Bleeding

Erin C. Nunnold, MD

Bleeding may potentially occur at any anatomic location in a hospitalized child. When evaluating a patient who has bled or is bleeding, the goals are simple: (1) stop the active bleeding, and (2) prevent further bleeding. How one achieves these goals depends on the answer to a basic question, "Is the bleeding secondary to an anatomically localized problem (e.g., trauma), or is it secondary to a generalized bleeding disorder (coagulopathy)?" Coagulopathies are further discussed in detail in Chapter 33, Anemia, Thrombocytopenia, and Coagulation Abnormalities. *Epistaxis, hemoptysis, hematemesis, melena, hematochezia, rectal bleeding, hemarthrosis,* and *hematuria* are terms used to describe bleeding from various locations. In addition, bleeding into the skin and soft tissues may produce ecchymoses, petechiae, or purpura. This chapter discusses bleeding that does not involve the gastrointestinal or urinary tract. These subjects are addressed in detail in Chapter 19, Gastrointestinal Bleeding, and Chapter 23, Hematuria.

PHONE CALL

Questions

1. What are the child's vital signs, including temperature?
2. Where is the bleeding?
3. What is the child's underlying illness and reason for hospitalization?
4. What medications is the child receiving?

The vital signs allow you to quickly determine whether the blood loss has been severe enough to result in depletion of intravascular volume. Tachycardia and/or hypotension might indicate such a state. If the child is febrile and has petechiae or purpura, one must immediately consider the possibility of sepsis with associated coagulopathy. The location of the bleeding obviously allows you to develop a more specific differential diagnosis, and the patient's underlying illness may give you clues regarding potential causes of the bleeding (e.g., liver disease or cystic fibrosis). Discovering that the patient is receiving a medication that might affect platelets or clotting factors is obviously of potential significance.

Orders

If the vital signs suggest shock, an intravenous (IV) bolus of either normal saline or lactated Ringer's solution should be given (10 to 20 mL/kg), and blood should be sent to the blood bank for typing and cross-matching. If bleeding is massive, type O-negative whole blood (as well as plasma and platelets if a coagulopathy is suspected) should be ordered immediately. A complete blood count, prothrombin time (PT), and partial thromboplastin time (PTT) should also be ordered to determine the degree of anemia and the potential need to correct deficiencies in platelets or clotting factors.

If active bleeding is apparent from an accessible site (e.g., skin, external nares, or oral cavity), firm pressure should be applied and held.

If the child is receiving anticoagulating medications, their use should be suspended.

Inform RN

Active bleeding, abnormal vital signs, and fever with purpura and petechiae all require immediate attention. In the absence of these concerns, the RN should be notified of when you will be at the bedside.

ELEVATOR THOUGHTS

Potential causes of bleeding depend on the site of the blood loss. Again, the basic question of whether the bleeding reflects a localized problem or a systemic one should be kept in mind. Local trauma to a blood vessel or vessels is in general far more common than a coagulopathy, particularly with epistaxis and hemoptysis. Generalized petechiae or ecchymoses should make you consider a systemic coagulopathy more carefully. Potential causes are listed by anatomic site:

Epistaxis	Blunt trauma
	Self-inflicted trauma (picking)
	Nasal congestion, crusting
	Excessive sneezing
	Foreign body
	Hypertension
	Polyp
	Tumor (e.g., angiofibroma)
	Nasal hemangioma
	Congenital syphilis ("snuffles")
	Wegener's granulomatosis
Hemoptysis	Aspiration of blood from the mouth and upper airway

Hemoptysis—
Cont'd
	Foreign body
	Infection
	   Tuberculosis
	   Pneumonia
	   Pneumonitis
	Lung abscess
	Bacterial tracheitis
	Cystic fibrosis
	Chest trauma
	Pulmonary vasculitis (lupus, Wegener's granulomatosis, Churg-Strauss syndrome, polyarteritis, Goodpasture's syndrome)
	Pulmonary embolus
	Pulmonary hypertension
	Severe congestive heart failure
	Idiopathic pulmonary hemosiderosis
	Heiner's syndrome
	Arteriovenous malformations

Petechiae, purpura, ecchymoses	Trauma (e.g., blood pressure cuff) Sepsis Septic emboli (endocarditis) Vasculitis (e.g., Henoch-Schönlein purpura) Viral infections Drugs (salicylates, steroids, nonsteroidal agents) Scurvy

Any site	Thrombocytopenia
	   Decreased platelet production (e.g., marrow failure, leukemia)
	   Increased platelet destruction (disseminated intravascular coagulopathy [DIC], idiopathic thrombocytopenic purpura [ITP], hemolytic-uremic syndrome [HUS], thrombotic thrombocytopenic purpura [TTP], splenic trapping)
	Abnormal platelet function (inherited defect, drugs)
	Clotting factor abnormality
	Hemophilia (factor VIII or IX deficiency)
	Other factor deficiency (inherited or from liver disease)
	Consumptive coagulopathy (DIC, cavernous hemangioma)
	Uremia
	Von Willebrand's disease
	Vitamin K deficiency

MAJOR THREAT TO LIFE

- Exsanguination
- Hypoxia from pulmonary hemorrhage or embolism
- Sepsis
- Intracranial hemorrhage secondary to a clotting abnormality
- Severe systemic necrotizing vasculitis

Exsanguination is always possible as long as bleeding remains active. Similarly, persistent or recurrent hemoptysis indicates active pulmonary bleeding and is very worrisome. A febrile child with petechiae and/or purpura needs immediate evaluation and empiric treatment of presumed sepsis. Severe clotting defects should be corrected as quickly as possible because they may lead to secondary bleeding in other locations, including intracranially. Vasculitides are rare but must be considered and treated promptly because they may quickly lead to multiorgan failure.

BEDSIDE

Quick-Look Test

Is the patient comfortable, alert, and in no distress, without any evidence of active bleeding?

If so, your evaluation may proceed in a more relaxed manner without the need for immediate intervention. However, if the child is actively bleeding or has persistent hemoptysis, particularly if the vital signs are abnormal, immediate intervention is necessary as you proceed with further evaluation. Similarly, if the patient is febrile and has petechiae or purpura, additional evaluation and treatment need to begin immediately.

Airway and Vital Signs

A child with epistaxis or hemoptysis may rarely have such excessive bleeding that the airway becomes compromised. Labored respirations, cyanosis, tachypnea, grunting, and retractions of accessory muscles may all be signs that the airway is compromised. In many instances, simple suctioning and turning the child to the side to clear the airway of blood alleviate the problem. However, if the airway cannot be maintained in this manner, the child needs to be intubated. Tachycardia and/or hypotension is indicative of shock secondary to either hypovolemia or sepsis and requires immediate management (see Chapter 25, Hypotension and Shock). Hypertension may result in rupture of small intranasal blood vessels and can thus lead to epistaxis. Fever may be associated with infection or vasculitis. Fever with petechiae or purpura should be treated as sepsis (e.g., meningococcemia) until proved otherwise.

Selective Physical Examination I

After a quick look and check of the airway and vital signs, the child should be examined briefly to determine the likelihood of a major threat to life, in which case immediate intervention is necessary before obtaining more historical information and reviewing the chart. The goal of this initial selective examination is to search for signs that (1) bleeding remains active (usually obvious), (2) pulmonary bleeding or emboli are causing significant hypoxia and/or respiratory distress, (3) sepsis is a possibility, or (4) the child is also bleeding intra-abdominally or intracranially.

HEENT	Pupil size and reactivity, papilledema (intracranial bleeding may lead to increased intracranial pressure [ICP]), persistent epistaxis, meningeal signs (sepsis with meningitis)
Chest	Grunting, retracting, breath sounds (respiratory distress); chest wall trauma
Abdomen	Distention, tenderness, bruising, rebound tenderness, rigidity
Skin	Multiple petechiae, purpura (meningococcemia); cyanosis (with hemoptysis would be concerning)
Neurologic	Alterations in consciousness, focality (suggestive of intracranial bleeding)

Management I

After the quick look, check of the airway and vital signs, and brief examination as described earlier, you may need to intervene if the patient is actively bleeding, if you suspect pulmonary embolism or hemorrhage, if sepsis is a concern, or if intracranial bleeding is suspected.

Active Bleeding

Bleeding from the nose, oral cavity, or mucocutaneous sites usually abates with the application of pressure. Pressure should be applied firmly for 5 minutes or longer while trying to avoid the temptation to frequently visualize the site of bleeding. With epistaxis, the child should be positioned on the side, gauze should be placed or packed within the nares, and pressure should be held over the bridge of the nose. Epistaxis most often occurs as a result of ruptured vessels in Kiesselbach's plexus, an area of anastomosed arterioles just within the nares on the septum. If the bleeding remains active or is profuse, blood should be sent to the laboratory for a stat complete blood count, platelet count, PT, and PTT and to the blood bank for typing and cross-matching. While these tests are performed, pressure should continue to be applied.

If bleeding is massive and/or the child is in shock, type O-negative blood should be requested from the blood bank and transfused as soon as possible. Depending on the site of bleeding, a general surgical or surgical subspecialty (ear, nose, and throat [ENT] for epistaxis) consultation is likely to be needed immediately because operative management may be necessary.

Coagulopathies detected by laboratory testing should be corrected if possible with appropriate blood products (platelets, fresh frozen plasma, or cryoprecipitate; see Chapter 33, Anemia, Thrombocytopenia, and Coagulation Abnormalities). If bleeding persists after correction of clotting abnormalities, surgical consultation should be considered.

Pulmonary Embolus

Pulmonary embolism is a rare childhood event that should be suspected in a child with hemoptysis who is tachypneic and hypoxic, although these signs are not invariably present. Pulse oximetry analysis or arterial blood gas determinations help establish the degree of hypoxia. If the child has a known deep venous thrombosis or hypercoagulable state, suspicion should be high and anticoagulation with heparin considered while further evaluation is proceeding. Once the child's airway and vital signs are stabilized, a helical computed tomographic (CT) scan of the chest should be performed as soon as possible to determine the probability of an embolus. If the diagnosis remains uncertain, pulmonary angiography should be considered to diagnose or exclude an embolus definitively. Once pulmonary embolism is diagnosed, anticoagulation is the treatment of choice. Large emboli may require surgical intervention.

Pulmonary Hemorrhage

Cystic fibrosis and vasculitides are conditions that may lead to acute pulmonary hemorrhage. With cystic fibrosis, persistent inflammation of the lung parenchyma may eventually lead to erosion into a major vessel and the sudden onset of massive pulmonary hemorrhage and hemoptysis. Emergency bronchoscopy, pulmonary angiography, and percutaneous catheter embolization of bronchial arteries may be necessary to localize and treat the involved vessels. If the patient has a history of systemic vasculitis or systemic lupus erythematosus or if such a diagnosis is being considered because of associated symptoms and physical findings, aggressive treatment of the underlying illness with corticosteroids and cytotoxic agents should be considered.

Sepsis

A child with fever and petechiae or purpura should be considered to have sepsis, and further evaluation and empiric treatment of sepsis should begin immediately. Blood, urine, and cerebrospinal fluid (if signs suggestive of meningitis are present) should be obtained and antibiotics administered as quickly as possible. If the child is critically ill, antibiotics should not be delayed while awaiting the performance of a lumbar puncture. Ceftriaxone, 50 mg/kg per dose every 12 hours empirically, covers pneumococcus, meningococcus, and

Haemophilus influenzae. Vancomycin should be added if there are concerns regarding resistant organisms. In a child younger than 2 months, the combination of ampicillin and cefotaxime should be used to provide additional coverage of the potential neonatal pathogens *Listeria monocytogenes*, group B streptococcus, and *Escherichia coli.*

Intracranial Bleeding

If intracranial bleeding is suspected because of focal neurologic findings or altered mental status, immediate CT scanning and neurosurgical consultation are required. If signs of increased ICP are present, management should proceed as outlined in Chapter 7, Altered Mental Status. Stat measurement of the platelet count, PT, and PTT are necessary with appropriate correction of deficiencies (see Chapter 33, Anemia, Thrombocytopenia, and Coagulation Abnormalities, for guidelines regarding the administration of blood products).

Selective Physical Examination II

If the child is not actively bleeding and your suspicion of pulmonary hemorrhage, pulmonary embolism, sepsis, or intracranial bleeding is not high, you should proceed with a more detailed physical examination:

HEENT	Fundi (retinal hemorrhage), hemotympanum, nasal deformity ("saddle nose" of Wegener's granulomatosis), palatal petechiae, dental trauma
Neck	Adenopathy (infection, malignancy, vasculitis), Kernig's and Brudzinski's signs
Chest	Breath sounds, rales, external trauma, friction rub
Heart	Murmurs (endocarditis), friction rub
Abdomen	Bowel sounds, tenderness (vasculitis), hepatosplenomegaly (malignancy, DIC, ITP, liver disease, secondary coagulopathy), rectal examination for occult blood
Musculoskeletal	Swollen joints (hemarthrosis, vasculitis), bone pain (malignancy), absent radii (thrombocytopenia–absent radii syndrome)
Genitourinary	Testicular swelling, tenderness (vasculitis)
Skin	Rashes, Osler's nodes, Janeway lesions, splinter hemorrhages (vasculitis, infectious), hemangiomas (Kasabach-Merritt syndrome)

| Neurologic | Abnormal sensation, motor deficits (peripheral neuropathy or weakness with vasculitis) |

Selective History and Chart Review

Has the child bled excessively before?

A history of previous episodes should raise suspicion of an inherited coagulopathy or chronic thrombocytopenia. Recurrent epistaxis may be self-inflicted and is also suggestive of a potential anatomic lesion (e.g., polyp or hemangioma).

Has the patient had a recent infection?

If the patient has been hospitalized with a bacterial infection, sepsis with associated DIC is a possibility. A recent viral infection might suggest idiopathic thrombocytopenic purpura or Henoch-Schönlein purpura. Recent diarrhea, particularly if bloody, might indicate HUS.

What drugs has the patient received?

Multiple drugs may be associated with thrombocytopenia or decreased platelet function, including salicylates, nonsteroidal anti-inflammatory drugs, and antibiotics. Oral contraceptives may increase the risk for pulmonary embolism.

Is there a family history of coagulopathies? Has there been bleeding after childbirth or circumcision, menorrhagia, or epistaxis in family members?

If yes, this is an obvious clue to a potential cause.

Is there any reason to suspect liver or renal failure, either secondary to the child's underlying illness or as a consequence of treatment?

Again, the answers to these questions may be diagnostically helpful.

If hemoptysis is present, has the child been exposed to tuberculosis? Have there been numerous upper and/or lower airway infections? Has the child undergone recent dental treatment? Is there any history of heart disease?

Numerous infections should raise suspicion of cystic fibrosis. Recent dental procedures might suggest lung abscess. A history of heart disease might increase the risk for endocarditis.

Has the child been hospitalized with severe traumatic injuries?

Chest trauma may result in hemoptysis. Crush injuries, burns, or severe head trauma may lead to DIC.

If the child is a newborn, is there a history of maternal thrombocytopenia or lupus? Has the mother been treated with any drugs that may cause vitamin K deficiency (e.g., anticonvulsants) or suppress platelet production? Has the neonate received vitamin K?

Neonatal immune thrombocytopenia may be the result of transplacental passage of maternal IgG antiplatelet antibodies such as those seen in lupus or ITP. Vitamin K deficiency typically results in bleeding on the second or third day of life.

Management II

After the selective history and physical examination, further laboratory testing may be necessary to determine the cause of the bleeding or to exclude possible diagnoses. In many instances, the bleeding is minimal, self-limited, and not life threatening. If epistaxis has occurred and resolved, additional testing may be unnecessary. It may be presumed that the bleeding was secondary to local trauma, and a simple "wait and see" approach may suffice. Similarly, self-limited bleeding localized to one area of the skin may often be presumed to be secondary to trauma and frequently does not require further evaluation. Excessive bleeding, hemoptysis, hemarthrosis, and generalized petechiae and purpura should be further evaluated with laboratory testing. Likewise, **recurrent** episodes of bleeding should be additionally evaluated. The following tests should be performed to assess the degree of anemia, possible thrombocytopenia, possible microangiopathy, or possible clotting factor abnormality:

1. Complete blood count
2. Platelet count
3. Peripheral blood smear
4. PT
5. PTT

Though not usually necessary immediately, a bleeding time may also be useful to determine whether abnormalities in platelet function are present.

For those with hemoptysis, a chest radiograph should be performed. Additional testing may be done selectively, depending on the clinical situation. If DIC is suspected, fibrinogen and D-dimer determination may be helpful. Hepatic enzyme, blood urea nitrogen, and creatinine determinations and urinalysis are indicated if liver or renal disease is a consideration. Blood cultures, echocardiography, or helical CT scanning should be performed if endocarditis or pulmonary embolism is suspected. Specific clotting factor assays should be performed if unexplained PT and/or PTT abnormalities are present.

Definitive management of bleeding depends on the cause. Management of life-threatening conditions has been outlined earlier. Less acute disorders should be managed as follows.

Infections

Pneumonia, tuberculosis, and lung abscess should be treated with appropriate antibiotics. Chest radiographic studies should be performed in all patients with suspected lung infection. If possible, sputum should be sent to the laboratory for culture (including mycobacterial), Gram staining, and acid-fast staining. A purified protein derivative skin test should be performed if tuberculosis is suspected. Empiric treatment of suspected pneumonia can be initiated with cefuroxime or ceftriaxone. The decision to empirically treat for *Mycoplasma pneumoniae* with erythromycin or azithromycin should be individualized as well. Cold agglutinins, often present in patients with *M. pneumoniae* infection, can be detected at the bedside by placing a small amount (2 to 3 mL) of blood in a purple-top tube and placing it on ice for several minutes. In the presence of cold agglutinins, clumping of cells can be seen along the glass walls of the tube as it is rolled in the hand. Lung abscesses should be treated with antibiotics effective against *Staphylococcus aureus* and anaerobes, such as clindamycin.

Vasculitis

Wegener's granulomatosis, Churg-Strauss syndrome, lupus, Goodpasture's syndrome, and less commonly, polyarteritis nodosa and Henoch-Schönlein purpura, among others, may result in pulmonary hemorrhage. Prompt treatment with corticosteroids may be life saving. Consideration should also be given to the use of cytotoxic therapy. Consultation with a rheumatologist is usually necessary.

Coagulopathies

Disorders of coagulation may be divided into thrombocytopenias, abnormalities in platelet function, and clotting factor deficiencies. Depending on the cause (or presumptive cause), the treatment of these conditions may vary (see Chapter 33, Anemia, Thrombocytopenia, and Coagulation Abnormalities).

10

Chest Pain

Rodney R. Mayhorn, MD

In contrast to a hospitalized adult patient, chest pain in childhood is rarely the result of cardiac pathology. Chest wall, esophageal, and psychogenic causes are much more common, and a call from a nurse regarding chest pain can usually be evaluated in a less urgent manner than can a similar call regarding an adult. Nonetheless, as with all problems arising in a hospitalized child, the major threats to life need to be considered, and in rare situations the possibility of myocardial ischemia or other cardiac causes of pain needs to be further evaluated.

It also needs to be emphasized that a child's definition of "pain" may be less precise than an older person's, and therefore palpitations, dysphagia, or heartburn may all be considerations when a child complains of chest pain.

PHONE CALL

Questions

1. What are the vital signs, including temperature?
2. How severe is the pain? How uncomfortable is the child?
3. What is the child's underlying illness and reason for hospitalization?
4. Has the child complained of chest pain before?

The vital signs and degree of severity allow you to gauge the urgency of the problem. Tachycardia may be present regardless of the cause of the pain, but extreme tachycardia (>200 beats per minute) suggests supraventricular tachycardia (SVT) or another tachydysrhythmia as a potential cause. Bradycardia in a patient with chest pain is an ominous sign that reflects impending cardiac arrest. Tachypnea may be present secondary to pneumonia, pleuritis, pneumothorax, pulmonary embolism, or hyperventilation and anxiety. Reviewing the recorded respiratory rates of the child during the period *preceding* the onset of the pain may allow you to determine whether a pulmonary process was "brewing" before the chest pain became apparent. Similarly, hypertension may reflect anxiety or may be associated with coarctation of the aorta, vasculitides such as Takayasu's arteritis, pheochromocytoma, and other systemic illnesses that may be associated with chest pain. As with bradycardia, hypotension is an ominous sign and may reflect a dissecting or ruptured aortic aneurysm or massive myocardial infarction. A fever should raise suspicion of an infectious cause for the chest pain, such as pneumonia, pleuritis, myocarditis, or pericarditis. The child's underlying illness and reason for hospitalization may offer clues to the cause of the pain. Sickle cell disease with acute chest syndrome, systemic juvenile rheumatoid arthritis (JRA) with pericarditis, and cystic fibrosis with pneumothorax are examples of illnesses associated with specific causes of chest pain.

Orders

If the vital signs reveal bradycardia or hypotension, an intravenous (IV) line should be placed, a relatively small bolus of normal saline or lactated Ringer's solution should be given (10 mL/kg), and the patient should be placed on a cardiac monitor. Additional fluid may be necessary; however, you should evaluate the patient first because of the risk of exacerbating congestive heart failure if it is present. When the IV line is placed, ask the nurse to send blood for a stat hematocrit, fractionated creatine phosphokinase (CPK), and troponin. If a hematocrit can be determined on the ward, this should be done because a decreasing hematocrit raises suspicion of hemorrhage, such as from a ruptured or dissecting aneurysm. Pulse oximetry (or arterial blood gas analysis) should be performed and oxygen administered, initially 100% by mask. Bedside electrocardiographic (ECG) and chest radiographic studies should be performed as soon as possible.

If the child does not have bradycardia or hypotension but is tachypneic, posteroanterior and lateral chest views should be ordered to specifically look for pneumonia, pleural effusions, an enlarged cardiac silhouette, pneumothorax, rib fracture, or pneumomediastinum. Keep in mind that tachypnea may be a sign of anxiety in reaction to pain rather than being directly related to the cause of the pain. An arterial blood gas revealing a very low P_{CO_2}, high pH, and normal P_{O_2} suggests hyperventilation.

Inform RN

Abnormal vital signs or severe discomfort requires **immediate** evaluation of the patient. Otherwise, let the nurse know when you plan to arrive.

ELEVATOR THOUGHTS

Potential causes of chest pain in children are most easily categorized according to organ system or anatomic location:

Cardiac	Pericarditis (bacterial, viral, inflammatory)
	Myocarditis (viral or secondary to JRA, systemic lupus erythematosus [SLE], rheumatic fever)

Cardiac— Cont'd	Dysrhythmias
	SVT
	Ventricular tachycardia
	Myocardial ischemia or infarction secondary to
	Sickle cell disease
	Kawasaki disease and coronary artery aneurysms
	SLE (with or without a lupus anticoagulant)
	Antiphospholipid antibodies
	Oral contraceptives
	Cocaine
	Severe aortic stenosis, pulmonary stenosis
	Anomalous coronary artery
	Cardiomyopathy
	Aortic dissection or rupture (e.g., from Marfan syndrome or Takayasu's arteritis)
Mediastinal	Mediastinitis (e.g., from caustic ingestion and ruptured esophagus or recent thoracic surgery)
	Pneumomediastinum
Pulmonary	Pneumonia
	Pneumothorax
	Pleuritis (infectious, JRA, SLE, familial Mediterranean fever)
	Pulmonary embolism
	Pulmonary infarction (e.g., acute chest syndrome in sickle cell disease)
Gastrointestinal	Esophagitis
	Esophageal reflux
	Gastritis
	Peptic ulcer
Musculoskeletal	Costochondritis
	Rib fracture
	Pectoral insertion pain or muscle strain
	Clavicle fracture
Psychogenic	Behavioral
	Hyperventilation

MAJOR THREAT TO LIFE

- Myocardial ischemia or infarction
- Pericarditis with tamponade
- Aortic dissection or rupture
- Pneumothorax, pneumomediastinum, or pneumopericardium
- Pulmonary embolism

- Pulmonary infarction
- Perforated or hemorrhaging peptic ulcer

All of these conditions are rare in children, but one must be aware of the possibility of one or more of these events in children with predisposing risk factors (e.g., aortic dissection with Marfan syndrome and pneumothorax with cystic fibrosis). The cardiac threats to life may result in cardiogenic shock, the pulmonary threats may produce severe hypoxia, and perforation or hemorrhage of an ulcer may lead to peritonitis and sepsis and to hypovolemic shock, respectively.

BEDSIDE

Quick-Look Test

Does the child appear well and comfortable, with no signs of distress?
If so, suspicion of a cardiac or pulmonary cause of the chest pain is low, as is suspicion of a perforated peptic ulcer. An ill-appearing child may have any of the potential causes listed earlier and requires prompt attention. Body position may offer clues to the source of the chest pain. Pericarditis and pericardial effusions may make it difficult for the child to lay supine; therefore, the child may prefer to sit and lean forward and is likely to appear anxious.

Airway and Vital Signs

Labored respirations, tachypnea, flaring, retracting, and grunting are signs of respiratory compromise. If there is any concern regarding the airway, intubation needs to be considered. As noted earlier, fever suggests infection-related causes of the pain. Tachycardia and tachypnea may occur *as a result* of the pain or may be indicative of cardiac or pulmonary processes. Extreme tachycardia suggests SVT, and an ECG study should be obtained immediately (see Chapter 22, Heart Rate and Rhythm Abnormalities). Hypotension may be present with pericarditis, myocarditis, SVT, myocardial infarction, aortic dissection, tension pneumothorax, pulmonary embolism, or a perforated peptic ulcer and peritonitis. Narrow pulse pressure suggests pericardial tamponade or tension pneumothorax. An exaggerated decrease in systolic arterial pressure during inspiration (>20 mm Hg), known as pulsus paradoxus, is also suggestive of these conditions. Normally, a slight decrease in filling of the left ventricle occurs during inspiration. This decrease may become exacerbated by the presence of a large amount of pericardial fluid or by tension pneumothorax. Pulsus paradoxus is measured by first determining systolic pressure during normal expiration. At this pressure, Korotkoff sounds are not heard with inspiration. One then listens as the manometer slowly falls to determine the point at which sounds are heard equally well during inspiration and expiration. The difference in the two determinations is the degree of pulsus paradoxus, normally less than 10 mm Hg (see Fig. 25-2).

Selective Physical Examination

General	Marfanoid body habitus: tall, thin, long arms and fingers
HEENT	Pupillary dilatation (cocaine), bulbar nonexudative conjunctivitis (Kawasaki disease), dislocated lenses (Marfan syndrome)
Neck	Distended neck veins with prominent venous pulsation (pericardial effusion), deviation of the trachea (tension pneumothorax)
Chest	Absent breath sounds (pneumothorax, pleural effusion); rales (pneumonia, congestive heart failure, pulmonary embolus); pleural rub (pleuritis); consolidation (pneumonia, infarction, acute chest syndrome); grunting, flaring, retracting (respiratory distress); chest wall tenderness (costochondritis); localized point tenderness (rib fracture); subcutaneous emphysema (pneumomediastinum); pectoral stress maneuvers (Fig. 10-1).
Heart	Muffled heart sounds (pericardial effusion, pneumopericardium), rub (pericarditis), murmur (aortic or pulmonary stenosis)
Abdomen	Rigid, rebound tenderness (peritonitis); epigastric tenderness (ulcer)
Pulses	Absent femoral pulses (aortic dissection)

Selective History and Chart Review

What does the pain feel like?

Pericarditis pain is usually sharp or stabbing and is frequently referred to the shoulder. Ischemic or infarctive pain is often crushing or squeezing. Tearing pain radiating to the neck suggests aortic dissection. Pleuritic pain is sharp rather than aching and is worse with inspiration. As mentioned previously, "pain" may also imply palpitations, dysphagia, or anxiety, and attempting to elicit the specific characteristics of what the child is feeling may be difficult.

What exacerbates the pain?

Pericarditis is worse in the supine position and is relieved by leaning forward. Pain primarily with inspiration suggests pleuritis or a musculoskeletal cause. Pain with palpation of the chest is consistent with musculoskeletal causes. Pain with swallowing (dysphagia) suggests esophagitis. Pain after eating may be secondary to esophageal reflux (heartburn).

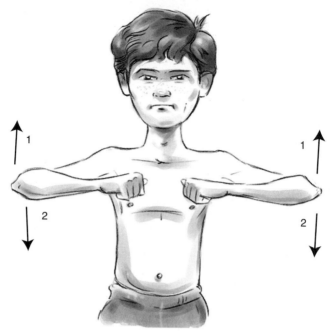

Figure 10–1 Pectoral stress maneuvers. With the patient's arms extended and elbows bent, ask the patient to move against resistance, first upward and then downward.

Does the pain radiate?

Pericarditis may cause pain in the left shoulder or the back. Aortic dissection may also radiate to the back.

What drugs has the child received?

Amphetamines may potentially cause tachyarrhythmias. Oral contraceptives may predispose to thrombosis and produce cardiac or pulmonary infarcts. Corticosteroids and nonsteroidal anti-inflammatory agents may cause esophagitis, gastritis, and peptic ulcer.

Has the child complained of chest pain previously?

A history of previous complaints and the results of previous evaluations, if any, may provide clues to the cause of the current complaints.

Management

Pericarditis

If your selective history, physical examination, and chart review suggest pericarditis as a possibility, chest radiographic studies may reveal an enlarged cardiac silhouette or a "water bottle"–shaped heart. The presence of excess fluid in the pericardial sac is confirmed by echocardiography. Various ECG abnormalities may be present. Excessive fluid may result in decreased voltage in the QRS complexes. Generalized ST-segment elevation in all leads is more indicative of pericarditis than myocardial infarction, which produces elevation in selected leads, depending on the coronary vessel involved. Management of pericarditis depends on the suspected cause. If infectious pericarditis is a possibility, diagnostic pericardiocentesis should be performed by the cardiologist to obtain fluid for Gram staining and culture. If tamponade is imminent (narrow pulse pressure, hypotension, pulsus paradoxus, and distended neck veins), therapeutic pericardiocentesis may be necessary, with placement of a drainage catheter for a short time. Pericarditis secondary to JRA may respond to IV ketorolac, 0.5 mg/kg per dose every 6 hours, indomethacin, 1 to 3 mg/kg/day divided into three doses, or prednisone, 1 to 2 mg/kg/day. Similarly, oral prednisone may be sufficient for pericarditis secondary to SLE, but if the pericarditis is severe, IV methylprednisolone, 30 mg/kg/day (maximum, 1 g) for 1 to 3 days, may be necessary for both JRA and SLE. Pericardial effusions secondary to thyroid disease or uremia should respond to treatment of the underlying condition.

Dysrhythmias

See Chapter 22, Heart Rate and Rhythm Abnormalities.

Myocardial Ischemia or Infarction

When myocardial ischemia or infarction is suspected, an ECG study should be obtained to look for patterns consistent with ischemia or infarction (Table 10-1). Serum fractionated CPK and troponin levels should also be determined. Oxygen should be administered, initially at 100%. Morphine, 0.1 to 0.2 mg/kg intravenously every 2 to 4 hours, may relieve the discomfort, but keep in mind that respiratory depression and/or hypotension may be exacerbated, and naloxone should be at the bedside in case these effects occur. Arrangements for immediate transfer to the pediatric intensive care unit (PICU) and consultation with a cardiologist should be made and the underlying cause of the ischemia or infarction addressed. Patients with sickle cell disease may require an exchange transfusion. Those with hypercoagulable states may require heparinization. Thrombolytic therapy or IV nitroglycerin may also be necessary.

Aortic Dissection

While arrangements are being made for transfer to the PICU, an emergency chest computed tomography (CT) scan or echocardiogram

TABLE 10-1 **Myocardial Infarction Patterns**

Type of Infarct	Patterns of Changes (Q Waves, ST Elevation or Depression, T-Wave Inversion)*
Inferior	Q in II, III, aVF
Inferoposterior	Q in II, III, aVF, and V_6 R > S and positive T in V_1
Anteroseptal	V_1 to V_4
Anterolateral to posterolateral	V_1 to V_5; Q in I, aVL, and V_6
Posterior	R > S in V_1, positive T, and Q in V_6

*A significant Q wave is greater than 40 msec wide or greater than a third of the QRS height. ST-segment or T-wave changes in the absence of significant Q waves may represent a non–Q-wave infarct.

From Marshall SA, Ruedy J: On Call: Principles and Practices, 2nd ed. Philadelphia, WB Saunders, 1993.

should be obtained to confirm the diagnosis. A widened mediastinum on a chest film raises suspicion but is not diagnostic. Blood for a complete blood count (CBC), prothrombin time, partial thromboplastin time, and typing and cross-matching should be sent to the laboratory immediately and large-bore IV access ensured. Urgent consultation with cardiothoracic surgeons is necessary if this diagnosis is suspected.

Pneumomediastinum or Mediastinitis

Pneumomediastinum most often occurs with pneumothorax as a result of ruptured alveoli and tracking of air into the mediastinal space. However, it may also occur with esophageal perforation or may have no identifiable underlying cause. In an older child beyond the neonatal period, pneumomediastinum is rarely a problem in itself because the air may escape into the neck or the abdomen. This does not occur as readily in a newborn, however, and air in the mediastinum at this age is therefore more likely to lead to compromise of cardiac output or rupture into the pleural space. Chest radiographs reveal a sharper cardiac border and may also disclose subcutaneous air. Treatment is directed at the pulmonary disease. Unless there is cardiovascular compromise, the air in the mediastinal space need not be evacuated and resolves spontaneously. Mediastinitis and/or pneumomediastinum after esophageal perforation requires urgent treatment. Esophageal perforation is usually seen in the context of ingestion of corrosive substances. Alkali ingestion places children at increased risk because it results in liquefactive necrosis affecting all layers of the esophagus. Perforation is also a potential complication of upper endoscopic examination. Surgical consultation for mediastinal evacuation and drainage, as well as

repair of the esophagus, is necessary. Broad-spectrum empiric antibiotic treatment covering both aerobes and anaerobes is also necessary
after collection of appropriate culture specimens.

Pneumothorax

Treatment of pneumothorax depends on its severity. Small pneumothoraces may resolve spontaneously without treatment. Oxygen,
100% by mask or by hood in an infant, may result in quicker resolution by increasing the pressure gradient for nitrogen between pleural
air and blood. Large pneumothoraces require closed thoracostomy
(chest tube), and tension pneumothoraces resulting in respiratory
distress may require emergency evacuation with an angiocatheter
and syringe. To accomplish emergency evacuation,

1. Either the second intercostal space in the midclavicular line or
   the third or fourth intercostal space in the midaxillary line
   (may be easier in infants) should be chosen and cleaned in
   sterile fashion.
2. If there is sufficient time, anesthetizing the skin and subcutaneous tissue with lidocaine may make the procedure easier for
   you and the patient.
3. A 20- or 22-gauge angiocatheter should then be inserted
   directly perpendicular to the rib surface *below* the intercostal
   space to be entered and the needle advanced over the *top* of
   the rib to avoid the nerves and vessels that run under the inferior margin of the ribs. Once the pleural space is entered, a
   "pop" may be felt, and a rush of air may be heard through the
   angiocatheter.
4. The needle should be withdrawn while keeping the catheter in
   place, and a stopcock and syringe can then be attached to the
   catheter and air withdrawn with the syringe and expelled by
   rotating the stopcock. If a chest tube is necessary, the procedure may require conscious sedation in a young child and
   should therefore be performed in a controlled setting where
   the child may be appropriately monitored. The procedure is
   similar to that described earlier but is modified so that a short,
   0.5-cm incision is made over the rib and a curved hemostat is
   used to puncture the pleura. Again, the hemostat is guided
   over the top of the rib. Once the tip of the hemostat is in the
   pleural space, the hemostat may be opened slightly and the
   chest tube inserted into the incision and guided to the proper
   position with the hemostat. The tube, once positioned, should
   be sutured in place and covered with a sterile dressing. The position should then be confirmed by chest radiographic study.

Pneumonia

If bacterial pneumonia is suspected from the clinical and radiographic
findings, antibiotics are required. A CBC with differential and blood
cultures, as well as sputum Gram stain and culture, if possible, should

be obtained before empiric treatment with IV cefuroxime or ceftriaxone. A purified protein derivative test should be conducted if exposure to tuberculosis is a possibility. Bedside cold agglutinin determinations (see Chapter 9, Bleeding) may help you decide whether azithromycin should be added to cover *Mycoplasma pneumoniae*. If pleural fluid is also present, aspiration of the fluid for Gram stain and culture may be considered before starting antibiotic treatment.

Pleural Effusion

Thoracentesis should be considered for diagnostic purposes, and if the effusion is large, thoracentesis may be therapeutic as well. The procedure is identical to that for pneumothorax, except that the pleural cavity is entered posteriorly with the patient sitting upright. As much fluid as possible is withdrawn and should be sent for culture, Gram stain, cell count, and total protein determination.

Pulmonary Embolism

Management is discussed in Chapter 9, Bleeding.

Esophagitis, Gastritis, or Peptic Ulcer

Antacids, an H_2 receptor antagonist, or a proton pump inhibitor may provide relief. Aluminum hydroxide, 5 to 15 mL orally every 3 to 6 hours, is one choice of antacid. Ranitidine, 2 to 4 mg/kg/day every 12 hours orally or 1 to 2 mg/kg/day every 8 hours intravenously, or omeprazole (Prilosec), 0.6 mg/kg per dose given twice a day, may be used. Consultation with a gastroenterologist and endoscopic examination may be required.

Costochondritis

Ibuprofen, 30 mg/kg/day divided in four doses, naproxen, 10 to 20 mg/kg/day twice a day, or ketorolac, 0.5 mg/kg per dose given every 6 hours, may provide relief.

Psychogenic

Reassurance and efforts aimed at relaxing the patient are the best approach. As with abdominal pain, headaches, and extremity pain, idiopathic chest pain is common in children, particularly during the preadolescent years. Concern regarding family members with heart disease may contribute to the child's fears and subsequent pain. Reassurance that they have a "normal heart" may be all that is required to result in resolution of the pain.

Constipation

Erica L. Kroncke, MD

Constipation is common in both hospitalized and otherwise healthy children. Although it is not usually an emergency, calls from a nurse regarding hard stool or absence of bowel movements in a hospitalized child are frequent. The appropriate evaluation and management of this problem differ with the age of the child. In a toddler or older child, functional causes are common, whereas in an infant, dietary causes are often the first consideration. Despite their relative rarity, potentially life-threatening causes need to be considered at any age, particularly during the neonatal period, when constipation may be one of the features of bowel obstruction secondary to congenital anomalies.

PHONE CALL

Questions

1. Is the stool hard and is defecation difficult, or has there been no stool for a some time? Exactly what has the frequency of stool been during the child's hospitalization?
2. How old is the child?
3. Are there any associated gastrointestinal signs or symptoms, such as abdominal pain, poor oral intake, nausea, vomiting (especially bilious), or abdominal distention?
4. Why is the child hospitalized?
5. Has the child been constipated in the past?
6. What medications has the child received?

Characterizing the "constipation" is the most important step. It may be normal for a formula-fed infant to go longer than 1 or 2 days without a stool, but such a pattern may be considered "constipation" by a parent or a nurse. Similarly, an older child who stools infrequently but has normal, soft stools without associated symptoms is unlikely to have a problem. Generally, the nature of the stool is much more indicative of constipation than the frequency is. "Straining" in infants is a common concern of parents and is often a function of uncoordinated abdominal and perineal muscle contractions during defecation. Straining alone usually requires no evaluation or intervention.

Once it is clear that the child does in fact appear to be constipated, the age of the child allows you to further consider possible causes. Associated symptoms and the reason for the child's hospitalization may suggest bowel obstruction or a systemic process affecting the gastrointestinal tract. A history of constipation suggests a chronic problem rather than one related to the current hospitalization. Finally, medications such as narcotics are frequent causes of constipation.

Orders

Most calls regarding infrequent or absent stooling do not require urgent action. If the problem is brought to your attention in the middle of the night and the child is stable with no associated symptoms, it may often be necessary to defer further evaluation until more urgent matters are addressed. In this situation, symptomatic treatment may be reasonable if it appears that it will be a while until you are able to evaluate the child further. For an infant who is passing small, hard stools, the addition of a small amount of sugar to the formula (e.g., corn syrup or juice) is sometimes successful. A child who has had constipation in the past may often be managed by prescribing the same regimen of cathartics and/or stool softeners that has previously been successful. For a child who is otherwise stable without previous constipation, a trial of a stool softener or a cathartic may be reasonable until either the constipation is relieved or time is available to evaluate further. Docusate sodium (Colace), lactulose, and polyethylene glycol (MiraLax) can be used as stool softeners, and senna concentrate (Senokot) and bisacodyl can stimulate defecation. It needs to be emphasized that the aforementioned orders should not simply be reflexively given. Once time permits and matters that have taken priority have been addressed, careful evaluation of the constipated child should proceed.

A child who has associated symptoms such as abdominal pain, vomiting, or abdominal distention obviously needs to be evaluated promptly because a significant intra-abdominal process is then more likely.

ELEVATOR THOUGHTS

Potential causes of constipation differ depending on the age of the child:

Neonate or infant	Dietary
	Insufficient volume
	Insufficient bulk
	Anatomic
	Imperforate anus or anal atresia
	Intestinal atresia or stenosis

Neonate or infant—Cont'd

Malrotation of the gut
    Hirschsprung's disease
Botulism
Hypothyroidism
Spinal cord lesions (meningomyelocele, spina bifida)
Amyotonia congenita
Meconium ileus (cystic fibrosis)
Pseudo-obstruction
Hypokalemia
Hypercalcemia
Syndromes
    Prune-belly syndrome
    Trisomy 21

Older child

Functional (e.g., withholding)
Dietary
    Insufficient fluid
    Insufficient bulk
Painful defecation (e.g., fissure)
Hirschsprung's disease
Hypothyroidism
Spinal cord lesions (e.g., tumor, diastematomyelia)
Amyotonia congenita
Guillain-Barré syndrome
Bowel obstruction
Food-borne botulism
Pseudo-obstruction
Scleroderma
Hypokalemia
Hypercalcemia
Drugs or toxins (antacids, anticholinergics, iron, lead, narcotics, among others)
Adynamic ileus
Abdominal or pelvic mass lesion

MAJOR THREAT TO LIFE

Constipation as the sole complaint is not suggestive of a life-threatening illness. The major threats to life are associated with other signs and symptoms, which should suggest the diagnosis.

- Bowel obstruction (abdominal pain, bilious vomiting)
- Botulism (weakness, hypotonia)
- Guillain-Barré syndrome (weakness, decreased deep tendon reflexes)
- Drugs or toxins
- Hypokalemia

BEDSIDE

Quick-Look Test

In nearly all cases, the infant or child appears comfortable. If an infant is irritable or an older child appears distressed, one of the aforementioned major threats to life should be further considered.

Airway and Vital Signs

A child with constipation and no associated signs or symptoms is expected to have normal vital signs and a stable airway. If such is not the case, a prompt search for signs to suggest one of the threats to life just listed should be undertaken. Fever, tachycardia, and hypotension suggest bowel obstruction with perforation and subsequent peritonitis. Labored respirations and/or tachypnea may be associated with bowel obstruction or may also be a sign of respiratory muscle weakness secondary to botulism or Guillain-Barré syndrome. Abnormal vital signs may be seen with hypokalemia or a number of toxic syndromes (narcotics, anticholinergics).

Selective History and Chart Review

Does the child have abdominal pain, nausea, vomiting, or abdominal distention?

Relatively mild pain or, rarely, severe pain may occur as a result of constipation. Other gastrointestinal symptoms should raise concern about bowel obstruction.

In a neonate, has there been a normal stool yet? Is there a history of a meconium plug?

Meconium plugs at birth suggest Hirschsprung's disease or cystic fibrosis. These disorders, as well as structural anomalies of the gastrointestinal tract, are possibilities if the neonate has not had a stool.

What is the infant's or child's diet?

Breast-fed infants should have several relatively loose, light yellow or green stools every day, often after each feeding; therefore, constipation in an exclusively breast-fed infant is rare and suggests either inadequate intake of breast milk or an explanation other than diet. Honey is a notorious source of *Clostridium botulinum* spores, the cause of infant botulism. Insufficient volume of intake because of either diet or intercurrent illness may cause stool desiccation and constipation. In both infants and older children, insufficient fecal bulk may result in an inadequate stimulus to peristalsis and subsequent constipation. A high-starch or high-protein diet, a lack of carbohydrate or fiber, or the continued use of puréed foods beyond infancy may not provide adequate roughage to promote defecation.

Has there been a history of constipation or fecal soiling?

Chronic constipation may lead to encopresis, characterized by retention of stool with leakage of fluid stool involuntarily around a large fecal mass. This may occur as a result of withholding secondary to a traumatic toilet-training experience, painful defecation because of anal fissures, or a psychological disturbance. Occasionally, Hirschsprung's disease is diagnosed late in a child after years of constipation. A history of *never* having a normal stooling pattern may suggest such an underlying anatomic defect.

Are the signs and symptoms suggestive of a systemic process?

In an infant, poor feeding, poor sucking, a weak cry, hypotonia, ptosis, and respiratory insufficiency may suggest botulism or hypothyroidism. An older child with growth delay, dry skin, myxedema, brittle hair, cold intolerance, and fatigue may also have hypothyroidism. Spinal cord lesions, static encephalopathy, and Guillain-Barré syndrome produce neurologic findings. Amyotonia congenita or scleroderma should be suggested by other clinical findings. Remember also that *any* acute illness may result in adynamic ileus.

What medications has the child received?

Constipation may be secondary to a long list of possible medications, most commonly narcotics and anticholinergics.

Selective Physical Examination

HEENT	Large anterior or posterior fontanelle (hypothyroidism), mydriasis (botulism, anticholinergics), meiosis (narcotics), dry mucous membranes (botulism, anticholinergics), large tongue (hypothyroidism)
Neck	Goiter (hypothyroidism)
Chest	Respiratory insufficiency (bowel obstruction with abdominal distention, botulism, Guillain-Barré syndrome)
Cardiovascular	Mild bradycardia (congenital hypothyroidism, narcotics), tachycardia (anticholinergics), hypertension (anticholinergics, Guillain-Barré syndrome), hypotension (narcotics, Guillain-Barré syndrome)
Abdomen	Bowel sounds, distention, tenderness, masses, rebound, rigidity (bowel obstruction)
Rectal	Impacted stool, patulous anus and rectum (functional constipation), absence of stool (Hirschsprung's disease), explosive fecal or gaseous discharge (Hirschsprung's disease), meconium plug in an infant (cystic fibrosis,

Rectal—Cont'd	Hirschsprung's disease), nonpatent rectum (imperforate anus), anal fissure
Skin	Dryness (hypothyroidism), myxedema (hypothyroidism), thickening, atrophy, pigment changes, tightening (scleroderma), jaundice (hypothyroidism)
Neurologic	Absent or delayed reflexes (hypothyroidism, Guillain-Barré syndrome, spinal cord lesions), calf muscle hypertrophy (hypothyroidism), hypotonia (hypothyroidism, botulism, spinal cord lesions)

Management

If a systemic illness is detected, appropriate management should relieve the cause of the constipation. In such a situation, symptomatic treatment of the constipation with dietary changes, suppositories, manual disimpaction, enemas, cathartics, and stool softeners may be used as an adjunct to definitive treatment of the underlying illness.

In most hospitalized children with constipation that becomes apparent while you are on call, proceed with symptomatic treatment while planning to address dietary or functional issues at a more convenient time. If a hard stool is present in the rectum, treatment should first be directed toward assisting passage of the stool. In an infant a glycerin suppository or enema may be used. In an older child, bisacodyl or senna may successfully relieve the impaction. A Fleet Children's Enema may also be tried. If these measures are unsuccessful, manual disimpaction may be necessary, although for most children (and physicians), this is considered one of the last resorts. Several options are available to increase bulk or soften stool. Increasing the volume of fluid intake, as well as dietary supplements such as prune juice, olive oil, or mineral oil (1 tbs orally), may be helpful. Green vegetables, fruits, bran, and whole grains add bulk. Stool softeners as described earlier may also be prescribed. If anal fissures are present, sitz baths may relieve some of the discomfort, and stool softeners may be the best initial choice of treatment.

Laboratory or radiographic evaluation of a constipated child is rarely necessary, except if one wishes to document the presence of large amounts of stool in the colon with a plain abdominal film. If bowel obstruction is suspected, the need for further evaluation and consultation with pediatric surgeons is obvious. Similarly, other tests are ordered only if one is suspicious of an underlying systemic illness or anatomic defect. Serum triiodothyronine, thyroxine, and thyroid-stimulating hormone should be measured if hypothyroidism is a consideration. Hirschsprung's disease may be suggested by barium enema or anal manometry but is confirmed by rectal biopsy. If Guillain-Barré syndrome is suspected, a lumbar puncture (looking for an elevated cerebrospinal fluid protein level) and nerve conduction studies may be appropriate before considering therapy with intravenous immunoglobulin. Botulism is diagnosed by detecting *C. botulinum* organisms or toxin in the feces. An enzyme-linked immunosorbent assay is available for detecting fecal toxin.

For most calls regarding constipation in the middle of the night, simple symptomatic treatment is often all that is necessary, and such management allows you to "move on" to other matters that often take priority.

Crying and the Irritable Infant

Lori A. Porter, MD

Crying and irritability may be considered expected findings in hospitalized infants because these signs are associated with any condition causing pain or discomfort. Usually it is clear that the infant is irritable because of an apparent underlying illness. In some hospitalized infants, however, the irritability or crying may be difficult to explain. There may not be an apparent cause for the irritability, or the character or degree of the irritability may differ from that present on admission. Evaluation of an irritable infant must be particularly thorough to search for clues that suggest a source of the irritability. Sepsis and other infections should always be at the top of the list of considerations, even in the absence of fever, but this should not keep you from thinking of other possible explanations. Crying in an infant in the absence of illness, such as that seen in infants with colic, should always be a diagnosis of exclusion.

PHONE CALL

Questions

1. What are the vital signs?
2. Has the infant's degree of irritability *changed* since admission? Is this a new sign or simply a persistent one?
3. Why is the infant hospitalized?

Fever and irritability are indicative of infection and require immediate action. Some tachycardia is expected in an infant who is irritable, but extreme tachycardia or abnormalities in the respiratory rate or blood pressure should also raise your level of concern. Because at least some degree of irritability is likely to be present in most hospitalized infants, it is important to determine whether the current status of the infant is **different**. For example, an infant admitted with bacterial meningitis who has received only a few doses of antibiotics may continue to be irritable for several days until the infection and meningeal inflammation begin to resolve. In contrast, in an infant who has been gradually responding to treatment and then becomes increasingly irritable, a new condition has probably developed to explain the change in status. It may be serious, such as a subdural effusion, or simple, such as an infiltrated intravenous (IV) site.

Orders

No orders should be given until the infant is further evaluated.

Inform RN

An infant with a change in the degree of irritability or new onset of irritability needs to be evaluated immediately.

ELEVATOR THOUGHTS

What might cause irritability in the infant? As mentioned earlier, almost **any** condition may be associated with irritability, and infection is a very common cause. The following list contains some of the more common possibilities, as well as some that may often be overlooked:

Infection	Sepsis
	Meningitis
	Encephalitis
	Brain abscess
	Lymphadenitis
	Pneumonia
	Gastroenteritis
	Myocarditis
	Pericarditis
	Viral syndrome
	Cellulitis
	Mastitis
	Otitis media
	Urinary tract infection
	Pyomyositis
	Osteomyelitis
	Septic arthritis
Gastrointestinal and intra-abdominal conditions	Gastritis
	Gastroesophageal reflux and esophagitis
	Intussusception
	Volvulus
	Bowel obstruction
	Appendicitis
	Peptic ulcer disease
	Constipation
	Anal fissure
	Inguinal hernia

Inflammatory disorders	Kawasaki disease
	Systemic juvenile rheumatoid arthritis
Metabolic and endocrine disorders	Hyponatremia or hypernatremia
	Hypocalcemia or hypercalcemia
	Hypokalemia
	Hypoglycemia
	Urea cycle disorders (early)
	Reye's syndrome (early)
	Zinc deficiency
	Protein malnutrition
	Scurvy
	Hyperthyroidism
Cardiac processes	Supraventricular tachycardia
	Congestive heart failure
	Pericarditis
	Anomalous left coronary artery from the pulmonary artery
Intracranial processes	Increased intracranial pressure (ICP)
	Subdural hematoma
	Subdural effusion with meningitis
	Brain tumor
	Seizures
Toxic processes	Lead ingestion
	Vitamin A poisoning
	Narcotic withdrawal
	Fetal alcohol syndrome
Other disorders	Trauma, including child abuse
	Respiratory failure
	Foreign body ingestion
	Teething
	Colic
	Hunger
Mechanical problems	Infiltrated IV site
	Entanglement in monitor wires or IV tubing
	Skin irritation from monitor lines
	Blood pressure cuff
	Too small a diaper
	Lying on a foreign body in the bed
	"Hair tourniquet" of a digit

MAJOR THREAT TO LIFE

- Infections (sepsis, meningitis)
- Intra-abdominal conditions (bowel obstruction, appendicitis)
- Metabolic disturbances
- Increased ICP
- Seizures
- Cardiac disorders (dysrhythmia, pericarditis, myocarditis)
- Respiratory failure

Immediate evaluation of an irritable infant should focus on searching for signs suggestive of one of the aforementioned threats and/or recognizing that the infant is at risk for one or more of these conditions because of an underlying illness or its treatment.

BEDSIDE

Quick-Look Test

An irritable infant, by definition, appears ill. If the infant is quiet by the time of your arrival, this is not necessarily reassuring. Irritability may be intermittent or may progress to lethargy if the underlying cause is significant. Intussusception, anal fissure, seizures, supraventricular tachycardia, gastroesophageal reflux, systemic juvenile rheumatoid arthritis, teething, and colic should be greater considerations if the irritability is intermittent.

Airway and Vital Signs

Fever and irritability are signs of sepsis in an infant until proved otherwise. Further evaluation and management should include blood, cerebrospinal fluid (CSF), and urine culture, followed by the empiric administration of antibiotics. Suspicion of sepsis should be particularly high in a very young infant (<2 months). Cultures should be obtained as efficiently as possible and antibiotics administered as soon as possible. In a critically ill infant, the risks of delaying antibiotic treatment need to be weighed against the benefit of obtaining as many of the cultures just mentioned as possible. In such a situation, it is sometimes best to administer antibiotics after the blood culture, assuming that blood can be obtained fairly readily. Subsequent CSF and urine cultures may be affected by this approach; however, one may use the CSF profile (white blood cells [WBCs], protein, glucose) and urinalysis (WBC count) to aid in determining the possibility of meningitis and a urinary tract infection, respectively. The choice of antibiotics depends on the infant's age, as well as any special considerations, such as the presence of a ventriculoperitoneal shunt, recent surgery, or immunodeficiency (for further discussion, see Chapter 18, Fever). Hypothermia in an infant may also be associated with infection. Extreme tachycardia should suggest supraventricular tachycardia (see Chapter 22, Heart Rate and Rhythm Abnormalities), as well as myocarditis. Keep in mind that tachycardia may occur secondary to the irritability and crying. Tachypnea should alert you to the possibility of pneumonia, respiratory failure, congestive heart failure, or metabolic acidosis associated with a metabolic disorder. Hypotension may be related to sepsis or to an intra-abdominal catastrophe.

Comprehensive Physical Examination

When evaluating an irritable infant, it is critical that the physical examination be especially thorough rather than selective. Given the limitations of the history at this age, it should also be the initial step in your evaluation rather than the usual approach of history-taking followed by physical examination. Particular attention needs to be paid to potential sources of infection (e.g., ears), the abdominal examination, and a careful examination of the extremities. It is very easy to overlook the fact that an infant is not moving an extremity normally because of pain. This may be seen with septic arthritis, osteomyelitis, "hair tourniquets," and trauma (including occult fractures). Carefully inspect any IV sites by removing tape and other coverings so that you can clearly visualize the skin. An infiltrated or infected IV site can easily be overlooked. Remember that meningeal signs are not reliable indicators of meningitis in an infant.

HEENT	Fontanelle (flat or bulging?), pupils, conjunctivitis (infections, Kawasaki disease), periorbital soft tissue (cellulitis), tympanic membrane (otitis), auditory canal (foreign body, trauma), nose (rhinorrhea), mouth, pharynx (stomatitis, trauma)
Neck	Adenopathy (Kawasaki disease); erythema, warmth (adenitis)
Chest	Breath sounds (pneumonia, foreign body aspiration, congestive heart failure); breast swelling, warmth (mastitis); erythema, tenderness (rib fracture)
Cardiovascular	Heart sounds (myocarditis, pericarditis, supraventricular tachycardia); thrills, heaves (congestive heart failure)
Abdomen	Bowel sounds, distention, masses (bowel obstruction)
Genitalia	Masses (inguinal hernia), testicular swelling or tenderness
Rectal	Masses, stool, bleeding
Extremities	Swelling, warmth (infections); bruising (trauma); cyanosis (respiratory failure, "hair tourniquet"); limited use, limited range of motion, tenderness (trauma, infection)

| Neurologic | Focal signs (brain abscess, tumor), seizures (metabolic disturbance) |
| Skin | Rash, petechiae, purpura (systemic juvenile rheumatoid arthritis, meningococcemia); wounds (trauma) |

Selective History and Chart Review

What has the infant's previous behavior been like? How is the infant described in previous notes?

As noted earlier, an attempt should be made to determine whether the infant's status has *changed*. If so, this suggests that either a new problem has developed or the underlying illness being treated during this hospitalization is progressing.

Does the infant have a known infection that is currently being treated?

If so, you need to consider the possibilities of inadequate treatment and/or a suppurative complication of the initial infection (e.g., mastoiditis following otitis; meningitis, osteomyelitis, or septic arthritis following bacteremia). Look carefully at the fever pattern during the hospitalization. A recurrence following initial defervescence suggests "seeding" of a distant site after bacteremia.

What has the infant's oral intake been? Has there been any vomiting, constipation, or diarrhea?

The answers may suggest a gastrointestinal cause of the irritability.

Has the infant received IV fluids?

Review the type and amount of fluids, as well as any recent electrolyte measurements, to determine the likelihood of a metabolic abnormality to explain the irritability.

What medications has the infant received?

Aspirin, as well as other drugs, may lead to Reye's syndrome. Numerous other medications may result in seizures or metabolic disturbances. Recent narcotic or benzodiazepine use raises the possibility of withdrawal symptoms.

Management

Further evaluation and management of an irritable infant depend on the differential diagnosis that you develop after the quick look, physical examination, and history and chart review. It may be apparent at this point that the infant's irritability is not a significant *change* in status and can easily be attributed to the underlying reason for admission. If this is the case, continuing the present management with continued observation of the infant may be the most appropriate next step. It needs to be emphasized, however, that **continued and frequent observation** is the key element of this approach and that further evaluation may become necessary if the irritability either changes in character or persists.

If the irritability of the infant is believed to be either "new" or different in character, further evaluation is necessary. As mentioned earlier, if fever is present, cultures should be obtained and antibiotics begun. If an intra-abdominal process is suspected, the infant should be given nothing orally, and radiographs and surgical consultation may be necessary (see Chapter 6, Abdominal Pain). If metabolic disturbances remain a possibility, serum electrolyte, calcium, glucose, and ammonia measurements are helpful, followed by appropriate correction of the disturbance if present. Neurologic signs suggesting seizures or increased ICP should be managed appropriately (see Chapter 7, Altered Mental Status).

In some cases, no other identifiable clues may be present to help guide further evaluation. In these circumstances, it may be best to pursue additional studies and management, with the goal being to **exclude** and empirically treat the major threats to life. What could be happening **tonight** that is potentially life threatening? Remembering that sepsis is always a possibility, blood, CSF, and urine cultures should be obtained and antibiotics begun empirically in a young infant (<2 months) and in an older infant who appears particularly ill. In an older infant, this decision requires clinical judgment and discussion with the senior resident and/or attending physician. Serum electrolyte, calcium, and glucose levels should be determined if a recent result is unavailable. As emphasized previously, **repeated evaluations** of the infant are necessary in this situation to ensure that the abdominal, cardiac, respiratory, or neurologic status is not changing. Additional studies depend on your findings as the process evolves.

Evaluation of an irritable infant requires a careful, thorough approach and is therefore often a time-consuming and potentially frustrating process. Remember that your goals while on call are to (1) identify a cause and treat it when possible and (2) exclude or empirically treat life-threatening illness. This should help you prioritize and prevent you from becoming as "irritated" as the patient.

13

Cyanosis

James J. Nocton, MD

As with many problems in pediatrics, appropriate evaluation of a patient with cyanosis depends on the age of the child. The diagnoses you consider when confronted with cyanosis in a newborn differ from those you consider when evaluating an older child or teenager. In all patients, a distinction should be made between peripheral cyanosis and central or generalized cyanosis. Peripheral cyanosis is, by definition, present in the extremities, with sparing of the central regions of the body. It is usually the result of localized vascular changes that lead to poor perfusion and/or venous stasis. Peripheral cyanosis may be secondary to vascular phenomena (e.g., "physiologic" acrocyanosis of the newborn, Raynaud's phenomenon, sepsis), obstructive processes (superior vena cava syndrome, deep venous thrombosis, tourniquets), or blood disorders such as hypercoagulability (with subsequent thrombosis) and hyperviscosity (e.g., polycythemia). The presence of peripheral cyanosis without generalization suggests that primary lung or heart disease is not present. In contrast, generalized cyanosis, indicative of a large amount of reduced hemoglobin (>5 g/dL) or oxygen saturation below approximately 90%, is more consistent with primary heart disease or respiratory insufficiency but may also occur if some of the processes that cause peripheral cyanosis are severe enough (e.g., sepsis). This chapter focuses on generalized cyanosis because it is more common, more likely to be life threatening, and more likely to require extensive evaluation when on call.

The many causes of central cyanosis can be broadly divided into two groups: (1) decreased oxygenation of hemoglobin as a consequence of either respiratory insufficiency or cardiac disease and (2) abnormalities of hemoglobin (methemoglobinemia or hemoglobin with reduced affinity for oxygen). Nearly all cases encountered in infants and children are a result of decreased oxygenation because of lung or heart disease, but hemoglobin abnormalities should always be considered. In a full-term newborn, cardiac and pulmonary disease should be considered equally, whereas in an older child, congenital heart disease is a less likely consideration. This chapter is divided into two sections, with evaluation of a newborn discussed separately from evaluation of an older child.

CYANOSIS IN A NEWBORN

PHONE CALL

Questions

1. What are the vital signs?
2. Is the infant alert and active and able to feed or lethargic and refusing to feed?
3. How old is the child?
4. Is the cyanosis central or peripheral?
5. Are there signs of respiratory distress (tachypnea, grunting, flaring, retracting)?
6. Are there signs of poor perfusion (delayed capillary refill, cold extremities)?

The vital signs and behavior of the infant allow you to determine the urgency of the situation and may also provide clues to the potential cause of the cyanosis. Unfortunately, it is often difficult, based on signs and symptoms alone, to distinguish the many potential causes of neonatal cyanosis. Tachycardia, tachypnea, signs of respiratory distress, poor perfusion, and/or hypotension may indicate sepsis, cardiogenic shock associated with congenital heart disease, or severe respiratory insufficiency. Fever or hypothermia may raise suspicion of septic shock. Lethargy is expected if central nervous system (CNS) depression and secondary respiratory insufficiency are occurring. Exacerbation of the signs of distress with feeding may suggest congestive heart failure. This occurs with congenital heart lesions that result in an increase in pulmonary blood flow (e.g., transposition of the great arteries, truncus arteriosus, and total anomalous pulmonary venous return) or with lesions associated with obstructed left heart outflow (as seen with coarctation of the aorta, valvular aortic stenosis, and hypoplastic left heart syndrome). The age of the infant may provide a clue to the cause. Because the ductus arteriosus normally closes functionally by the third day of life, the onset or worsening of cyanosis at this age may indicate the presence of a congenital heart lesion that depends on ductal flow to perfuse the lungs (i.e., obstructions to pulmonary blood flow, such as with tricuspid atresia or pulmonary atresia) or to provide oxygenated blood to the systemic circulation (e.g., transposition of the great arteries with an intact ventricular septum). Peripheral cyanosis in the early newborn period may be "physiologic."

Orders

1. If possible, an arterial blood gas sample should be obtained from a site distal to the ductus arteriosus (i.e., the left arm or the legs) while the infant is breathing room air, and the infant then placed on 100% oxygen. After at least 10 minutes, a second

TABLE 13-1 **Hyperoxia Test Interpretation**

	Pao$_2$ in Room Air* (mm Hg)	Pao$_2$ in 100% Fio$_2$ (mm Hg)*
Healthy	70	>200
Lung disease	50	>150
Cyanotic heart disease		
Decreased pulmonary blood flow	<50	<100
Increased pulmonary blood flow	50	<150
Methemoglobinemia	70	>200

*Values are approximations.

arterial blood gas sample should be obtained. This test, the **hyperoxia test**, may help distinguish primary cardiac disease from lung disease and other potential disorders. In cyanotic congenital heart disease, the Pao$_2$ is not expected to rise to a value greater than 150 mm Hg for mixing lesions or 100 mm Hg in the case of severely restricted pulmonary blood flow (Table 13-1). Remember that pulse oximetry (oxygen saturation analysis) cannot be a substitute for measurement of Pao$_2$ because saturation reaches the maximum of 100% at approximately 90 mm Hg (see Appendix D, The Oxyhemoglobin Dissociation Curve of Normal Blood). Caution should be used in interpreting the hyperoxia test too strictly. Exceptions to the generalization may occur, and therefore the results should always be interpreted in conjunction with other clinical information.

2. A serum glucose (or Dextrostix) measurement, chest radiograph, and 12-lead electrocardiogram (ECG) should be ordered stat. Additional laboratory measurements that should be obtained include a complete blood count and serum electrolyte determinations.
3. The infant should be placed on a cardiorespiratory monitor with continual pulse oximetry.
4. An intravenous (IV) line should be placed, and the infant should be maintained without oral intake.

Inform RN

A newborn with cyanosis needs to be evaluated immediately.

ELEVATOR THOUGHTS

What is the differential diagnosis of cyanosis in a newborn?

Central cyanosis	See Table 13-2
Peripheral cyanosis	Physiologic acrocyanosis
	Arterial thrombosis
	Vasomotor instability

TABLE 13-2 **Differential Diagnosis of Neonatal Cyanosis**

Disease	Mechanism
Pulmonary	
Respiratory distress syndrome	Surfactant deficiency
Sepsis, pneumonia	Inflammation, pulmonary hypertension, shunting R → L
Meconium aspiration pneumonia	Mechanical obstruction, inflammation, pulmonary hypertension, shunting R → L
Persistent fetal circulation	Pulmonary hypertension, shunting R → L
Diaphragmatic hernia	Pulmonary hypoplasia, pulmonary hypertension
Transient tachypnea	Retained lung fluid
Cardiovascular	
Cyanotic heart disease with decreased pulmonary blood flow	R → L shunt as in pulmonary atresia, tetralogy of Fallot
Cyanotic heart disease with increased pulmonary blood flow	R → L shunt as in d-transposition, truncus arteriosus
Cyanotic heart disease with congestive heart failure	R → L shunt with pulmonary edema and poor cardiac output, as in hypoplastic left heart syndrome and coarctation of the aorta
Heart failure alone	Pulmonary edema and poor cardiac contractility, as in sepsis, myocarditis, supraventricular tachycardia, or complete heart block; high-output failure, as in patent ductus arteriosus, vein of Galen, or other arteriovenous malformation
Central Nervous System	
Maternal sedative drugs	Hypoventilation, apnea
Asphyxia	CNS depression
Intracranial hemorrhage	CNS depression, seizure
Neuromuscular disease	Phrenic nerve palsy, hypotonia, hypoventilation, pulmonary hypoplasia
Hematologic	
Acute blood loss	Shock
Chronic blood loss	Congestive heart failure
Polycythemia	Pulmonary hypertension
Methemoglobinemia	Low-affinity hemoglobin or red blood cell enzyme defect
Metabolic	
Hypoglycemia	CNS depression, congestive heart failure
Adrenogenital syndrome	Shock (salt losing)

R → L, right-to-left intracardiac (foramen ovale), extracardiac (ductus arteriosus), or intrapulmonary shunting.

From Behrman RE: Nelson Textbook of Pediatrics, 14th ed. Philadelphia, WB Saunders, 1992, p 464.

MAJOR THREAT TO LIFE

Cyanosis in a newborn is nearly always a threat to life, and all of the conditions just listed and in Table 13-2 (with the exception of methemoglobinemia and physiologic acrocyanosis) are potentially fatal. In particular, cardiac conditions that depend on a patent ductus arteriosus for pulmonary or systemic circulation may be fatal within the first few days of life.

BEDSIDE

Quick-Look Test

Is the infant alert, active, and breathing comfortably?
   If so, you may proceed with slightly less urgency. An infant in obvious distress may need urgent intervention, such as intubation, blood pressure support, and/or initiation of a prostaglandin infusion (see later).

Airway and Vital Signs

Severe compromise of the airway by congenital masses (e.g., goiter, cavernous hemangioma, tumor) is an unusual cause of cyanosis and is obvious. **Hypotension** is the most significant sign and suggests cardiogenic or septic shock (or rarely, salt-wasting congenital adrenal hyperplasia). If hypotension is present, support of blood pressure should proceed while you are pursuing your evaluation (see Chapter 25, Hypotension and Shock). In addition to standard support with maintenance of intravascular volume and vasopressors if necessary, consideration may need to be given to the use of prostaglandin E_1 infusion if any ductus-dependent lesion (e.g., hypoplastic left heart syndrome or critical coarctation of the aorta) is a possibility (see "Management," later). As noted earlier, tachypnea and/or tachycardia can be expected in many cardiac and pulmonary disorders. Weak respiratory effort may suggest CNS depression from maternal drugs or birth asphyxia.

Selective Physical Examination

When evaluating a cyanotic newborn, you should ask three questions to help guide your further evaluation and treatment:

1. *Are there signs of respiratory distress?*
   If none are present, primary lung disease is unlikely.

2. *Are there signs of congestive heart failure and/or hypotension and poor perfusion?*
   Congestive heart failure suggests congenital heart disease associated with increased pulmonary blood flow; the additional findings of poor perfusion and/or hypotension suggest obstruction to

left heart outflow. Sepsis, myocarditis, supraventricular tachycardia, adrenal insufficiency, or complete heart block may also produce these signs, but the degree of cyanosis is not usually as great in these conditions.

3. *Are there signs of CNS depression?*

The infant's mental status should be assessed immediately, with simultaneous questioning regarding irritability, lethargy, and general responsiveness. Any sign of a depressed level of consciousness is concerning.

General	Evaluation of a cyanotic newborn requires a fairly quick but complete physical examination
	The presence of any dysmorphic features or extracardiac congenital malformations, especially midline defects (e.g., cleft lip or palate), increases the likelihood of congenital heart disease
HEENT	Pupillary constriction (maternal narcotics); cyanosis of the oral and mucous membranes, usually the most easily recognized sites, implies generalized cyanosis; nasal flaring (respiratory distress)
Neck	Masses (airway compromise), deviation of the trachea (congenital heart disease, tension pneumothorax)
Chest	Grunting, retractions (respiratory distress); abnormal breath sounds (pneumonia, congestive heart failure)
Cardiac	Hyperdynamic precordium, thrills, heaves (ventricular hypertrophy, volume overload from left-to-right shunting); point of maximum impulse (situs inversus, cardiomegaly); silent precordium (pericardial effusion, cardiomyopathy); murmurs (congenital heart disease)
Lungs	Breath sounds (pneumonia, respiratory distress syndrome, meconium aspiration), absent breath sounds (pulmonary hypoplasia, diaphragmatic hernia)
Abdomen	Scaphoid (diaphragmatic hernia); location of the liver, spleen (situs inversus)
Pulses	Weak (coarctation, hypoplastic left heart, aortic stenosis, sepsis), femoral and brachial pulses unequal (coarctation)
Genitalia	Ambiguous (congenital adrenal hyperplasia)
Neurologic	Lethargy, hypotonia, lack of response to stimuli (CNS depression from maternal drugs, birth asphyxia)
Skin	Cyanosis, petechiae, purpura (sepsis)

Selective History and Chart Review

Review the maternal history. Did the neonate's mother have any illnesses during pregnancy? What is the gestational age of the infant? Did the mother receive antibiotics or narcotics during labor and delivery? If so, why?

A maternal infection perinatally is a risk factor for neonatal sepsis. Maternal narcotics may be passed transplacentally and affect the infant postnatally, especially if administered close to the time of delivery. Maternal systemic lupus erythematosus is a risk factor for congenital heart block in a neonate.

Was the delivery complicated? Was meconium present, and if so, was it visualized below the vocal cords of the infant at the time of delivery? Was the infant's trachea appropriately suctioned? What were the Apgar scores?

Meconium aspiration, which may lead to pneumonia and/or persistent fetal circulation, should be specifically investigated. The Apgar scores may suggest birth asphyxia and subsequent CNS impairment.

Is there a family history of congenital heart disease?

A previous family history increases the risk for disease in the child being evaluated.

Management

By the time you have completed the quick-look test, check of the airway and vital signs, and selective physical examination and history, it may remain unclear whether the newborn has a primary respiratory problem, cardiac disease, or one of the other potential causes of cyanosis. An algorithm for the further evaluation of a cyanotic newborn is presented in Figure 13-1. An abnormal hyperoxia test result (failure to detect an appropriate rise in Pao_2) effectively excludes causes other than lung or heart disease, makes congenital heart disease most likely, and allows you to concentrate on further differentiating heart from lung disease. The chest radiographic findings and ECG results can be extremely valuable tools to help differentiate congenital heart disease from lung disease and also to allow preliminary discrimination of the various forms of cyanotic heart disease. The presence of a specific congenital heart lesion can then be confirmed with echocardiography.

Abnormal Hyperoxia Test Result

CHEST RADIOGRAPH

When interpreting the chest radiograph, several questions should be asked.

1. Is a primary lung process responsible for the cyanosis?

Infiltrates and/or consolidation, suggesting pneumonia or meconium aspiration, may be present. A diaphragmatic hernia may not be obvious by physical examination and should be ruled out. If meconium aspiration, pneumonia, or a diaphragmatic hernia is

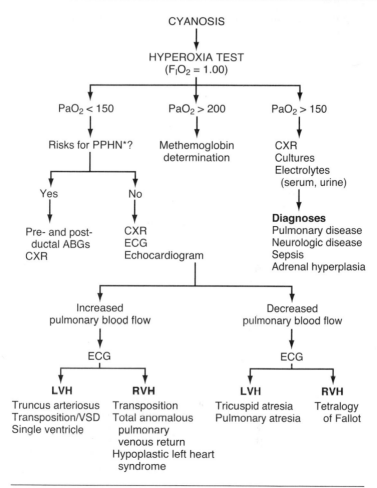

Figure 13–1 Approach to cyanosis in a newborn.

present, persistent fetal circulation (persistent pulmonary hypertension) should be strongly suspected. This condition can be detected by obtaining arterial blood gas samples from both a preductal (right arm) and a postductal (left arm or legs) vessel. A decrease in Pao_2 in the postductal sample relative to the preductal sample suggests right-to-left shunting across the ductus as a result of pulmonary hypertension. If both determinations are extremely low (<40 mm Hg) and the other clinical findings suggest persistent fetal circulation, there may be significant intracardiac right-to-left shunting across the foramen ovale as a result of the same process.

If the lung fields do not reveal signs of inflammation, consolidation, or diaphragmatic hernia, heart disease is more likely (if the hyperoxia test result is abnormal), and one should then ask the next question.

2. *Are there increased pulmonary markings, suggesting increased pulmonary blood flow, or is there a paucity of markings, suggesting diminished pulmonary blood flow?*

As shown in Figure 13-1, increased pulmonary blood flow is associated with a different set of congenital heart lesions than decreased pulmonary blood flow is.

3. *What is the shape of the heart?*

A few lesions may result in a characteristic cardiac silhouette (Fig. 13-2).

Shape	Defect
Boot	Tetralogy of Fallot
	Tricuspid atresia
Egg on a string	Transposition of the great arteries
Snowman	Total anomalous pulmonary venous return

4. *Where is the aortic arch?*

A right-sided aortic arch is associated with intracardiac defects 40% of the time.

ELECTROCARDIOGRAM

The most distinguishing features of the ECG in the various forms of congenital heart disease are the presence and pattern of ventricular hypertrophy (see Fig. 13-1).

ECHOCARDIOGRAM

Once congenital heart disease is suspected, you should consult with a pediatric cardiologist and arrange for an echocardiogram to confirm the diagnosis.

Normal Hyperoxia Test Result

If the hyperoxia test result is normal and the infant has no signs that suggest heart or lung disease, other potential causes need to be

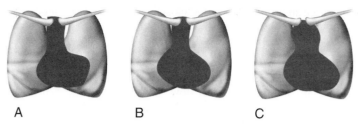

Figure 13–2 Abnormal cardiac silhouette. **A,** "Boot-shaped" heart seen in a cyanotic child with the tetralogy of Fallot or tricuspid atresia. **B,** "Egg-shaped" heart seen in transposition of the great arteries. **C,** "Snowman" sign seen in total anomalous pulmonary venous return (supracardiac type). (From Park MK: Pediatric Cardiology for Practitioners, 2nd ed. Chicago, Year Book, 1988, p 54.)

considered further. In this case, sepsis remains a possibility and appropriate cultures should be obtained before starting broad-spectrum antibiotic coverage for the most common neonatal pathogens (see Chapter 18, Fever). CNS disease should be easily excluded if there are no signs of CNS depression in the infant and the maternal and delivery history is unremarkable. Hypoglycemia should have been detected by Dextrostix testing and corrected appropriately. The salt-wasting variant of congenital adrenal hyperplasia in a female infant is suggested by the presence of abnormal genitalia. Because a male infant with this disorder may have normal genitalia, the diagnosis depends on laboratory measurement of serum and urine electrolytes. Methemoglobinemia should be suspected if the cyanotic infant appears well, the infant has an otherwise normal examination, and the infant's blood appears "chocolate brown" when exposed to room air.

Treatment

Further management depends on the diagnosis made after the evaluation just presented.

CYANOTIC HEART DISEASE

If the clinical findings, arterial blood gas results, chest radiogram, and ECG findings are consistent with congenital heart disease, immediate consultation with a pediatric cardiologist is necessary. Admission to an intensive care unit, where appropriate monitoring can occur, is also necessary. If the infant has significantly decreased pulmonary blood flow or poor perfusion secondary to a left heart outflow defect, consideration should be given to initiation of a prostaglandin E_1 infusion. Prostaglandin E_1 vasodilates the ductus arteriosus and improves pulmonary or systemic blood flow. The infusion can be initiated at 0.05 to 0.1 µg/kg/min and increased to 0.2 µg/kg/min if necessary. The rate of infusion should be titrated according to the response in PaO_2 or the improvement in peripheral perfusion.

The infant should be monitored closely because apnea is a potential complication. The infusion often adequately stabilizes the infant's condition until a surgical procedure can be performed. Oxygen should be administered with caution to an infant with congenital heart disease because increasing the Pao_2 may induce vasoconstriction of the ductus and worsening of cyanosis in those with ductal-dependent pulmonary blood flow. Increasing the Pao_2 may also cause pulmonary vasodilatation, thereby decreasing pulmonary vascular resistance and resulting in increased pulmonary blood flow at the expense of systemic blood flow.

PNEUMONIA OR RESPIRATORY DISTRESS

Ventilatory support, antibiotics, selective pulmonary vasodilators, and extracorporeal membrane oxygenation may all be required. Admission to an intensive care unit and neonatology consultation may be necessary (see Chapter 28, Respiratory Distress). If a diaphragmatic hernia is present, surgical consultation is also necessary.

SEPSIS

As mentioned earlier, appropriate cultures and broad-spectrum antibiotic coverage are required.

HYPOGLYCEMIA

Hypoglycemia may be seen alone or in connection with one of the other disorders causing cyanosis and should be appropriately corrected (see Chapter 35, Glucose Disorders).

CNS DISORDERS

Brain or spinal cord injury from birth trauma can be confirmed by computed tomography (CT) or magnetic resonance imaging (MRI). Hypoxic-ischemic injury (asphyxia) may also result in cerebral edema that can be detected by CT scanning. Care should be supportive.

Narcosis causing cyanosis, hypotonia, and slow, shallow respirations is a result of heavy doses of morphine, meperidine, or barbiturates taken by or given to the mother shortly before delivery. It can be treated with naloxone, 0.1 mg/kg, intravenously, intramuscularly, subcutaneously, or intratracheally. If the initial dose is unsuccessful, repeated doses may be given at 2- to 3-minute intervals.

METHEMOGLOBINEMIA

Methemoglobin is the product of oxidation of hemoglobin to the ferric state. It is present in healthy people, but the erythrocytic reducing system maintains amounts at less than 2% of the total hemoglobin content. Methemoglobinemia may be hereditary (a deficiency of the reducing enzyme NADH cytochrome b_5 reductase) or may occur secondary to exposure to a toxin (aniline dye, nitrobenzene, nitrites). Methylene blue, 1 to 2 mg/kg intravenously, can be used to treat both hereditary and toxin-related methemoglobinemia.

CONGENITAL ADRENAL HYPERPLASIA

The salt-losing form of 21-hydroxylase deficiency causes virilization, vomiting, dehydration, and potentially, cyanosis in the newborn period. As noted earlier, male infants may have normal genitalia. Low serum sodium and chloride and high potassium levels may be present. Plasma renin levels are elevated, as are serum levels of 17-hydroxyprogesterone and urinary 17-ketosteroids. Contrast imaging of the urogenital tract in virilized females may be helpful when the genitalia are particularly ambiguous. Treatment is aimed at replacing glucocorticoid and mineralocorticoid, as well as sodium. A dehydrated infant needs volume and sodium replacement initially (see Chapter 15, Diarrhea and Dehydration) and then hydrocortisone (10 to 20 mg/m^2/day orally in two or three divided doses), 9α-fluorohydrocortisone (0.05 to 0.3 mg/day), and sodium chloride (1 to 3 g/day) as maintenance therapy.

CYANOSIS IN AN OLDER CHILD

PHONE CALL

Questions

1. Are there signs of respiratory distress?
2. Are there signs of altered mental status?
3. Is the cyanosis generalized or localized?
4. Why is the child hospitalized? Is there a history of lung or heart disease?

Cyanosis in an older child is seen most often in the context of lung disease, such as pneumonia, reactive airway disease, or an exacerbation of cystic fibrosis. Changes in mental status may suggest a neurologic cause for hypoventilation and secondary cyanosis. Alternatively, mental status changes may be a result of hypoxia. Remember, cyanotic older children frequently become acidotic and symptomatic more quickly than newborns do because they lack the adaptations that allow newborns to tolerate lower levels of oxygen, such as fetal hemoglobin, higher hematocrit, and increased levels of 2,3-diphosphoglycerate (2,3-DPG).

Orders

1. An arterial blood gas determination should be done as soon as possible. Oxygen should be administered and the patient placed on continuous cardiorespiratory monitoring and pulse oximetry.
2. An IV line should be placed if not already present.
3. A complete blood count and serum glucose (or Dextrostix) measurement should be obtained and extra blood drawn into a red-top tube and saved (if toxicology screening studies or serum chemistry studies are thought to be necessary after your further evaluation).
4. A stat chest radiograph and ECG should be obtained.

Inform RN

Cyanotic patients should be evaluated immediately.

ELEVATOR THOUGHTS

What are the causes of cyanosis beyond the newborn period?

Pulmonary	Pneumonia
	Cystic fibrosis
	Bronchiectasis
	Pulmonary embolism
	Foreign body
	Chemical aspiration
	Reactive airway disease
	Primary pulmonary hypertension
	Lymphoid interstitial pneumonia
	Pneumothorax
	Pulmonary hemorrhage
Cardiac	Congenital heart disease
	Myocarditis
	Tetralogy of Fallot "spells"
	Dysrhythmia
	Cardiomyopathy
Neurologic	Encephalopathy
	Encephalitis
	Toxins
	Metabolic disease
	Neuromuscular disease
Hematologic	Polycythemia
	Hypercoagulable state
	Methemoglobinemia
Peripheral or localized	Arterial thrombosis
	Raynaud's phenomenon
	Compartment syndrome (traumatic)
	Superior vena cava syndrome

MAJOR THREAT TO LIFE

Cyanosis in an older child nearly always indicates a critical underlying process. With the exception of Raynaud's phenomenon and methemoglobinemia, the other possibilities are all life threatening.

BEDSIDE

Quick-Look Test

A cyanotic older child commonly has other signs of respiratory distress or may also appear lethargic or obtunded if neurologic disease is present or the hypoxia is severe and prolonged. The paroxysmal hypercyanotic episodes experienced by young children with the tetralogy of Fallot ("tet spells") may result in syncope after a short period of respiratory distress.

Airway and Vital Signs

Because most older children with cyanosis have lung disease, particular attention should focus on the airway and the presence of tachypnea. If there is any compromise, intubation may be required. Bradycardia and hypotension are ominous signs in a cyanotic child. Shallow, slow respirations suggest neurologic dysfunction and hypoventilation.

Selective Physical Examination

HEENT	Edema, proptosis, localized cyanosis (superior vena cava syndrome); pupillary constriction (narcosis); ptosis (neuromuscular disease); nasal flaring (respiratory distress)
Neck	Distended neck veins (congestive heart failure, superior vena cava syndrome), deviation of the trachea (tension pneumothorax), use of accessory muscles
Lungs	Breath sounds, grunting, retracting (respiratory distress, congestive heart failure, pneumothorax, foreign body); stridor; wheezing; weak respiratory effort (neuromuscular disease, CNS disease)
Heart	Rate and rhythm (dysrhythmias), single loud S_2 sound (pulmonary hypertension), murmurs (a temporary *decrease* in the intensity of a systolic murmur is associated with hypercyanotic spells in the tetralogy of Fallot)
Extremities	Weak pulses (myocarditis or cardiomyopathy and congestive heart failure, arterial thrombosis, compartment syndrome), edema (congestive heart failure), local cyanosis (thrombosis, vasospasm, compartment syndrome), clubbing (chronic lung or cyanotic heart disease), transient pallor of the digits changing to cyanosis and then hyperemia (Raynaud's phenomenon), muscle tenderness (compartment syndrome)
Neurologic	Weakness, decreased reflexes (neuromuscular disease); altered mental status (encephalitis, toxin)

Selective History and Chart Review

Has the cyanosis been chronic or recurrent, or is this an acute episode? Is there a history of chronic heart or lung disease?

Mild cyanotic heart disease may go undetected for years; therefore, a history of previous cyanosis may be helpful. The same is true of chronic lung disease, such as cystic fibrosis or primary pulmonary hypertension. Suspicion of a "tet spell" is obviously high in those with a known history. Cyanotic heart disease may be associated with polycythemia. Pneumothorax may occur in those with known lung disease, such as reactive airway disease or cystic fibrosis.

In a patient with respiratory distress, is the history suggestive of foreign body or chemical aspiration?

This should be considered, especially in a toddler.

Has the patient had fever, upper respiratory symptoms, or "flu" symptoms?

This raises suspicion of lung infection, myocarditis, or in a child with neurologic findings, encephalitis or postinfectious Guillain-Barré syndrome and secondary respiratory insufficiency.

What medications has the patient received? Has there been exposure to dyes or chemicals?

One should specifically look for narcotics, barbiturates, or substances known to produce methemoglobinemia.

Is the patient predisposed to a hypercoagulable state?

This may cause pulmonary embolism or arterial thrombosis. Oral contraceptive use, antiphospholipid antibodies, and immobilization are risk factors for hypercoagulability.

If cyanosis is localized to the distal end of an extremity and is associated with pain, is the patient at risk for compartment syndrome?

Trauma (e.g., fractures) or excessive exercise and muscle swelling can precipitate compartment syndrome.

Management

In nearly all cases of cyanosis in an older child, a respiratory, cardiac, or neurologic cause is readily apparent, and management should proceed as indicated by the underlying disorder (see Chapter 7, Altered Mental Status; Chapter 10, Chest Pain; Chapter 22, Heart Rate and Rhythm Abnormalities; and Chapter 28, Respiratory Distress). Management of a few selected processes that are associated with hypercyanosis and are not discussed elsewhere is presented here.

Tetralogy of Fallot

Placement of the child in the knee-chest position compresses the femoral arteries and increases systemic vascular resistance, thereby decreasing right-to-left shunting across the ventricular septal defect and improving pulmonary blood flow. Oxygen should be administered and the child calmed as much as possible. Morphine, 0.2 mg/kg subcutaneously, may aid in relaxing a young child. If these measures are unsuccessful or if the attack is particularly severe, administration of IV sodium bicarbonate should be considered to correct the metabolic acidosis that quickly develops as the Pao_2 is maintained below 40 mm Hg. IV propranolol (0.1 to 0.2 mg/kg) may also be considered to alleviate the tachycardia that often accompanies episodes and may impede adequate pulmonary blood flow. IV phenylephrine (5 to 10 µg/kg every 10 to 15 minutes) may also help increase systemic vascular resistance.

Polycythemia

If polycythemia is severe enough (hematocrit of 65% to 70%) and associated with hyperviscosity, plethora, and/or cyanosis, consideration should be given to phlebotomy and replacement of whole blood with plasma, 5% albumin, or normal saline solution. The volume replaced can be calculated as follows:

$$Volume\ (mL) = \frac{Estimated\ blood\ volume\ (mL) \times Desired\ hematocrit\ change}{Starting\ hematocrit}$$

Arterial Thrombosis

Heparinization may relieve the clot and prevent further thrombosis in those with a hypercoagulable state. An initial IV bolus of 50 U/kg should be followed by a maintenance infusion of 10 to 25 U/kg/hr. The partial thromboplastin time should be maintained at 1.5 to 2.5 times normal.

Raynaud's Phenomenon

An episodic, triphasic (white-blue-red) color change of the digits, usually bilateral and symmetrical, associated with cold exposure or anxiety should suggest vasospasm. Most cases can be managed by simple rewarming. Refractory cases can be treated with nifedipine, 10 mg one to three times a day.

Compartment Syndrome

Immediate surgical consultation is required because fasciotomy is necessary to relieve pressure and restore adequate blood flow.

SUMMARY

Cyanosis is a challenging problem and usually represents a true emergency. A stepwise approach as outlined here that combines a selective physical examination and a few laboratory and radiographic studies usually allows you to determine a cause in an efficient manner and begin appropriate treatment. It should be clear that by thinking logically about the problem, you can take the actions necessary to ensure that neither you nor the patient is "blue."

14

Delivery Room Problems

Lacy E. Taylor, MD

A call requesting the presence of a pediatrician at the delivery of a newborn may be received for a limited number of reasons. The call may be "routine" (e.g., request for a pediatrician to be present for cesarean section or forceps delivery), it may be for premature delivery or multiple births, or it may be because fetal monitoring during labor reveals fetal distress. For any type of call, you should always be prepared to resuscitate the newborn and to manage the several other potential problems discussed in this chapter.

PHONE CALL

Questions

1. What is the gestational age?
2. Are there signs of fetal distress?
3. Does there appear to be any meconium?
4. Are there any known complications of pregnancy (e.g., infection, poor weight gain, no prenatal care)?
5. Is there more than one fetus?

Obviously, the younger the gestational age, the more likely the presence of immature lungs in the newborn and subsequent respiratory distress at birth. Fetal tachycardia (>160 beats per minute [bpm]) or bradycardia (<120 bpm) or a fetal scalp blood pH less than 7.25 suggests fetal distress. Tachycardia may be seen with fetal hypoxia, maternal fever, or anemia. Bradycardia may be seen with hypoxia, inadvertent administration of anesthetic to the fetus, or congenital heart block. Understanding the relationship of bradycardia to uterine contractions (**decelerations**) may be helpful (Fig. 14-1). **Late decelerations** reflect fetal hypoxia from lack of sufficient uteroplacental blood flow, whereas early and variable decelerations are less worrisome. Hypoxia results in acidosis and a fall in fetal scalp blood pH. A value lower than 7.20 indicates significant distress and is generally a reason for immediate early delivery. Passage of meconium

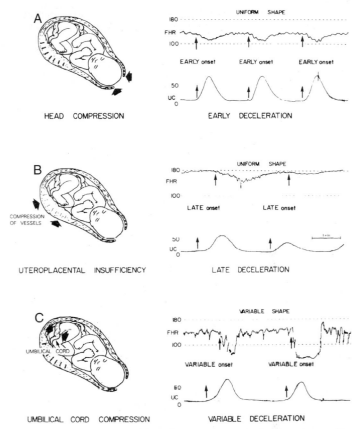

Figure 14–1 Three types of decelerations. **A**, Early decelerations reflect head compression with contractions of the uterus. **B**, Late decelerations occur when there is uteroplacental insufficiency as a result of compression of the blood supply to the placenta during uterine contraction. **C**, Variable decelerations occur with umbilical cord compression during uterine contraction. FHR, fetal heart rate; UC, uterine contraction.

into amniotic fluid may be a sign of fetal distress and presents an added risk to the infant because this meconium may be aspirated into the lungs at delivery and result in obstruction of small airways and perhaps secondary complications (persistent fetal circulation, pneumonia).

Several maternal illnesses may potentially complicate delivery. Maternal infections may place the newborn at risk for sepsis, diabetes may result in macrosomia and a difficult delivery, and maternal systemic lupus erythematosus may give rise to congenital heart block.

Orders

You should ask the delivery room nurse to make sure that the infant warming table is prepared in the event that resuscitation is necessary. A laryngoscope, laryngoscope blades, several sizes of endotracheal tube (sizes 2.5 to 4.5), an umbilical catheterization tray, intravenous (IV) angiocatheters, butterfly needles, and syringes, in addition to oxygen and wall suction, should be present. Naloxone as well as epinephrine, atropine, sodium bicarbonate, surfactant, and dopamine should be readily available.

Inform RN

You need to go directly to the delivery room. It is optimal to arrive well before the delivery so that you have time to briefly review the mother's chart.

ELEVATOR THOUGHTS

What possibilities do I need to anticipate?

Respiratory failure

- Hyaline membrane disease (in a premature infant)
- Secondary to birth asphyxia or central nervous system (CNS) depression
- Meconium aspiration
- Sepsis
- Choanal atresia
- Diaphragmatic hernia
- Mandibular hypoplasia
- Pneumothorax
- Cystic adenomatoid malformation
- Phrenic nerve paralysis
- Pulmonary hypoplasia

Severe anemia (and secondary hydrops fetalis)
Plethora (polycythemia)
Seizures
Congenital malformations (e.g., cleft lip or palate)
Birth injury
Shock

Ideally, you are present to witness the delivery of a healthy newborn, and you should therefore be prepared to congratulate the parents on the birth of their very beautiful baby.

MAJOR THREAT TO LIFE

All of the aforementioned are major threats.

BEDSIDE

Quick-Look Test

You should look to see whether delivery is imminent. If not, you should find and review the maternal history.

Selective Maternal History

Does the mother have any medical illnesses?

　　Specifically, diabetes, hypertension, systemic lupus erythematosus, chronic renal disease, chronic lung or heart disease, and sickle cell anemia may affect the developing fetus and potentially predispose to problems at birth.

Does the mother use narcotics, alcohol, cocaine, tobacco, or other drugs? Has the mother received narcotics during labor?

　　All may affect the fetus and newborn infant. Narcotics administered within 1 hour of delivery may result in significant CNS depression in the newborn.

Is there a history of previous high-risk pregnancies?

　　Such a history may increase the risk associated with the current pregnancy.

Has the mother had any infections during pregnancy? Does she have a current infection? Is she receiving or has she received antibiotics? Has a cervical culture for group B streptococci been performed, and if so, what are the results?

　　Rubella, human parvovirus B19, human immunodeficiency virus, cytomegalovirus, toxoplasmosis, herpes simplex, syphilis, tuberculosis, varicella, and hepatitis C may all be transmitted transplacentally and affect the newborn if present during pregnancy. Group B streptococci, *Escherichia coli*, hepatitis B, and herpes simplex may be acquired perinatally.

Have the maternal membranes ruptured, and for how long? What is the maternal white blood cell count?

　　The risk for neonatal infection secondary to ascension from the cervix and genital tract is greater if the membranes have been ruptured for 18 hours or more and/or maternal leukocytosis is present.

What is the mother's blood type and Rh status?

　　ABO or Rh incompatibility may result in hemolytic anemia in the newborn.

Has polyhydramnios or oligohydramnios been present?

Polyhydramnios is associated with anencephaly, hydrocephaly, bowel atresia, tracheoesophageal fistula, cleft lip or palate, cystic adenomatoid malformation, and diaphragmatic hernia. Oligohydramnios is associated with pulmonary hypoplasia, renal agenesis, growth retardation, twin-twin transfusion, and fetal anomalies.

Has amniocentesis been performed?

Chromosome abnormalities, neural tube defects (elevated α-fetoprotein level), and the degree of fetal lung maturity (a lecithin-sphingomyelin ratio >2:1 generally indicates maturity) may all be determined with amniocentesis.

Has a nonstress test, a contraction stress test, or a biophysical profile been performed?

Abnormal results of such testing may indicate fetal hypoxia. Interpretation of the nonstress test and contraction stress test may be difficult because of high false-positive rates with these tests.

Fetal Vital Signs

As noted earlier, tachycardia or bradycardia may indicate fetal distress. The pattern of decelerations and the beat-to-beat variability of the fetal heart rate should also be observed. Decreased beat-to-beat variability reflects fetal distress. Maternal fever may indicate infection, in which case the newborn is also at risk.

Management I

At the majority of deliveries, the newborn is crying and vigorous once removed from the perineum. These infants do not require any immediate intervention other than drying and bulb suctioning of the nose and mouth, but they may need a period of observation (e.g., if there is prematurity, congenital malformation, or any question of meconium aspiration or sepsis). All infants whose delivery you attend should have an Apgar score assigned (see later) and should be examined thoroughly.

Newborns who are not breathing, are not vigorous, or are in distress obviously need intervention. The key is to be an astute observer of the transition period in order to judge which infants need help and which do not.

Respiratory Failure

If the infant is received from the obstetrician and is not crying, is cyanotic, is limp, and has not initiated respirations, initial efforts should be directed toward suctioning the mouth and nose and vigorously stimulating the infant in an effort to provoke respiration, **unless thick meconium is present**. If meconium is present, immediately proceed to intubate the infant and note whether meconium is present at or below the level of the vocal cords. Once the endotracheal tube is positioned, suction should be applied and the tube slowly withdrawn. If necessary (when particularly thick meconium is suctioned into the tube), this procedure should be repeated until you are satisfied that as much meconium as possible has been removed. You should then return to clearing the upper airway of secretions and vigorously stimulating the infant. This is best accomplished by rubbing the back of the torso while the infant is in a supine position. Throughout this time, another person should be monitoring the newborn's pulse. Monitoring of the pulse is most easily accomplished by holding the umbilical stump with the thumb and forefinger. This person can help your evaluation by tapping out the heart rate on the surface of the warming table. If the infant does not respond with a spontaneous breath, improved color, and improved muscle tone within several seconds or if the heart rate is less than 100 bpm, bag-and-mask ventilation with 100% oxygen should be administered while you continue to stimulate. You should be looking for spontaneous respirations and improved color and tone while bagging. If the infant does not respond within 10 to 15 seconds or if the heart rate falls below 60 bpm, intubation plus endotracheal ventilation is necessary. For a heart rate below 60 bpm, chest compressions should also be started. If the newborn's mother received narcotics during labor, naloxone, 0.1 mg/kg, should be given to the infant either intravenously, endotracheally, or intramuscularly. This dose may be repeated every 3 to 5 minutes. If the heart rate and color of the infant do not improve quickly with endotracheal ventilation, additional resuscitation measures are necessary. At this point, you need to call for more "hands" because an umbilical venous catheter or peripheral IV line should be placed and samples drawn for arterial blood gas measurement. Fluid volume, epinephrine, sodium bicarbonate, and vasopressors may all be necessary to resuscitate the infant. Remember to listen to the lungs for adequate ventilation and to look for symmetrical rise of the infant's chest. Pulmonary hypoplasia, diaphragmatic hernia, or pneumothorax may interfere with adequate ventilation.

If the infant begins to breathe spontaneously and does not require immediate intubation, you should carefully observe the pattern of respiration and look for signs of respiratory distress. Labored breathing, intercostal and subcostal retractions, and tachypnea are worrisome signs and can quickly evolve in a newborn who is initially breathing comfortably. These signs may indicate any of the problems associated with respiratory failure in the newborn, and you should then proceed with a physical examination to determine the probable cause.

Shock

Internal hemorrhage from birth trauma, fetomaternal transfusion, placental abruption, hemolytic anemia, or umbilical cord trauma may result in shock in the newborn. Pallor, poor perfusion, cyanosis, respiratory distress, and cold extremities may all be present at birth. Resuscitation should begin immediately by maintaining the airway and respirations (see earlier) and supporting the circulation. Hypovolemia can be corrected with normal saline solution, plasma, or type O-negative blood after placement of a peripheral IV line or, ideally, umbilical catheters (both arterial and venous). Vasopressors may be necessary to support the blood pressure. Once the infant is stabilized, further evaluation, with a complete physical examination and laboratory studies, can proceed.

Physical Examination

HEENT	Swelling (caput succedaneum, cephalohematoma), indentations (skull fracture), subconjunctival hemorrhages (often considered a "normal" event with delivery), colobomas, ear anomalies, encephaloceles (may obstruct the nose or airway), cataracts, dysmorphic facies
Neck	Masses (goiter, cystic hygroma), tracheal position
Chest	Symmetry and adequacy of chest rise; equal breath sounds; rales; rhonchi; grunting, flaring, retracting (respiratory distress)
Heart	Location of heart sounds (right-sided sounds may indicate congenital heart disease or a shift secondary to diaphragmatic hernia, tension pneumothorax, or a lung mass), murmurs (congenital heart disease), bradycardia (congenital heart block, hypoxia)
Abdomen	Scaphoid, flat, distended (scaphoid suggests diaphragmatic hernia); liver and spleen position (situs inversus may be associated with cyanotic heart disease); umbilical cord inspection for two arteries and one vein (lack of a vessel may be associated with other congenital anomalies, including cardiac defects)
Genitalia	Testes palpable and descended in a male, external genitalia normal in a female
Extremities	Tone (generalized decrease associated with asphyxia or hypoxia, poor perfusion, or neuromuscular disorder), movement (nerve palsy secondary to birth injury), presence of all digits, color (cyanosis, plethora), perfusion
Neurologic	Alert, active, moving all extremities, responsive to stimuli

An Apgar score should be assigned at 1 and 5 minutes of life for all infants (Table 14-1). In those requiring resuscitation, 10-, 15-, and 20-minute scores may also be necessary. The first Apgar score indicates the need for resuscitation, and later scores are more indicative of the potential for morbidity and mortality.

TABLE 14-1 **Apgar Evaluation of a Newborn Infant**

Sign	0	1	2
Heart rate	Absent	Below 100	Over 100
Respiratory effort	Absent	Slow, irregular	Good, crying
Muscle tone	Limp	Some flexion of extremities	Active motion
Response to catheter in nostril (tested after the oropharynx is clear)	No response	Grimace	Cough or sneeze
Color	Blue, pale	Body pink, extremities blue	Completely pink

Sixty seconds after complete birth of the infant (disregarding the cord and placenta), the five objective signs above are evaluated, and each is given a score of 0, 1, or 2. A total score of 10 indicates an infant in the best possible condition. An infant with a score of 0 to 3 requires immediate resuscitation.

Modified from Apgar V: A proposal for a new method of evaluation of the newborn infant. Curr Res Anesth Analg 32:260-267, 1953.

Management II

Severe Anemia

If the infant is born with pallor and shock and appears to be in distress, acute blood loss from a perinatal problem (abruption of the placenta, placenta previa, internal hemorrhage) is more likely than chronic intrauterine anemia. Chronic intrauterine anemia is more likely to produce fetal hydrops and signs of congestive heart failure at birth. In contrast to acute blood loss, laboratory measurements of hemoglobin, the reticulocyte count, and mean cell volume are often abnormal. A newborn infant who is symptomatic and anemic is likely to require a transfusion. Additional evaluation of a newborn with anemia is outlined in Figure 14-2 and should include a complete blood count, reticulocyte count, Coombs test, peripheral smear review, and a determination of infant and maternal blood types.

Plethora (Polycythemia)

Delayed umbilical cord clamping, twin-twin transfusion, maternal diabetes, and chromosomal abnormalities are a few of the conditions that may result in polycythemia in the newborn, which is defined as a central hematocrit greater than 65%. Many newborns are asymptomatic, but respiratory distress, cyanosis, lethargy, and seizures may all occur. An infant who appears ruddy or reddish purple should be suspected of having polycythemia and should have a hematocrit determination immediately. If polycythemia is present, a partial exchange transfusion should be performed with the aim of

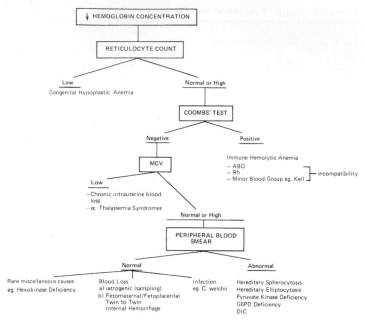

Figure 14–2 Algorithm for the evaluation of a newborn with anemia. DIC, disseminated intravascular coagulation; G6PD, glucose-6-phosphate dehydrogenase; MCV, mean cell volume.

reducing the hematocrit to 50%. The volume of the exchange is calculated as follows:

$$\text{Volume (mL)} = \frac{\text{Estimated blood volume (mL)} \times \text{Desired hematocrit change}}{\text{Starting hematocrit}}$$

Seizures

Seizures in the delivery room are most likely secondary to asphyxia and hypoxic or ischemic injury to the CNS. Other possibilities include a structural anomaly of the brain, intracranial bleeding, electrolyte disturbance, hypoglycemia, drug withdrawal, and meningitis or sepsis. A Dextrostix blood glucose determination and hematocrit, arterial blood gas analysis, and serum electrolyte measurements should be obtained, oxygen administered, and the neonate treated with anticonvulsants (see Chapter 29, Seizures). Blood cultures, a lumbar puncture, and administration of antibiotics to empirically treat potential causes of meningitis in the neonatal period are also necessary.

Congenital Malformations

Any malformations of the infant noted should be discussed **immediately** with one or, ideally, both of the parents. If you are unsure of the presence of an anomaly, you should state this to the parents and let them know that you will be discussing it with other physicians (senior residents, neonatologists, the infant's pediatrician) who will be available to examine the infant. If you are unsure of the **significance** of an anomaly, you should also say so to the parents and again let them know that other physicians will be available to them to fully discuss the particular anomaly and its implications. As the first physician to evaluate their child, the parents will be looking to you for an initial confirmation that all is "perfect" with their newborn. Despite the extreme pressure to satisfy their wishes, it is imperative that **any** potential problem be discussed with them at the time. If this is not done, their initial sense of reassurance will be crushed by bad news sometime in the next few days.

As mentioned earlier, many trips to the delivery room end with your handing over a swaddled infant to a mother or father and declaring the infant healthy, with little or no intervention required on your part. If there has been a problem, you should remember to phone and inform the infant's pediatrician-to-be (if one has been identified) of the problem.

Diarrhea and Dehydration

Nosheen N. Shaikh, MD

Diarrhea is defined as frequent, watery stools and is a common problem in infants and children. In most cases, diarrheal illnesses are mild and self-limited; however, the potential for dehydration secondary to diarrhea is great. Hypovolemia and electrolyte abnormalities may occur, which in turn may lead to significant morbidity or even mortality. When called regarding a child with diarrhea, your priorities should be to (1) quickly evaluate the volume status of the child and recognize the clinical signs of dehydration, (2) appropriately correct volume deficits, (3) appropriately correct electrolyte abnormalities, and (4) identify the most likely cause of the diarrhea. This chapter discusses diarrhea, as well as the general fluid management of hospitalized children. Specific electrolyte abnormalities are discussed in detail in Chapter 34.

PHONE CALL

Questions

1. Clarify whether *diarrhea* is present. Both increased frequency *and* increased water content define diarrhea.
2. What are the child's vital signs?
3. How old is the child?
4. How long has the child had diarrhea?
5. Is there blood, mucus, or pus in the stool?
6. Why is the child in the hospital?

Hypotension implies significant hypovolemia and requires urgent attention and intervention (see Chapter 25, Hypotension and Shock). The infant may be able to maintain normal blood pressure in the face of significant hypovolemia; tachycardia may be the only finding initially. The duration of diarrhea may allow you to estimate the risk for dehydration. Blood or pus in the stool and the reason for admission may provide clues to the cause of the diarrhea.

Orders

1. If hypovolemia is a concern, the child should have an intravenous (IV) line placed. If the child is hypotensive, an immediate 10- to 20-mL/kg bolus of normal saline or lactated Ringer's solution should be ordered (see Chapter 25, Hypotension and Shock).
2. Electrolyte, blood urea nitrogen, creatinine, venous pH determinations, and a complete blood count with differential should be ordered. The serum sodium concentration is necessary for you to plan appropriate rehydration if the child is found to be dehydrated. Ask the nurse to check urine specific gravity as well.
3. The child should not receive any oral intake until you evaluate further.

Inform RN

"I will arrive at the bedside in … minutes." A child with abnormal vital signs or bloody diarrhea should be evaluated immediately.

ELEVATOR THOUGHTS

What causes diarrhea?
Mild diarrhea without dehydration is a nonspecific finding that may be present with nearly any illness in childhood. Diarrhea as a manifestation of a pathologic condition of the gastrointestinal tract is usually more severe and has greater potential to lead to dehydration.

Infections

Diarrhea in children may result from infection of the gastrointestinal tract itself (gastroenteritis, colitis) or from acute infections elsewhere, such as an upper respiratory infection, pneumonia, hepatitis, or a urinary tract infection.

Viral gastroenteritis	Rotavirus
	Norwalk virus
	Adenovirus
	Influenza
	Enteroviruses
Bacterial colitis	*Salmonella, Shigella, Yersinia,* or *Campylobacter* ("SSYC")
	Enteropathogenic *Escherichia coli*
	Staphylococcal food poisoning
	Clostridium difficile (pseudomembranous colitis)
	Vibrio cholerae
	Mycobacterium tuberculosis

Parasitic infection
    Giardiasis
    Amebiasis
    Cryptosporidiosis
    Worms (strongyloidiasis, ascariasis, trichuriasis, hookworm, tapeworms)

Malabsorption

Secondary lactase deficiency (e.g., after gastroenteritis)
Cystic fibrosis
Celiac disease
Primary immunodeficiencies (including human immunodeficiency virus)
Schwachman-Diamond syndrome
Abetalipoproteinemia

Diarrhea in the Neonate

Milk protein intolerance
Necrotizing enterocolitis
Overfeeding

Miscellaneous Causes

Drugs
Laxative abuse
Starvation stools
Inflammatory bowel disease
Typhlitis

MAJOR THREAT TO LIFE

- Dehydration
- Electrolyte abnormalities
- Sepsis

BEDSIDE

Your initial goal should be to determine the degree and type of dehydration, if any. Dehydration can be classified as hyponatremic, isonatremic, or hypernatremic, depending on the serum sodium concentration. The appropriate management of each type of dehydration differs; therefore, it is critical to identify which type is present. Determining the degree of dehydration can usually be accomplished with a brief physical examination and a few selected questions. If dehydration is present, you should initiate therapy before returning to perform a more detailed physical examination, history, and chart review.

Quick-Look Test

Does the child look well (comfortable), sick (uncomfortable or distressed), or critical (about to die)?

Infants are often irritable or lethargic if dehydration is present. Older children generally appear ill if the diarrhea is significant.

Airway and Vital Signs

Look carefully at the heart rate and blood pressure. These values provide you with a quick assessment of the degree of hypovolemia, if any. A child with a normal heart rate and blood pressure is unlikely to have severe hypovolemia. Orthostatic blood pressure should be determined in older children if tachycardia is present in the absence of hypotension. Fever suggests gastroenteritis or colitis.

Selective Physical Examination I

What is the child's volume status?

In addition to the vital signs, estimation of the hydration status of the child can be made by selectively examining the following:

1. Mucous membranes

   Are they moist or dry? How dry? Absence of tears suggests severe dehydration, as do very sunken eyes.

2. Skin turgor

   Normal or decreased? Is there "tenting"? Is the skin "doughy"? Skin turgor can be assessed by gently pinching and releasing the skin over the abdomen between the thumb and forefinger. Normally, in an adequately hydrated person, the skin retracts immediately and quickly. Slow retraction suggests moderate dehydration, and "tenting," or the lack of retraction, suggests severe dehydration. "Doughy" skin is suggestive of hypernatremic dehydration, a condition in which intracellular volume decreases as a means of attempting to maintain equal osmolality between the extracellular and intracellular spaces. In the case of hypernatremic dehydration, the child's appearance may be deceptive. Clinical signs of dehydration may not be as obvious as in the other two forms of dehydration, hyponatremic and isonatremic dehydration, which result in a decrease in extracellular volume and have an insignificant effect on intracellular volume.

3. Capillary refill and temperature of the extremities

   Normal or delayed (>2 seconds) refill? Warm or cool extremities? Delayed capillary refill and/or cool extremities imply inadequate distal perfusion secondary to hypovolemia.

4. Anterior fontanelle (in an infant)

   Flat or sunken?

5. Weight

   Determining the current weight of the child is necessary, and comparing it with a previous recent weight (if known) is

TABLE 15-1 **Estimation of Volume Deficit in a Dehydrated Child**

Infant	5%	10%	15%
Child	3%	6%	9%
Mucous membranes	Normal	Dry	Parched
Tears	Present	Decreased	Absent
Eyes	Normal	Slightly sunken	Severely sunken
Skin turgor	Normal	Slow retraction	Tenting
Skin temperature	Normal	Slightly cool	Cool, clammy
Capillary refill	<2 sec	2-3 sec	>3 sec
Heart rate	Normal	Mild tachycardia	Severe tachycardia
Fontanelle	Flat	Slightly depressed	Sunken
Urine output	Normal	Decreased	Severe oliguria, anuria

also very useful. It is conventional to assign a "percent dehydration" to a dehydrated child (Table 15-1). Either a known amount of weight loss or the estimated percentage can then be used to determine the volume deficit.

Selective History and Chart Review I

Has a previous weight been recorded with which you can compare the current weight?

This allows you to most accurately estimate the volume deficit.

What has the child's urine output been?

Normal urine output (approximately 1 to 2 mL/kg/hr and similar to recent intake) suggests that the child is either euvolemic or only mildly dehydrated. Severe oliguria or anuria suggests a large volume deficit. In infants, you may need to base an estimate of urine output on the number of wet diapers per day that the child has had.

Has the child also been vomiting?

Vomiting and diarrhea often coincide, thereby potentially adding to the volume deficit.

Are there other factors that may contribute to volume loss, such as fever or recent surgery?

Management

Principles

Fluid therapy can be divided into three categories:
1. Maintenance therapy
2. Deficit replacement
3. Replacement of ongoing losses

Maintenance therapy is aimed at providing the body's normal daily requirements for fluid and electrolytes. In a healthy person, water is physiologically "lost" through urine, stool, and so-called insensible losses (pulmonary and cutaneous losses). Electrolytes (primarily sodium and potassium) are also lost in urine and stool. These water and electrolyte losses are usually replaced through eating and drinking; however, in those who are ill and hospitalized, oral intake is often greatly reduced or absent, and therefore IV replacement of maintenance fluids is necessary. Several methods are available for estimating a person's maintenance requirements. The simplest method is based on caloric requirements and assumes that 100 mL of water, 2 to 4 mEq of sodium, and 2 to 4 mEq of potassium are necessary for each 100 calories expended. The calories expended for a 24-hour period depend on body weight and are estimated by using the following rules for a hospitalized child:

100 cal/kg for the first 10 kg

50 cal/kg for the next 10 kg

20 cal/kg for each kg above 20

Therefore, a 30-kg child would expend approximately 1700 cal/day and require 1700 mL of water and 34 to 68 mEq each of sodium and potassium. A solution of 5% dextrose and 0.2 normal saline with 20 mEq of potassium per liter at a rate of 70 mL/hr adequately approximates these requirements (0.2 normal saline solution contains 0.2×154 mEq/L = 31 mEq/L of sodium). This method can be used to calculate the maintenance requirements for a child of any weight, and by determining the appropriate volume (with the rules just presented), appropriate amounts of sodium and potassium can also be provided.

Deficit replacement is aimed at replacing the amount of water and electrolytes that have already been lost. A deficit is present when physiologic and pathologic losses are greater than oral or IV intake. As noted earlier, your initial goal when evaluating a potentially dehydrated child is to determine the severity and type of dehydration.

The severity of dehydration, or the percentage of body weight lost, is determined either by the known difference in weight or by the estimated "percent dehydration" based on clinical findings (see Table 15-1). In infants, total body water is a larger percentage of body weight than in children, and therefore clinical estimates of mild, moderate, or severe dehydration represent a slightly larger deficit.

The type of dehydration (hyponatremic, isonatremic, or hypernatremic) depends on the relative losses of water and sodium, as well as on attempts that have already been made to correct a deficit (e.g., replacement of losses with free water). Hyponatremic dehydration can be defined as a serum sodium concentration less than 130 mEq/L, isonatremic dehydration as a serum sodium concentration of 130 to 150 mEq/L, and hypernatremic dehydration as a serum sodium concentration greater than 150 mEq/L. Most infants and children with diarrhea and dehydration have the isonatremic form (approximately 70%), but certain clues may lead you to suspect either hyponatremia or hypernatremia. An infant who has been given large amounts of free water to replace diarrheal losses is probably hyponatremic. Conversely, an infant with fever and diarrhea who has ingested an inappropriately mixed, highly concentrated formula may have hypernatremia.

Replacement of ongoing losses is appropriate when there are reasons to believe that these losses are significant. For example, a patient with excessive vomiting may continue to lose large amounts of gastric fluid. A child with an ileostomy or excessive burns may also continue to have large fluid losses. These losses must be considered when determining appropriate fluid therapy, or the amount of water and electrolyte replacement may be significantly underestimated.

Treatment

For all but the most mildly dehydrated patients, management should begin with an initial IV fluid bolus of 10 to 20 mL/kg of normal saline solution. The goal is to rapidly expand the extracellular fluid volume, particularly intravascular volume. In severely affected children, the bolus may need to be repeated until signs of improved peripheral perfusion and stable hemodynamics are present. This initial approach is appropriate for hyponatremic, isonatremic, and hypernatremic dehydration and therefore should not be delayed while waiting for the serum sodium result. Hypotonic solutions and those containing potassium should not be used during this initial phase of therapy because the goal is to provide fluid that remains intravascular and potassium may be dangerous if renal function is abnormal or hyperkalemia is already present.

After the initial replenishment of intravascular volume, subsequent therapy is aimed at replacing the calculated deficits of water and electrolytes while also providing ongoing maintenance requirements and replacement of ongoing losses. When determining appropriate subsequent therapy, it is assumed that sodium is the only electrolyte to be replaced. Because calculations are based on the sodium deficit, the extracellular space is preferentially replenished (which is desirable).

The water deficit is determined by a known weight loss (1 kg = 1 L) or estimated by your clinical examination. For children with hyponatremic or isonatremic dehydration, the sodium deficit can be calculated by using the following formula, once the current serum sodium concentration is known:

$$\text{Deficit (mEq)} =$$
$$(135 - Na)(0.6)(\text{Normal weight in kg}) + (\text{Weight loss in kg})(Na)$$

where Na is the current measured serum sodium concentration (in mEq) and weight loss is either known or estimated from clinical findings.

Subsequent management depends on the type of dehydration present and is discussed in the following sections.

ISONATREMIC AND HYPONATREMIC DEHYDRATION

Isonatremic and hyponatremic dehydration are clinical states resulting primarily from loss of extracellular volume. They should be managed as follows:

1. Calculate or estimate the volume deficit (based on weight or clinical examination, respectively).
2. Calculate the sodium deficit with the formula presented earlier.
3. Estimate the daily maintenance requirements (based on normal weight) and add these to the deficit determination (step 1).
4. Subtract the amounts of fluid and sodium already given as boluses to determine the amount of fluid and sodium to be administered over the next 24 hours.
5. Replace half of these amounts in the first 8 hours and half in the remaining 16 hours with a concentration of saline that provides the appropriate amounts of water and sodium as determined by your calculations.
6. Add potassium to the fluids only after the child has voided and you have established that renal function is normal.
7. Replace ongoing losses at 8-hour intervals if they continue to be significant. Table 15-2 lists the estimated electrolyte composition of various body fluids that may be lost abnormally; such charts can be used to determine the concentration of replacement fluids.
8. Check the serum sodium and potassium concentration again in 4 to 6 hours. Also monitor the child's clinical findings and urine output and specific gravity closely as a guide to hydration status.

This plan assumes that symptomatic hyponatremia (altered mental status, seizures) is not present. If the child has symptoms secondary to severe hyponatremia, hypertonic saline infusion may be required initially (see Chapter 34, Electrolyte Abnormalities). As noted earlier, the amount of sodium administered should then be subtracted when calculating the deficit to be replaced.

TABLE 15-2 **Estimated Electrolyte Composition of Body Fluids**

Fluid	Na (mEq/L)	K (mEq/L)	Cl (mEq/L)
Gastric	20-80	5-20	100-150
Pancreatic	120-140	5-15	40-80
Bile	120-140	5-15	80-120
Small bowel	100-140	5-15	90-130
Ileostomy	40-135	3-15	20-115
Diarrhea	10-90	10-80	10-110
Burns	140	5	110

HYPERNATREMIC DEHYDRATION

Hypernatremic dehydration results from an excessive loss of free water in the absence of a significant sodium deficit. In contrast to the other types of dehydration, replacement of the water deficit must occur **slowly**, over a period of 48 hours or more. Rapid decreases in the extracellular fluid sodium concentration may lead to cerebral edema secondary to a large intracellular shift of fluid. For this reason, the goal should be to reduce the serum sodium concentration by no more than 10 mEq/L/day. Management should proceed as follows:

1. Calculate the free water deficit. As noted previously, clinical findings in those with hypernatremic dehydration can be deceptive and may not reflect the severity of dehydration. Therefore, it is often reasonable to estimate a 10% loss of weight unless the weight loss is known. The free water deficit can also be calculated by using the following formula:

Deficit (L) = Normal total body water – Current total body water
where

$$\text{Normal total body water} = \frac{(\text{Current total body water})(\text{Current osmolality})}{\text{Normal osmolality}}$$

$$\text{Osmolality} = 2(\text{Na}) + \frac{\text{BUN}}{2.8} + \frac{\text{Glucose}}{18}$$

Therefore,

$$\text{Deficit (L)} = \frac{(\text{Current weight in kg})(0.6)(\text{Current OsM})}{290} - (\text{Current weight in kg})(0.6)$$

2. Subtract the amount of water given as boluses. Add maintenance requirements for 48 hours.
3. Replace the remaining water deficit over a 48-hour period with a solution that is either a one-fourth or one-third normal saline solution initially and check the serum sodium level frequently (i.e., every 2 to 4 hours initially). It is usually necessary to make frequent adjustments in the concentration and/or rate to ensure an appropriate, slow steady fall in the serum sodium concentration.
4. Add potassium to the IV fluids only after the child has voided and you have established that renal function is normal.
5. Replace ongoing losses every 8 hours if they are significant.

After initiating therapy, you should return to perform a more detailed physical examination, history, and chart review to look for clues to the cause of the diarrhea.

Selective Physical Examination II

General	Wasted appearance (starvation stools, laxative abuse, immunodeficiency)
Chest	Rales, wheezes, cough (cystic fibrosis, tuberculosis)
Abdomen	Bowel sounds, distention, tenderness, masses (gastroenteritis, colitis, inflammatory bowel disease, typhlitis); protuberance (celiac disease)
Lymph nodes	Adenopathy (immunodeficiency, tuberculosis)
Skin	Rashes (viral gastroenteritis)

Selective History and Chart Review II

Has the child been exposed to others with diarrhea?

If so, a common infection or perhaps staphylococcal food poisoning is suggested.

Is there blood, leukocytes, or eosinophils in the stool?

Blood and/or fecal leukocytes are more consistent with a bacterial cause than a viral one but may also be present with inflammatory bowel disease or some parasitic infections. The stool can be examined easily for leukocytes by preparing a thin smear on a slide and adding a drop of methylene blue. A Wright stain allows you to identify eosinophils, which may lead to a diagnosis of milk protein allergy in an infant or a parasite in an older child.

In addition to these bedside tests, stool cultures should be considered if bacterial colitis is suspected. A stool sample for ova and parasite detection should also be considered if there is any possibility of this diagnosis.

Has the child received antibiotics? What other drugs has the child received?

Clostridium difficile infection should always be considered in a child in whom diarrhea develops while in the hospital or if the child has received antibiotics recently, and a low threshold should exist for sending stool to the laboratory for toxin assays. Diarrhea is a common adverse effect of many drugs but is usually mild when drugs are the cause.

Is there a history of recent gastroenteritis?

Secondary lactase deficiency is a common sequela of gastroenteritis and may lead to persistent mild diarrhea.

REMEMBER

1. Your primary goal should be to assess the degree of dehydration and begin appropriate rehydration when dehydration is present.

2. All of the management strategies discussed in this chapter are based on multiple **estimations**. The most critical aspect of managing a dehydrated infant or child is frequent monitoring and reassessment, with appropriate adjustments in therapy. This is especially true in cases of hypernatremic dehydration.

3. Initial management is aimed at rapidly replenishing intravascular volume. Once this has been accomplished, you have time to plan your subsequent management.

Extremity Pain

David E. Melbye, MD

Extremity pain is a frequent complaint in children, as are headaches and abdominal pain. The list of potential causes of extremity pain is extensive; however, very few of these causes are immediately life threatening. When called regarding a child with extremity pain, your primary goal should be to determine the likelihood of an illness that is either life threatening or associated with significant morbidity if the diagnosis is delayed.

PHONE CALL

Questions

1. How old is the child?
2. What is the severity of the pain?
3. Is there pain in one site or in multiple sites?
4. Is there swelling, warmth, or erythema at the affected site?
5. Is the child febrile?
6. Why has the child been hospitalized?

The age of the child may help you narrow the list of possible causes. For example, benign nocturnal leg pains, commonly referred to as "growing pains," are more common in younger children. Similarly, the various malignancies that may produce extremity pain tend to affect children of different ages (e.g., neuroblastoma and leukemia in a younger child, osteogenic sarcoma in an adolescent). The severity of the pain helps you determine the need for an urgent evaluation, but it may not necessarily reflect the seriousness of the underlying problem, particularly in a young child. Multiple painful sites should raise suspicion of a systemic process, whereas a single site makes a localized process more likely. If the affected area appears erythematous and swollen, trauma or infection is suggested. Fever increases the likelihood of an infectious cause, and the child's reason for hospitalization allows you to consider some specific causes (e.g., sickle cell crisis, deep venous thrombosis in a postoperative patient, hypertrophic osteoarthropathy in those with chronic lung disease).

Orders

If not recently administered, acetaminophen or ibuprofen may be given in an attempt to relieve the pain.

Inform RN

A child in severe pain, with fever, or with an extremity that appears abnormal should be seen immediately.

ELEVATOR THOUGHTS

What causes extremity pain? It may help to think anatomically and classify causes according to whether bone, muscle, joint, nerve, blood vessel, or skin and connective tissue are involved. Benign nocturnal pains (growing pains) and behavioral causes of pain are diagnoses of exclusion.

Bone	Osteomyelitis
	Infarction (e.g., in sickle cell crises)
	Malignancy (leukemia, neuroblastoma, primary bone tumor)
	Fracture
	Avascular necrosis
	Osteoid osteoma
	Hypertrophic osteoarthropathy
	Histiocytosis
Joint	Septic arthritis
	Slipped capital femoral epiphysis (hip) (9 to 16 years old)
	Legg-Calvé-Perthes disease (hip) (4 to 9 years old)
	Transient synovitis (hip)
	Serum sickness
	Traumatic arthritis
	Hemarthrosis (e.g., hemophilia)
	Juvenile rheumatoid arthritis
	Rheumatic fever
	Benign hypermobility
	Viral arthritis
	Lyme disease
	Spondyloarthropathy (inflammatory bowel disease, psoriatic arthritis, reactive arthritis)
	Systemic lupus erythematosus
Muscle	Myositis
	Infectious
	Traumatic

Muscle—Cont'd	Inflammatory (dermatomyositis, polymyositis)
	Electrolyte disturbances
	Cramps
	Muscle strain
Nerve	Neuropathy
	Radiculopathy
	Reflex sympathetic dystrophy
	Guillain-Barré syndrome
Vascular	Coarctation of the aorta
	Arterial thrombosis
	Deep venous thrombosis
	Vasculitis (which may also cause secondary neuropathy, arthritis, or myositis)
Connective tissue	Fasciitis
	Compartment syndrome
Skin and subcutaneous tissue	Herpes zoster
	Cellulitis
	Trauma
	Infiltrated intravenous (IV) line
	Restrictive tape or bandages
	"Hair tourniquet" (infants)
Other causes	Benign nocturnal pain
	Behavioral or psychogenic

MAJOR THREAT TO LIFE

1. Infection

   Either a localized infection (e.g., osteomyelitis, pyomyositis, or septic arthritis) or a systemic infection (e.g., meningococcemia, Rocky Mountain spotted fever, or toxic shock syndrome) may result in significant extremity pain.

2. Malignancy

   Malignancy is not usually an immediate threat unless cell lysis results in severe hyperuricemia, hyperkalemia, and other metabolic disturbances.

3. Sickle cell crisis

   If the crisis is accompanied by signs and symptoms of infection or acute chest syndrome, it may be life threatening.

4. Compartment syndrome (compromising the vascular supply)

5. Deep venous thrombosis leading to pulmonary embolism

6. Arterial thrombosis leading to peripheral gangrene

7. Vasculitis

   If also involving major organ systems (lungs, heart, central nervous system [CNS], gut, kidneys), vasculitis may threaten life. Kawasaki disease may result in coronary artery aneurysms and a subsequent risk for rupture or myocardial infarction.

8. Rheumatic fever
   If carditis is also present, congestive heart failure may ensue.
9. Guillain-Barré syndrome (may compromise respiratory function)

BEDSIDE

As noted earlier, your primary goal while on call is to determine whether the child has one of the major threats just listed. If you can exclude a life-threatening possibility, a secondary goal should be to narrow the extensive differential diagnosis for extremity pain to a few likely possibilities. Regardless of the cause, improving the comfort of the child should be a priority.

Quick-Look Test

Does the child look well (comfortable), sick (uncomfortable), or critical (about to die)? Is the child moving the affected extremity or extremities?

If the child appears critically ill, you should immediately suspect a multisystem illness (sepsis, vasculitis). With most causes of extremity pain, the child appears well or only mildly uncomfortable. In a young child, however, the response to even minimal discomfort may be severe. Note the posture of the child. The child may protect or position the extremity in a way that minimizes discomfort. For example, children with a septic hip usually prefer to hold the hip flexed, externally rotated, and abducted (Fig. 16-1).

Airway and Vital Signs

As with any pain, mild tachycardia and tachypnea may be expected. Severe abnormalities in the heart rate or respiratory rate or abnormal blood pressure should not be expected and may be clues that the extremity pain is only one manifestation of a systemic process. Similarly, a compromised airway suggests a more significant problem affecting the lungs, heart, CNS, and/or abdomen. Fever may indicate infection or any inflammatory condition (e.g., vasculitis, lupus, dermatomyositis, rheumatic fever).

Selective History and Chart Review

Where is the pain?

In a young child, this question may not be easy to answer. Young children may not be able to localize pain well or may give inconsistent answers. In many instances, you need to rely on a careful examination to localize the affected area or areas. Remember also that pain may be referred from other sites. Knee or thigh pain may represent a pathologic condition of the hip. Hip pain may be a symptom of lower back or intra-abdominal disease.

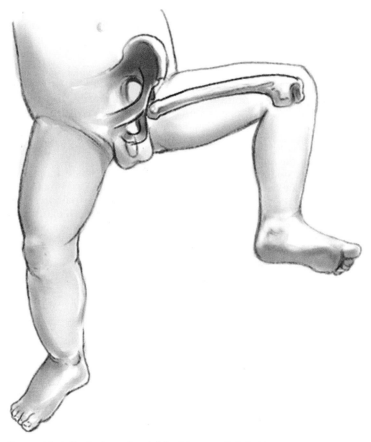

Figure 16–1 Posturing of a child with a septic left hip. In an attempt to relax the joint capsule, the child holds the affected hip flexed, externally rotated, and abducted.

You should therefore fully examine the joints proximal and distal to the site of pain.

Is the pain felt at a single site or at multiple sites? Is the pain well localized or diffuse?

Osteomyelitis, septic joints, fractures, pyomyositis, osteoid osteomas, hemarthroses, traumatic injuries, primary bone tumors, and cellulitis are most often well localized and at a single site. Isolated, unilateral hip pain (or referred thigh or knee pain) is suggestive of a septic hip, transient synovitis, slipped epiphysis,

Legg-Calvé-Perthes disease, avascular necrosis, or a spondyloar-thropathy (in an older child), but you should also consider the other localized processes just listed. Pain in multiple sites usually indicates a systemic process.

Has the child been irritable, lost weight recently, or had intermittent fever, malaise, and poor appetite?

These findings should raise suspicion of a systemic inflammatory condition such as infection or rheumatic disease, inflammatory bowel disease, or malignancy.

Is there a history of sickle cell disease or hemophilia, either in the patient or in the family?

Painful vaso-occlusive crises are the most frequent manifestation of sickle cell disease. These patients tend to have recurrences of pain in the same sites; therefore, the development of pain in a new site should raise suspicion of an alternative cause. Hemarthrosis may be the initial manifestation of hemophilia, and these patients also tend to have recurrences in the same joints.

Is there a history of recent extremity trauma?

Such a history raises suspicion of a fracture, hematoma, or compartment syndrome.

Has the child undergone prolonged immobilization?

Immobilization may predispose to deep venous thrombosis.

Is there a hypercoagulable state (birth control pills, lupus anticoagulant, protein C or S deficiency, antithrombin III deficiency, or nephrotic syndrome)?

A hypercoagulable state is a risk factor for venous or arterial thrombosis.

Has there been a recent upper respiratory infection or pharyngitis?

This may suggest Guillain-Barré syndrome or rheumatic fever.

Selective Physical Examination

Your examination should initially focus on the affected extremity. The source of the pain may often be unclear from the history alone, and your goal should be to determine whether the pain is the result of a problem in the bone, joint, muscle, nerve, vasculature, or skin and soft tissue. You should first inspect and note the position of the extremity and whether the child is willing to move the extremity spontaneously. Look for swelling, erythema, warmth, or deformity at all the joints, as well as over the long bones and the surface of the skin. Without moving the extremity, attempt to palpate over each of the bones and muscles and around the joints and carefully localize any tenderness as best as you can. Osteomyelitis, bone tumors, and bone infarctions should cause discrete point tenderness. A septic joint may also be tender, but the tenderness may not necessarily be severe unless the joint is moved. Because the hips and shoulders are deep joints surrounded by muscle and soft tissue, it is frequently not possible to appreciate tenderness or warmth at these sites. Compartment syndrome, myositis, and thrombosis (venous or arterial) may all result in exquisite muscle tenderness. Neuropathies may result in dysesthesia, paresthesia, or hyperesthesia. The passive range of motion of all of the joints of the extremity should be evaluated to determine whether limitations suggestive of arthritis are present. Muscle strength testing in the affected extremity should also be performed and the findings compared with strength elsewhere. If pain is in the lower extremity, your examination should include an assessment of the ability to bear weight and an observation of gait. Weakness is a clue that the underlying process may involve muscle and/or nerve. Deep tendon reflexes should also be measured to further evaluate this possibility. Pulses in the extremity should be palpated and tests of distal sensation performed, particularly if compartment syndrome or arterial thrombosis is suspected. Homans' sign is suggestive of deep venous thrombosis in the calf and is detected by flexing the knee with the patient supine and then quickly dorsiflexing the ankle to assess whether the patient experiences pain in the calf muscle. A negative finding does not rule out the diagnosis, however.

After your evaluation of the extremities, a general physical examination should be performed to look for signs that may indicate a systemic process. If the child has hip pain, a careful abdominal examination, as well as examination of the spine and lower part of the back, should be performed because pathologic conditions in these sites may result in referred pain (e.g., psoas abscess).

HEENT	Conjunctivitis (Kawasaki disease); pharyngitis (viral, streptococcal, rheumatic fever); oral ulcers (lupus, inflammatory bowel disease); swollen, cracked lips (Kawasaki disease)
Neck	Stiffness (meningitis)
Lungs	Respiratory distress (pulmonary embolism from deep venous thrombosis, acute chest syndrome with sickle cell disease)
Heart	Murmurs of aortic or mitral insufficiency (rheumatic fever)
Abdomen	Tenderness, mass (psoas abscess, appendicitis, vasculitis)
Back	Tenderness (diskitis, vertebral osteomyelitis), scoliosis
Skin	Rashes, vesicles, nodules (sepsis, herpes zoster, vasculitis, juvenile rheumatoid arthritis, rheumatic fever, dermatomyositis); pustules (disseminated gonococcal infection); erythema, warmth, edema (cellulitis, fasciitis); cyanosis (arterial thrombosis, compartment syndrome); inspection of IV sites for infiltration or restrictive taping; inspection of fingers and toes ("hair tourniquet," foreign body, paronychia)

Management

Further evaluation and management of major threats to life and other selected causes of extremity pain are discussed here.

Septic Arthritis

A child with fever and a single swollen, painful joint should be considered to have a septic joint until proved otherwise. Septic polyarthritis is also possible but much less common, and other signs and symptoms of sepsis are usually apparent. *Staphylococcus aureus* is the most common cause in young children. *Streptococcus pneumoniae* is also prevalent. In neonates, group B streptococci, *Escherichia coli*, *Listeria monocytogenes*, and *Candida albicans* are likewise common pathogens. *Neisseria gonorrhoeae* infection is an additional consideration in sexually active adolescents. Most septic joints are swollen, erythematous, and warm and have limited range of motion. However, if the affected joint is the hip, pain and limitation of motion may be the only objective signs of arthritis. Remember that the subjective pain may be referred to the thigh or the knee; therefore, any patient with fever and pain in these areas needs to undergo a careful evaluation of the ipsilateral hip. Plain radiographs or ultrasound studies of the hip may be helpful when it is unclear from your physical examination whether a hip effusion is present. Once you suspect septic arthritis, the synovial fluid needs to be aspirated immediately, before starting antibiotic treatment. You should proceed as follows:

1. Obtain radiographs of the affected area, a peripheral blood culture, complete blood count (CBC) and differential, C-reactive protein level, and an erythrocyte sedimentation rate. The blood tests may help you monitor the response to treatment. They may also help you distinguish a septic hip from transient synovitis, a postinfectious inflammatory synovitis that may produce fever and a sterile hip effusion in young children. The radiographs should be reviewed to look for evidence of a contiguous osteomyelitis.

2. Aspirate synovial fluid. You may need to consult a rheumatologist or orthopedic surgeon to help with this procedure, and the child may need sedation. If the affected joint is a hip, assistance from the radiologist to perform the aspiration under fluoroscopy may also be necessary. The orthopedic surgeon on call should be notified of any potential septic hip because if it is confirmed, open drainage of the hip in the operating room is necessary.

3. The fluid obtained at aspiration should be sent for the following:
   Gram stain
   White blood cell (WBC) count and differential
   Glucose

Aerobic and anaerobic culture

Mycobacterial culture

Acid-fast staining

Gonococcal culture (in those who are sexually active)

The appearance of the fluid should be noted. Septic joints usually result in cloudy or purulent fluid. WBC counts in the fluid are generally greater than 50,000/mm^3, with predominantly neutrophils, and the glucose concentration may be low. Exceptions to these generalizations are common with gonococcal arthritis.

4. After the foregoing procedures have been implemented, IV antibiotics should be empirically started. In children younger than 5 years, the combination of nafcillin and cefotaxime provides adequate coverage until culture results are available. In older children, nafcillin alone should be sufficient. If the Gram stain is positive, the choice of antibiotics can be more directed. The use of vancomycin instead of nafcillin should be considered if resistant organisms have been prevalent in the community.

5. A sexually active adolescent should also have throat, rectal, and cervical or urethral cultures obtained before starting antibiotics to further evaluate the possibility of gonococcal infection. The organism is more often cultured from these sites than from synovial fluid.

6. If tuberculosis is suspected from the exposure history, a tuberculin skin test and chest radiographic studies should be performed.

7. If your physical examination (point tenderness) or radiographs suggest osteomyelitis adjacent to the joint, the bone itself should also be aspirated, with any fluid obtained sent for the same studies as listed earlier for synovial fluid. Bone scanning may also be helpful in distinguishing osteomyelitis from septic arthritis. This distinction is important because the duration of antibiotic therapy is longer if osteomyelitis is present.

Osteomyelitis

The distal metaphysis of the long bones is a common site for osteomyelitis to develop. Localized point tenderness of a bone in a febrile child should be considered osteomyelitis until proved otherwise. Warmth and soft tissue swelling may be apparent if the periosteum has been penetrated and the infection has spread to adjacent soft tissue. If osteomyelitis is present without contiguous septic arthritis, passive range of motion of the joint is normal. Further evaluation of osteomyelitis is similar to that for septic arthritis, except that bone should be aspirated. Bone scanning may aid in identifying the optimal site to be aspirated and should be considered if physical examination fails to adequately localize the area of maximal tenderness. Plain radiographs are often unhelpful because changes are rarely seen within the first week of onset of osteomyelitis.

The most common pathogens are the same as those that cause septic arthritis. *Salmonella* should be considered in children with sickle cell disease, and *Pseudomonas* should be suspected in those with foot osteomyelitis after puncture wounds through shoes. After aspiration of the bone, IV nafcillin and cefotaxime (or ceftazidime if *Pseudomonas* is suspected) should provide adequate empiric coverage for the most likely pathogens.

Pyomyositis

Localized muscle abscesses containing staphylococci may occur either from hematogenous spread or from penetrating trauma to the muscle (including immunizations). Local warmth, tenderness, and a palpable mass within the muscle should raise suspicion of this disorder. Plain radiographs or ultrasonography of the muscle may be helpful. Surgical consultation for drainage is necessary before starting IV antibiotics.

Systemic Infections

Diffuse arthralgias and myalgias may be associated with numerous bacterial and viral systemic illnesses. You need to carefully and thoroughly evaluate the child for other signs of sepsis and potential sources of infection (see Chapter 18, Fever). Treatment depends on the specific cause. Influenza A may frequently cause severe pain and tenderness in the calf muscles, often associated with extreme elevations in muscle enzymes (creatine phosphokinase, aldolase). This process is self-limited and usually resolves within a few days. Other viral illnesses, Rocky Mountain spotted fever, or leptospirosis may result in similar findings.

Malignancy

Primary bone tumors (Ewing's sarcoma, osteogenic sarcoma), leukemia, and neuroblastoma may all cause extremity pain. The severity may range from mild pain and limping to severe, debilitating pain. Symptoms are often chronic but may be deceptively intermittent. Pain is frequently worse at night, and symptoms may be out of proportion to the objective findings. Plain radiographs may reveal lytic bone lesions, periostitis, or metaphyseal radiolucency. If you suspect malignancy, your goal while on call is to prevent any potential complications until the diagnosis can be confirmed and definitive treatment begun. Potential complications include metabolic disturbances (e.g., hyperuricemia, hyperkalemia), hematologic abnormalities (especially thrombocytopenia or neutropenia), infection (particularly if neutropenia is present), and the effects of space-occupying lesions (e.g., spinal cord compression). You should determine whether the CBC, electrolytes, calcium, uric acid, and phosphate have been checked recently. Consultation with the oncologist on call is necessary, with arrangements made for further diagnostic tests (biopsy, bone marrow aspiration) in the morning.

Sickle Cell Crisis

Dactylitis in an infant, also known as hand-foot syndrome, may be the first clinical manifestation of sickle cell anemia. Painful swelling of the hands, feet, and digits is most often symmetrical. In a young child, extremity pain is a frequent manifestation of the disease and is due to ischemic necrosis of bone as a result of vaso-occlusion from sickled cells. Affected sites tend to remain the same in the individual child, and the frequency of episodes can vary considerably. Your first goal should be to confirm that the current episode is secondary to vaso-occlusion and not another process. Osteomyelitis may mimic a vaso-occlusive crisis, and if there is any concern regarding infection, you should arrange to aspirate the affected site as described earlier before starting IV antibiotics. Careful evaluation of the child's respiratory status is mandatory to exclude a concurrent acute chest syndrome, and if the child is febrile, a thorough search for sources of infection is necessary. A CBC and reticulocyte count should be obtained, along with appropriate cultures if the child is febrile. If the diagnosis of sickle cell disease has not been confirmed, a peripheral blood smear should be reviewed and hemoglobin electrophoresis performed. Treatment consists of IV hydration and analgesia. Dehydration and acidosis should be corrected when present (see Chapter 15, Diarrhea and Dehydration). You need to re-evaluate the child frequently, and adjustments to the rate of hydration may be necessary because fluid overload may lead to pulmonary edema and the potential for acute chest syndrome. Oxygen should be administered if the patient is hypoxic. Vaso-occlusive crises often require narcotic analgesics, but acetaminophen and/or non-steroidal anti-inflammatory drugs may sometimes be sufficient. Ketorolac may be given in a dose of 0.5 mg/kg (maximum of 30 mg) every 6 hours. IV morphine or hydromorphone (Dilaudid) are the most commonly used narcotics. Morphine may be given at 0.1 to 0.2 mg/kg per dose intravenously every 2 to 4 hours and Dilaudid at 0.015 to 0.03 mg/kg per dose every 3 to 4 hours. Alternatively, patient-controlled analgesia (PCA) may be used, with a continuous infusion at a basal rate, a bolus amount, and a lock-out interval preprogrammed. A child receiving narcotics also needs frequent re-evaluation. Remember that respiratory depression is a serious potential consequence of narcotic administration, and acute chest syndrome may ensue quickly.

Compartment Syndrome

A recent arm or leg fracture or other trauma to an extremity can lead to compartment syndrome. Injury to muscles gives rise to swelling, which if severe enough, becomes limited by the tight-fitting fascia encasing some of the muscle groups in the arm or leg. Increased pressure within this compartment may compress blood vessels and lead to decreased circulation to the muscles and nerves. Pain, tenderness, distal sensory loss and/or weakness, and overlying tension, erythema, or edema may all occur. Pulses are not necessarily affected. If the patient has been placed in a cast for a recent fracture and is experiencing pain, the cast needs to be removed to adequately evaluate the extremity. Immediate surgical consultation and fasciotomy are necessary because irreversible necrosis may occur.

Deep Venous Thrombosis

Deep venous thrombosis is unusual in the pediatric age group but may occur in children who have been immobilized, are on prolonged bed rest, or have a hypercoagulable state. The goals of treatment are to prevent embolization and potential pulmonary infarction. Heparinization should be implemented if the child has any of these risk factors and physical examination reveals tenderness, warmth, edema, distended veins, and/or a positive Homans' sign suggestive of thrombosis. A 50-U/kg IV loading dose should be followed by a continuous infusion at 10 to 25 U/kg/hr and the dose adjusted to produce a partial thromboplastin time of 1.5 to 2.5 times the control value.

Arterial Thrombosis

Also unusual in childhood, arterial thrombosis or embolism is suggested by the four P's: pain, pallor, pulselessness, and paresthesias. Hypercoagulable states are the major risk factors in childhood, along with complications of indwelling catheters or attempts at placement of arterial lines. Heparin should be initiated as described earlier for venous thrombosis and vascular surgery consultation obtained immediately.

Vasculitis

Vasculitis may result in extremity pain for a number of reasons, including vaso-occlusion (similar to other thromboses), neuropathy (ischemic as a result of effects on the blood supply to the nerve), myositis, skin and soft tissue involvement, and arthritis. The vasculitis may be life threatening if other organ systems are also involved. Consultation with a pediatric rheumatologist is necessary, with consideration given to "pulse" steroids or cytotoxic agents.

Rheumatic Fever

Migratory polyarthritis or arthralgias and a history of recent pharyngitis or known streptococcal pharyngitis should raise your suspicion of rheumatic fever. A careful cardiac examination should be performed to listen for murmurs of aortic or mitral insufficiency. You should also look for signs and symptoms of associated congestive heart failure. A chest radiograph, echocardiogram, and streptococcal antibody tests (antistreptolysin-O [ASO], anti-DNAse B) may be useful. The arthritis of rheumatic fever tends to affect large joints; the pain is often severe and disproportionate to objective findings and responds dramatically to salicylates or other nonsteroidal agents.

Prednisone (if severe congestive heart failure is present) may also be necessary.

Guillain-Barré Syndrome

Pain and tenderness of muscles may be a feature accompanying the ascending weakness or paralysis of Guillain-Barré syndrome. The deep tendon reflexes should be carefully evaluated if the diagnosis is suspected, as should the airway and respiratory status. Cerebrospinal fluid analysis is necessary, with an albuminocytologic dissociation (protein greater than twice normal with <10 WBCs/mm^3) in a patient with a subacute polyneuropathy being diagnostic for Guillain-Barré syndrome. Consultation with a pediatric neurologist is usually necessary, and consideration should be given to treatment with IV immunoglobulin, steroids, or plasmapheresis.

REMEMBER

When evaluating an inpatient with extremity pain, first isolate the site and then organize your approach: bones, joints, muscles, blood vessels, nerves, skin. Use the opposite extremity as a control for your physical examination. When on call, concentrate on two goals:

1. Exclude a life- or limb-threatening process.
2. Make the child more comfortable.

Eye Problems and Visual Abnormalities

Marlene Peng, MD

Acute eye problems in children are less common than most of the other problems discussed in this book, and isolated problems of the eye are rarely life threatening. However, any problem involving the eye must be evaluated promptly for two reasons. First, eye and/or visual complaints may herald significant central nervous system (CNS) disease, including meningitis, encephalitis, and increased intracranial pressure (ICP). Second, any process involving the eye may potentially threaten vision.

PHONE CALL

Questions

1. Does the child appear well or sick?
2. How old is the child?
3. Is there drainage from the eye? What is the appearance of the drainage?
4. Is there periorbital swelling and erythema?
5. Is vision affected?
6. Is there pain or photophobia?
7. What was the reason for admission?

A child who appears ill should be suspected of having a systemic illness with associated conjunctivitis, orbital cellulitis, or periorbital cellulitis. A number of systemic infections (viral, bacterial, rickettsial) may produce conjunctivitis in addition to other signs and symptoms. The age of the child, the appearance of any drainage, the presence of periorbital swelling, and any pain or loss of vision help you to begin to differentiate the possible causes of eye inflammation. Pain or photophobia in a normal-appearing eye suggests photophobia, migraine, or early uveitis. If the call is regarding a newborn with eye drainage, ophthalmia neonatorum is a major consideration.

Orders

None.

Inform RN

"Will arrive at the bedside in … minutes." Ill-appearing children, those with swelling or erythema around the eye, those with pain or abnormal vision, and newborns all need to be seen immediately.

ELEVATOR THOUGHTS

What causes eye redness, drainage, pain, or swelling?
> Conjunctivitis or keratoconjunctivitis
>> Bacterial (*Neisseria gonorrhoeae* and *Chlamydia trachomatis* in the newborn)
>> Viral (herpes simplex in the newborn)
>> Other infections (e.g., Rocky Mountain spotted fever, leptospirosis)
>> Chemical (silver nitrate in the newborn)
>> Allergic
>> Kawasaki disease
> Uveitis
> Photophobia
> Traumatic corneal injury (abrasion, foreign body)
> Nasolacrimal duct obstruction (infant)
> Glaucoma
> Periorbital or orbital cellulitis
> Panophthalmitis

What causes abnormal or acute loss of vision?
> Many of the conditions just listed may lead to abnormalities in vision, but in the absence of any of these causes, you should consider the following:
> Retinal artery thrombosis
> Migraine
> Increased ICP
> Optic neuritis
> Retinal detachment (e.g., traumatic)
> Psychogenic

MAJOR THREAT TO LIFE OR VISION

- Infectious conjunctivitis or keratoconjunctivitis in the newborn
- Periorbital or orbital cellulitis
- Panophthalmitis
- Severe trauma
- Increased ICP

- Retinal artery thrombosis (secondary to vasculitis, emboli, or hypercoagulability)
- Meningitis (if photophobia is the primary complaint)

Treatment of each of these conditions should begin as soon as possible after diagnosis. Empiric treatment of *N. gonorrhoeae* conjunctivitis (in a newborn) and periorbital or orbital cellulitis (in an older child) should be considered if these conditions cannot be immediately excluded.

BEDSIDE

Quick-Look Test

Does the child look well (comfortable), sick (uncomfortable or distressed), or critical (about to die)?

A child who looks ill needs an immediate, thorough evaluation for a systemic illness.

Airway and Vital Signs

The vital signs should not be affected by a localized eye problem unless the child is also systemically ill. Fever should prompt a search for other potential sources and increase your concern about potential cellulitis or ophthalmitis.

Selective History and Chart Review

When did the eye inflammation begin?

In a newborn, onset within 12 hours of birth suggests chemical conjunctivitis from silver nitrate rather than an infectious cause. You should determine whether the infant received silver nitrate or erythromycin ocular prophylaxis (or neither). Gonococcal conjunctivitis typically begins 2 to 5 days after birth, although it may be delayed by partial treatment with ocular prophylaxis. Conjunctivitis secondary to *C. trachomatis* may not appear for 5 to 14 days.

If the child is a newborn, were there any maternal infections during pregnancy?

A history of gonorrhea, chlamydia, or herpes infection should raise your suspicion of these infections as causes.

Has the child been systemically ill or had a recent infection?

Periorbital and orbital cellulitis, as well as panophthalmitis, may occur secondary to hematogenous spread of bacteria, direct extension from sinusitis, or penetrating trauma and subsequent infection. *Staphylococcus aureus*, pneumococcus, and group A streptococcus are the most common pathogens. Conjunctivitis and uveitis may be associated with a number of systemic illnesses.

Are there other associated symptoms?

The presence of headache or neurologic symptoms may suggest migraine or CNS disease with increased ICP or associated optic neuritis.

Is there a history of trauma to the eye?

Corneal abrasions may easily occur from trauma that is unrecognized or is thought to be insignificant. If the child has recently undergone surgery, incorrect taping of the eyelids during surgery may lead to eye dryness and/or pain during the recovery period. Cellulitis may also develop after infection of a relatively minor abrasion or laceration of the skin near the eye.

Selective Physical Examination

Look carefully at the eyes and surrounding soft tissues, and note the characteristics of the drainage, if any. Observe the sclerae, conjunctivae, and extraocular movements of the child. The presence of pus (hypopyon) or blood (hyphema) in the anterior chamber may produce a visible fluid level between the inferior pole of the iris and the cornea and suggest infection and trauma, respectively. Visualize the retina as best as you can to look for papilledema, hemorrhages, and venous pulsations. If necessary, dilate the pupils so that you can adequately examine the retina. Remember to tell the nurse and document that you have dilated the pupils, lest their dilation be misinterpreted. In an infant who appears well, with clear, thin drainage or small amounts of mucoid drainage from the eye, you should suspect nasolacrimal duct obstruction. Thick, purulent drainage with marked injection and hyperemia of the sclerae and conjunctivae suggests gonococcal conjunctivitis in a neonate and other bacterial causes (*Haemophilus influenzae*, pneumococcus, staphylococcus, or streptococcus) in an older child. *C. trachomatis* may result in similar drainage but is generally less severe than that seen with gonococcus. Swelling and erythema of the soft tissues around the eye suggest periorbital cellulitis, especially if the child is febrile. Proptosis or any abnormalities in extraocular movement should make you very suspicious of orbital cellulitis. Papilledema warrants a computed tomography (CT) scan of the orbits to rule out a mass lesion, hemorrhage, cerebral edema, and hydrocephalus.

An eye that is injected but without mucopurulent drainage in an irritable child should raise your suspicion of uveitis, keratitis, glaucoma, trauma, or Kawasaki disease. Childhood glaucoma is rare and produces the classic triad of tearing, photophobia, and spasm of the eyelids secondary to corneal irritation. Corneal abrasions may be detected by instilling fluorescein dye onto the surface of the cornea and visualizing it with a Wood lamp. If herpes is a consideration, consultation with an ophthalmologist is necessary to determine whether characteristic dendritic lesions of the corneal epithelium are present.

Visual acuity should be tested with a Snellen chart, and visual field testing should be performed if the child is old enough to cooperate. Objective abnormalities in vision should be an indication to consult with an ophthalmologist.

Management

Any eye drainage should be Gram stained and cultured. Additional laboratory evaluation depends on the suspected diagnosis. Urgent ophthalmologic consultation should be obtained if you cannot adequately examine the eyes, if there are abnormalities in vision, or if the diagnosis is unclear. Definitive management of many conditions involving the eye needs the expertise of an ophthalmologist. A few of the most likely diagnoses you may need to address while on call are discussed here.

Ophthalmia Neonatorum

If the Gram-stained drainage reveals gram-negative diplococci characteristic of *N. gonorrhoeae*, ceftriaxone, 25 to 50 mg/kg/day intravenously for 7 days, and irrigation of the eye with normal saline solution at 15-minute to 2-hour intervals are necessary. Blood should be drawn for culture and additional cultures considered before instituting antibiotic treatment if the infant appears ill. *Chlamydia* infection can be treated with oral erythromycin for 14 days. Remember that coinfection with other sexually transmitted diseases must be suspected in an infant with gonococcal or chlamydial infection, including syphilis and human immunodeficiency virus (HIV).

Conjunctivitis in an Older Child

Distinguishing viral from bacterial conjunctivitis may be difficult, and many physicians elect to treat all cases of isolated conjunctivitis that are believed to be infectious. "Pink eye" may be treated with topical antibiotics such as bacitracin–polymyxin B or erythromycin for 5 to 7 days.

Herpetic Keratitis

Intravenous acyclovir should begin immediately in a newborn in whom herpetic keratitis is suspected because the infant may also be at risk for disseminated herpes infection. The addition of topical antiviral therapy should be considered and discussed with an ophthalmologist. Older infants and children may be treated with topical antivirals alone.

Periorbital and Orbital Cellulitis

If periorbital cellulitis is suspected, blood should be obtained for culture and empiric intravenous antibiotic treatment directed against the most likely pathogens begun. The combination of nafcillin and ceftriaxone or ampicillin-sulbactam is a reasonable choice. Cerebrospinal fluid (CSF) should be obtained for culture before starting antibiotics in an infant who appears ill. If proptosis or any abnormality in eye movement is noted, an emergency CT scan of the orbits should be obtained to look for orbital cellulitis or a frank orbital abscess. After obtaining blood for culture (and possibly CSF and urine if the infant appears ill), intravenous antibiotics similar to those used for periorbital cellulitis should be started. Otolaryngologic and ophthalmologic consultations should be obtained immediately and surgical drainage of the infected orbit considered. When in doubt, perform the CT scan. Orbital cellulitis is not something to be missed because it has tremendous potential for severe complications. Pressure within the orbit may affect the optic nerve and lead to visual loss. Alternatively, extension of the infection may result in cavernous sinus thrombosis or epidural or cerebral abscess.

Trauma

Corneal abrasions can be treated with topical antibiotics such as erythromycin or tobramycin applied three times a day. If the abrasion is large, the eye should be patched for 24 hours to promote healing. More severe forms of trauma should be managed by an ophthalmologist.

REMEMBER

1. Eye complaints may indicate a systemic or a CNS process.
2. Infection, trauma, and vascular occlusion of the eye are major threats to vision and should be excluded or appropriately managed.
3. Urgent ophthalmologic consultation may frequently be necessary and should be obtained if you suspect a process that may threaten life or vision.

Fever

Heather L. Toth, MD

One of the most common and potentially serious problems that the pediatric house officer deals with on call is fever. Fever can represent mild self-limited infections, serious infections, malignancies, or inflammatory illness. In a child who has already been hospitalized with appropriate evaluation, fever may be an expected finding that can be anticipated and treated. However, fever should never be ignored.

Generally, the accepted temperature that constitutes fever is 38.5°C, which corresponds to about 101.5°F. Regardless of age, this temperature is considered above normal and worthy of investigation and treatment. In neonates we often consider 38°C worrisome and an indication for evaluation to rule out sepsis. Therefore, fever must be considered in the context of the specific patient, the child's age, and the underlying diagnosis that led to the child's admission to the hospital.

Fever is a sign of potentially life-threatening illness and deserves hands-on evaluation.

PHONE CALL

It is important that the house officer obtain accurate information when notified about a child with fever. This allows prioritization of the call. The following questions are suggested:

1. How old is the child?
2. What is the child's admitting diagnosis?
3. What are the child's vital signs, including blood pressure?
4. What is the child's appearance? How is the child acting? Is the child alert? Oriented? Distressed? Agitated? Are the extremities well perfused? Pink?
5. Has the child been febrile previously?
6. Are there standing orders for an antipyretic and/or laboratory tests in the event of fever?
7. Does the child have any underlying condition that may compromise the immune system (e.g., cancer, sickle cell disease, rheumatologic diseases)?

High fevers (>39.5°C) warrant immediate hands-on evaluation in any child younger than 36 months. This is the age group at highest risk for occult bacteremia, and other sources of the fever must be ruled out by a thorough physical examination. Appropriate tests and an antipyretic (see Chapter 8, Analgesics and Antipyretics) should be ordered immediately over the telephone, and the nurse should be informed of the house officer's intent to evaluate the child immediately. The nurse can then have the chart readily available, medicate the child's fever, and be ready to assist the physician with the physical examination, especially if no parent or other caretaker is present with the child.

If the child, regardless of age, shows any signs of hemodynamic decompensation, a normal saline intravenous (IV) fluid bolus of 10 to 20 mL/kg should be started, and the nurse should be asked to page the senior pediatric resident to assist in the evaluation. If the child does not have adequate IV access, it is imperative to obtain at least one reliable IV line, preferably two.

In an older child (>3 years) the same questions should be asked, and the antipyretic should be administered. Confusion occasionally arises regarding the administration of antipyretics. Regardless of whether laboratory tests will be performed, it is important to give the antipyretic to control the febrile response and make the child more comfortable. An antipyretic does not affect a blood culture or a complete blood count, and antipyretics do not cause significant physical findings to disappear.

ELEVATOR THOUGHTS

The approach to fever in children is very age dependent in that neonates are far more susceptible to bacterial illness and have greater vulnerability to morbidity and mortality. In addition, the pathogens most commonly encountered in neonates differ from those found in older children. This difference is caused by two phenomena. The first is passive transmission of immunity via the placenta in the third trimester of pregnancy. This immunity conveys relative protection from viral illnesses such as varicella, rubella, and rubeola. Humoral factors transmitted in breast milk may also be protective and can last up to 2 to 3 months. The second major reason for the difference in pathogenic flora is immunization against both viral and bacterial pathogens, especially *Haemophilus influenzae* type B (HIB), *Bordetella pertussis*, *Clostridium tetani*, and hepatitis B virus. Since HIB immunization became routine, the incidence of invasive HIB infection has decreased dramatically (including meningitis, facial and orbital cellulitis, and invasive sinusitis).

If the child is a neonate and has been admitted to "rule out sepsis," cultures and other tests must be reviewed. Antibiotics are commonly started empirically in neonates, and it is important to know the antibiotics, the doses, the dosing interval, and their spectrum of anti-bacterial coverage. Could the antibiotic therapy already begun be inappropriate or inadequate?

It is important to carefully consider the vital signs in infants. Is the child appropriately tachycardic for the fever? Tachypnea must be distinguished from hyperpnea, which may indicate respiratory compensation for metabolic acidosis. Because blood pressure is generally preserved, it must be viewed in the context of the child's peripheral perfusion, urine output, and mental status. The child's hydration status must be assessed as well to add to the circulatory context. Circulatory collapse and shock, with their resultant metabolic acidosis and end-organ failure, must be avoided.

In an older child with any underlying conditions that predispose to infection, the same considerations apply. For example, a child with sickle cell disease who is older than 3 years should be considered functionally asplenic and therefore more susceptible to encapsulated bacteria. These children should be receiving daily penicillin (amoxicillin) prophylaxis against such organisms. Noncompliance has potentially serious consequences. Many older children have underlying conditions that may directly affect their immune system or their general health and nutrition status. Congenital heart disease, cystic fibrosis (CF), inflammatory bowel disease, short-gut syndrome, and neuromuscular disorders are chronic illnesses that can have a profound, if indirect effect on the immune system of older children and adolescents.

Therefore, while on the way to evaluate the child, organize the approach according to the child's age and the urgency of the vital signs. Always prioritize to rule out life-threatening conditions first: septic shock and meningitis.

MAJOR THREAT TO LIFE

- Septic shock
- Meningitis

The cascade of humoral factors released in response to fever can cause hemodynamic instability and jeopardize the function of multiple organ systems. Meningitis by its very location can compromise central nervous system function and result in altered mental status, seizures, deafness, and permanent disability.

BEDSIDE

Quick-Look Test

Does the child appear well (comfortable or playful), sick (distressed, agitated), or critical (lethargic, unresponsive)?

Toxic signs generally reflect hemodynamic instability and always include alteration in mental status.

Airway and Vital Signs

What are the heart rate, respiratory rate, and blood pressure?

Bradycardia in a febrile child is an ominous sign of impending circulatory collapse. Likewise, tachycardia out of proportion to the level of fever can be a sign of the child's desperate effort to preserve cardiac output.

Tachypnea and hyperpnea can reflect primary pulmonary disease, as well as respiratory compensation for metabolic acidosis.

Blood pressure must be viewed in the context of the child's perfusion, urine output, mental status, and volume status. Multiple mechanisms in the body interact to preserve blood pressure.

Selective Physical Examination I

What is the volume status? Are there signs of shock? What is the child's mental status?

Repeat vital signs, including temperature.

HEENT	Fundi, photophobia, mucous membranes, presence of tears
Neck	Stiffness
Cardiovascular	Heart rate, blood pressure, perfusion, murmurs, pulses (upper and lower)
Lungs	Quality of breath sounds and respiratory effort
Neurologic	Sensorium change
Skin	Turgor

Traditional teaching of clinical medicine always begins with history-taking. In actual practice, physical examination begins on first glance or at least simultaneously. Even at night, turn on the lights to adequately see the child as you ask the nurse or other caretaker for additional history. Again review the questions asked on the telephone. In addition, when did the child last eat or drink (very important if any surgical diagnosis or intervention is considered)? What has the child's fluid status been for the last 8 to 12 hours? Has the nurse or caretaker noticed any other changes in behavior, mood, or feeding? What laboratory studies were performed at the time of admission and what are the results? What medications is the child currently receiving (with dose and interval for each)?

Vital signs should be determined again at the time of your evaluation. This is especially critical if any of the initial vital signs were abnormal. Retake the temperature as well, preferably a rectal temperature. Other methods are adequate for screening but lack both the sensitivity and specificity of a rectal temperature. A thorough age-appropriate physical examination should follow, including funduscopic examination, pneumatic otoscopy, and rectal and/or pelvic examination if appropriate. Regardless of the findings of previous examinations, a complete examination must be performed *and documented thoroughly*. Special consideration should be given to general appearance and mental status, quality and rate of respirations, quality and rate of pulses, capillary refill time, hydration of the mucous membranes, and skin turgor. Remember that the major threat to life is septic shock and/or meningitis.

Management I

What measures need to be taken to prevent septic shock or to recognize meningitis?

Any known source of infection should be reassessed. Such assessment may require laboratory studies in the case of a child with bacteremia, pneumonia, or meningitis. Venous blood should be obtained for culture, preferably two samples, from virtually any febrile patient hospitalized for more than 24 hours, especially if the child is already receiving antibiotic therapy. Resistance to obtaining blood for culture is encountered among both nurses and parents, but it remains the standard and the best means of detecting occult bacteremia. Frequently, a complete blood count is also obtained and can yield helpful information regarding the white blood cell count and differential, platelet count, and hemoglobin and hematocrit, which can often indicate the presence of underlying chronic illness or malnutrition. The yield of blood culture is greatest in the setting of a patient with fever higher than 39.5° C and a total white blood cell count greater than 15,000.

Any sign of hemodynamic compromise must be addressed immediately. Perfusion, capillary refill, pulses, blood pressure, and heart rate, along with urine output, help determine the need for fluid resuscitation. Normal saline or lactated Ringer's solution is appropriate, generally in volumes of at least 10 to 20 mL/kg. If signs of circulatory compromise persist, the patient should be transferred expeditiously to the pediatric intensive care unit (PICU) for inotropic support.

In a neonate or toxic-appearing child, antibiotics should be promptly given as soon as samples for culture have been obtained. If there is difficulty in obtaining samples for culture quickly and the child appears toxic, empiric antibiotics should be started. In a neonate with fever and no known source, ampicillin and either gentamicin or cefotaxime are given. Older children may receive cefotaxime or ceftriaxone alone. The use of aminoglycosides must be accompanied by assessment of peak and trough levels, as well as blood urea nitrogen and serum creatinine levels, to monitor for nephrotoxicity.

If meningitis is suspected, a lumbar puncture is indicated. However, especially in infants, this procedure is not without risk. Be sure that the patient is hemodynamically stable and in no respiratory distress before placing the patient in a compromising position. (See Appendix A for how to perform a lumbar puncture.) Be sure that oxygen and airway support supplies are readily available. If there are any lateralizing signs on neurologic evaluation or suspicion of a space-occupying lesion, antibiotics should be given and an emergency head computed tomography (CT) scan obtained before the lumbar puncture. Whenever possible, record an opening pressure as soon as cerebrospinal fluid (CSF) is obtained, especially in an older child.

Further laboratory studies are frequently unnecessary, especially at night. Radiologic studies may be indicated, however. A chest radiograph is prudent in any patient with respiratory distress. For a toddler or preschool child with a sore throat and dysphagia, a lateral neck film should be performed to evaluate the retropharyngeal space, as well as the epiglottis, tonsils, and adenoids. CT scan of the head may be useful if there is a mental status change or lateralizing signs on neurologic evaluation. CT is also important in the setting of periorbital or orbital cellulitis if the fever persists, which is an indication that surgical intervention may be required.

Above all, a careful, thorough physical examination of the child determines what further work-up is necessary. Likewise, careful, thoughtful documentation of the house officer's findings and conclusions is critical to directing the work-up and treatment of a febrile patient.

Selective Chart Review

If the patient is stable and does not have signs of meningitis, look for localizing clues in the patient's history and physical examination, progress notes and/or consultations, and laboratory results. Other points worth checking include the following:

Temperature graph since admission

Recent white blood cell count and differential

Evidence of immunodeficiency (e g , sickle cell disease, asplenia, malignancy, human immunodeficiency virus [HIV] infection, use of steroids)

Allergies to antibiotics

Current medications

Selective Physical Examination II

Target areas suggested by the chart review of the patient's current complaints.

Vital signs	Repeat now
HEENT	
Fundi	Check for papilledema (intracranial abscess), Roth's spots (infective endocarditis)
Ears	Otitis media
Nose	Purulent drainage (sinusitis, foreign body)
Mouth	Dental abscess, pharyngitis, peritonsillar abscess
Neck	Stiffness (meningitis), cervical adenopathy (adenitis, retropharyngeal abscess)

Lungs	Crackles, wheezes, friction rub, consolidation (pneumonia, empyema)
Cardiac	New murmur (infective endocarditis)
Abdomen	Localized tenderness
Rectal	Tenderness, masses, blood
Musculoskeletal	Erythema, masses, swelling, effusion
Skin	Rash, petechiae, purpura, embolic phenomena, cellulitis, IV sites
Pelvic	If indicated

Management II

Besides blood, urine, sputum, and CSF cultures if indicated, cultures should be obtained from central lines, affected bones and/or joints, bullous skin lesions, the leading edge of cellulitis, the pharynx, middle ear, urethra, vagina or cervix, and any other site of apparent inflammation or infection. In addition, a Gram stain should be performed on any such culture material. Examination of the Gram stain can be very useful in making decisions regarding antibiotic coverage. In small children, sputum can rarely be obtained except from deep suctioning or from a tracheostomy.

Which patients need antibiotics now?
1. Patients with signs of sepsis, with or without shock, need broad-spectrum antibiotic coverage promptly.
2. Patients who are immunocompromised (i.e., neutropenic patients, patients receiving chemotherapy, HIV-positive patients, and asplenic patients, e.g., sickle cell patients).

Which patients need specific antibiotics now?
1. Patients with meningitis or any other localized infection that tends to have specific associated bacterial flora benefit from more specific antibiotic therapy.
2. Patients with a known positive culture.
3. Patients with specific antibiotic allergies.

Which patients do not need antibiotics until a specific pathogen is diagnosed?
    Patients older than 60 days who are not toxic, who are immunocompetent, and who have no specific source identified for their fever.

What antibiotic should be administered?
    In a neonate, ampicillin is chosen to cover *Listeria monocytogenes* and group B streptococci and gentamicin or cefotaxime to cover gram-negative enteric pathogens. Coverage for *Staphylococcus* species is needed in any postoperative patient; patients with indwelling catheters, gastrostomy tubes, or tracheostomies; and young patients with CF. Older children with CF require *Pseudomonas* coverage. Likewise, immunocompromised patients

require *Staphylococcus* coverage, as well as gram-negative coverage and frequently *Pseudomonas* coverage also.

REMEMBER

1. Fever requires hands-on assessment and can be an ominous finding in a small child.
2. Noninfectious sources of fever (i.e., drug-associated fever) are diagnoses of exclusion.
3. Antipyretics do not alter the yield of blood cultures or the white blood cell count or differential.
4. Fever in an immunocompromised patient can be an ominous sign.
5. Any sign of hemodynamic compromise must be treated quickly and then reassessed promptly for improvement. If no improvement is seen, strongly consider transfer to the PICU for inotropic support.
6. Seizures are commonly associated with a rapidly rising temperature in small children and do not, by themselves, suggest meningitis or other more serious infection.
7. Base selection of antibiotics on the probable organisms for that patient's age and localizing signs, if present.
8. Document your findings thoroughly, explain them to the parent or family, and notify everyone from the nurse to the attending physician of the patient's condition and your diagnosis and plan.

19

Gastrointestinal Bleeding

David G. Mueler, MD

In the pediatric population, gastrointestinal (GI) bleeding can occur at any age and from a variety of causes. As with adults, GI bleeding is generally approached by distinguishing upper and lower GI bleeding. It is equally important to consider the age of the child because the differential diagnosis for a newborn is quite different from that for a toddler or adolescent.

PHONE CALL

Questions

1. **How old is the patient?**
2. **Why is the patient in the hospital?**
3. **Clarify where the blood is coming from. Is it fresh (bright red blood) or old (melena, "coffee grounds")?**

    Vomiting of bright red blood or "coffee grounds" and most melena results from upper GI bleeding, whereas bright red blood from the rectum indicates lower GI tract bleeding. (There can occasionally be bright red blood with rapid upper GI bleeding.)
4. **How much blood has been lost?**

    Estimates of blood loss may be very inaccurate, but it is helpful to get a rough idea.
5. **What are the current vital signs?**

    Watch for tachycardia (early sign of hemodynamic instability) before hypotension (late sign).
6. **Is the bleeding a new problem or issue?**

    Acute infectious illnesses (salmonellosis and shigellosis) cause blood in the stool, as do chronic inflammatory conditions such as Crohn's disease and ulcerative colitis.
7. **What was the patient's last hemoglobin or hematocrit and platelet count?**
8. **Is the patient receiving an anticoagulant, such as heparin, warfarin (Coumadin), aspirin, nonsteroidal anti-inflammatory drug (NSAID), or fibrinolytic therapy?**

9. **Does the child appear to be in pain? Appear to be ill?**

Orders

1. If the patient does not have an intravenous (IV) line, the nurse should be instructed to place as large an IV line as possible or at least assemble supplies for IV line placement. You may need to consider two peripheral IV lines in situations in which the blood loss is significant and ongoing.
2. If the patient is hypotensive or the volume of blood loss is large, a 10- to 20-mL/kg bolus of normal saline or lactated Ringer's solution should be given immediately over a 5- to 10-minute period.
3. If the last complete blood count was more than 24 hours ago, another should be ordered and obtained immediately.

Inform RN

"Will arrive at the bedside in … minutes." Patients who are hemo-dynamically unstable (tachycardic, hypotensive, poorly perfused) or in pain must be examined *without delay*, and the senior resident should be informed immediately.

ELEVATOR THOUGHTS

Upper GI bleeding	Nosebleed
	Nasal trauma (vigorous suctioning, "picking")
	Oral or pharyngeal trauma (including dental)
	Esophagitis or gastritis
	Esophageal varices (liver disease, portal hypertension)
	Mallory-Weiss tear, prolapse gastropathy (vomiting)
	Peptic ulcer, duodenitis
	Swallowed maternal blood (newborn)
	Hemorrhagic disease of the newborn (confirm that vitamin K was given)
	Foreign body ingestion
Lower GI bleeding	Anorectal fissure (complication of constipation)
	Colitis (ulcerative, ischemic, infectious)
	Hemorrhoids
	Meckel's diverticulum
	Intussusception

Lower GI bleeding— Cont'd	Hemolytic-uremic syndrome
	Crohn's disease
	Milk protein allergy (infants)
	Necrotizing enterocolitis (prematurity)
	Polyps
	Henoch-Schönlein purpura (and other vasculitides)
	Vascular malformation
	Hirschsprung's enterocolitis

MAJOR THREAT TO LIFE

- Hypovolemic shock
- Ischemic bowel with secondary perforation, peritonitis, and sepsis

Although it is unusual for a child to lose a catastrophic amount of blood from GI bleeding, large-volume blood loss can occur, especially with ulcers, which can erode into arteries. Blood loss into the GI tract is generally insidious and results in anemia, sometimes severe, but it does not usually cause hemodynamic compromise. However, intussusception in particular can be associated with circulatory collapse. Likewise, in a premature infant, lower GI bleeding from necrotizing enterocolitis can be accompanied by septic shock. Children with chronic liver dysfunction before or after liver transplantation may have the potentially fatal combination of esophageal varices and coagulopathy.

BEDSIDE

Quick-Look Test

Does the child appear well (comfortable), sick (uncomfortable), or critical (about to die)?

Children who have had significant blood loss appear pale and poorly perfused and frequently have other signs of shock, such as tachycardia, cold clammy extremities (increased sympathetic tone), and tachypnea.

Airway and Vital Signs

Are there postural changes in the heart rate or blood pressure?

Vital signs should be obtained in the supine and sitting positions, except in infants. There should be less than a 15–beat per minute difference in heart rate and less than a 15–mm Hg fall in systolic blood pressure. Likewise, diastolic blood pressure should not fluctuate with position changes. Such changes suggest significant blood loss or distributive shock secondary to sepsis.

Selective Physical Examination

What is the child's volume status? Is the child in shock?

Cardiovascular	Pulse quality, capillary refill
Abdomen and rectum	Rigidity, guarding, rebound tenderness, masses and abnormal bowel sounds, heme-positive stool versus visible blood
Central nervous system	Mental status

Shock is a clinical diagnosis featuring inadequate peripheral perfusion, decreased urine output, and acidemia, with or without significant changes in blood pressure. A rectal examination with heme testing of the stool is absolutely necessary regardless of age or suspected cause of GI bleeding.

Management

What must be done immediately to treat shock or prevent it from occurring?

Placement of a reliable and reasonably large IV line should be accomplished quickly, and a 10- to 20-mL/kg bolus of normal saline or lactated Ringer's solution should be given. In premature infants and neonates, 5% albumin is expensive but preferred if readily available. Because the magnitude of the blood loss must be assessed, a complete blood count and platelet count should be obtained, as well as electrolyte, blood urea nitrogen, creatinine, amylase, and liver transaminase levels. If the amount of blood loss is large, typing and cross-matching should be done immediately. In a crisis situation, non–cross-matched type O-negative blood can be given, although this is rarely necessary. If there is any suggestion of sepsis, a bleeding disorder, and/or a hypoxic or ischemic insult, coagulation studies should also be performed (screening for disseminated intravascular coagulation). Also consider blood cultures and empiric broad-spectrum antibiotics if the child appears septic.

What can be done to stop the source of the bleeding?

Active GI bleeding is difficult to localize and treat. You must treat or prevent hypovolemia immediately and then pursue the underlying cause.

Upper GI Bleeding (Hematemesis and Most Melena)

Examine the child for sources of bleeding in the nose, mouth, and throat. Keep in mind that small children put all sorts of objects in their mouths and frequently walk around and fall with objects in their mouths, which can result in significant trauma. Chopsticks, rulers, pens or pencils, and various other items can cause lacerations and/or puncture wounds to the tongue, lips, or pharynx when children fall with these objects in their mouths. Consider iatrogenic trauma as well, such as suctioning and nasal prongs.

Esophageal bleeding can result from caustic ingestion, varices, or Mallory-Weiss tears and prolapse gastropathy associated with vomiting. The history should suggest the cause. H_2 blockers such as cimetidine and ranitidine or proton pump inhibitors usually help in alleviating esophagitis and gastritis. In children with liver disease and known varices, vasopressin may be used to control variceal bleeding.

Lower GI Bleeding (Usually Bright Red Blood per Rectum and Occasionally Melena)

The classic description of a "currant jelly" stool in an infant or toddler who appears uncomfortable strongly suggests intussusception. A mass may sometimes be palpable in the right lower quadrant or on rectal examination. Immediate surgical consultation should be followed by a contrast enema, which is frequently both diagnostic and therapeutic.

If there is associated diarrhea, stool should be obtained for culture of *Salmonella, Shigella, Yersinia, Campylobacter,* and other bacterial species. Stool should be examined for the presence of leukocytes, ova, and parasites, especially *Giardia lamblia.* Eosinophils seen on Wright stain of the stool suggest milk protein allergy in infants. Endoscopic study should be considered for inflammatory bowel disease.

In infants, careful examination of the perineum may reveal estrogen-withdrawal vaginal bleeding in females or the presence of small fissures around the anus. The use of a small test tube as a "poor man's proctoscope" can be helpful for finding internal fissures.

Abnormal Coagulation

Coagulopathies can result in heme-positive stools or overt bleeding. Correction of the prothrombin time (PT) or partial thromboplastin time (PTT) and thrombocytopenia and discontinuation of anticoagulant therapy should be undertaken immediately.

Selective History and Chart Review

What was the reason for admission? Has a cause of GI bleeding been identified during this admission? Is the child taking any medication that might worsen the bleeding? Is there any history of prolonged antibiotic use (Clostridium difficile)?

Medications that may result in bleeding or exacerbate GI bleeding include streptokinase, NSAIDs, steroids, heparin, and warfarin.

In a newborn, the records should be examined for the method of delivery and any birth asphyxia. Newborns who vomit blood have frequently swallowed maternal blood during the delivery. In addition, neonates may have swallowed maternal blood from breast-feeding. Asphyxiated infants are at greater risk for necrotizing enterocolitis, as are premature infants (<35 weeks). Also in newborns, passage of stools can cause small tears in anorectal tissue and give rise to fissures that result in small amounts of blood coating the stool.

Painless lower GI bleeding implies a Meckel diverticulum, whereas associated abdominal pain suggests intussusception in infants and toddlers, inflammatory bowel disease in children and adolescents, or infectious causes if associated with diarrhea.

A history of the last oral intake is important if emergency surgical intervention is indicated. In addition, some idea of urine output provides important information regarding cardiac output and volume status.

Laboratory Data

As noted earlier, several laboratory studies should be performed if not recently done, including the following:

Complete blood count and platelet count

Electrolytes, blood urea nitrogen, creatinine

Amylase, liver transaminases

PT, PTT

Flat and upright abdominal films, especially if the child is uncomfortable

An Apt test to distinguish maternal blood from the infant's blood (because of the presence of fetal hemoglobin in the infant)

If these studies have not been obtained within 24 hours of a significant change in the child's status, they should be obtained now.

Management II

When is surgical consultation appropriate?

Significant bleeding

Persistent bleeding requiring transfusion

Presence of signs and symptoms of bowel obstruction (Intussusception or volvulus) or ischemia

Consider a GI consultation and endoscopy to confirm the source of GI bleeding. Resuscitate with fluids and have all the laboratory and radiologic studies available before consultation whenever possible.

What other studies are available to localize the site of bleeding?

Endoscopic assessment is the test of choice for upper GI bleeding. Before endoscopy the child must be kept without oral intake (NPO) and must be hemodynamically resuscitated. Lower GI bleeding may require endoscopy, as well as possibly a radio-labeled red blood cell scan to detect mesenteric bleeding. Other tests to be considered include a Meckel scan and angiography.

REMEMBER

1. Give the child NPO orders and document when the last oral intake was in case surgical intervention or endoscopy is indicated.
2. Resuscitate the child before you pursue diagnostic studies.

3. Insertion of a nasogastric tube after examination of the nose, mouth, and pharynx is important if there are signs of bowel obstruction. Saline lavage can be helpful in localizing the source of bleeding to the stomach. A negative finding on lavage does *not* rule out upper GI bleeding. Remember that a nasogastric tube can be a source of trauma and bleeding.

4. Bismuth compounds (e.g., Pepto-Bismol) and iron supplements can turn stools black. True melena is pitch black, tar-like, and sticky and has an odor that is not soon forgotten. Iron supplements can also make stools test heme positive.

5. False-positive guaiac tests can result from red meat, turnips, bananas, and tomato skins.

Genitourinary Problems

James J. Nocton, MD

Several problems related to the genitourinary system may arise while a child is hospitalized and require prompt attention. Some of these problems, such as hematuria (Chapter 23) and urine output problems (Chapter 30), are reviewed elsewhere in this book. In this chapter, the approach to evaluating dysuria, scrotal pain, and vaginal bleeding while on call is discussed.

DYSURIA

PHONE CALL

Questions

1. Is the child febrile?
2. What is the child's diagnosis?
3. How old is the child?
4. Is the child a boy or a girl?
5. Is there gross hematuria?

The answers to these questions will allow you to begin to think about potential explanations for the problem. If fever is present, a urinary tract infection is much more likely. The child's diagnosis or gross hematuria may suggest specific causes (such as hemorrhagic cystitis related to cyclophosphamide treatment as part of chemotherapy protocols). Likewise, some problems may be more common at different ages (e.g., sexually transmitted diseases) or occur only in boys (balanitis).

Orders

Ask the nurse to collect the next urine for urinalysis and culture. If the child is an infant, the nurse will need to collect the urine by catheter.

Inform RN

"Will arrive at the bedside in … minutes." A child with fever or gross hematuria should be seen immediately.

ELEVATOR THOUGHTS

What causes dysuria?
  Urinary tract infections
      Cystitis (bacterial, adenoviral, drugs)
      Pyelonephritis
  Urethritis
      Sexually transmitted infection (STI) (gonococcus)
      Inflammatory (reactive arthritis, Kawasaki disease)
  Vaginitis
      STI
      Group A streptococcus
      Foreign body
  Passage of renal calculi
  Passage of a blood clot (trauma)
  Urethral irritation
      Girls
          Bubble bath
          Pinworms
          Urethral prolapse
          Sexual abuse
          Hypercalciuria
      Boys
          Hypercalciuria
          Urethral stricture
          Balanitis
          Foreign body insertion

MAJOR THREAT TO LIFE

Few life-threatening problems are associated with dysuria. If infection is present, it may progress to sepsis and shock. If hemorrhage from bleeding along the genitourinary tract is present, it could eventually lead to hypovolemia and shock.

BEDSIDE

Quick-Look Test

Most children will appear well. If they are distressed, lethargic, or unresponsive, shock from sepsis or hemorrhage and hypovolemia may be imminent.

Airway and Vital Signs

Tachycardia, if present, will most likely be secondary to pain or fever. An increased respiratory rate may also be related to pain or may reflect acidosis from infection. Hypotension will indicate potential shock.

Selective Physical Examination

HEENT	Conjunctivitis may be seen with reactive arthritis or with Kawasaki disease, both of which may cause urethritis
Abdomen	Flank tenderness (pyelonephritis), suprapubic tenderness (cystitis)
Genitals	Urethral or vaginal discharge, ulcerations, penile lesions (balanitis), vesicles (herpes simplex)

Selective History and Chart Review

Is the child at risk for STIs?

If the child is sexually active or has previously had such infections, the potential for an STI to be the cause is increased.

Is the child at risk for renal calculi?

A family history of renal calculi or conditions leading to potential hypercalcemia (see Chapter 34, Electrolyte Abnormalities) increase the risk.

Has there been a history of trauma or kidney tumor?

Trauma to the kidney or Wilms' tumor can lead to bleeding into the urinary tract and the passage of blood clots.

Has the child received medications that can cause hemorrhagic cystitis?

Management

Your priority while on call is to establish whether infection or hemorrhage is a probable cause of the dysuria because these are the two potential threats to life. Urinalysis should be performed as quickly as possible. A quick dipstick test at the bedside will determine whether there is heme in the urine, potentially from hemorrhage in the urinary tract, or whether leukocytes and nitrites are present, potentially indicative of infection. The presence of nitrites is more specific for bacteria in the urine because leukocytes may be present with noninfectious urethritis, as well as with urinary tract infections.

Microscopic analysis of urine will allow you to determine whether red blood cells are present, indicative of hemorrhage, rather than hemoglobinuria from hemolysis or myoglobinuria from rhabdomyolysis as the cause for heme in the urine. It will also allow quantitation of the number of white blood cells in the urine, with large numbers being more indicative of infection.

Urinary Tract Infection

If the child has fever, flank pain and tenderness, and large numbers of white blood cells in the urine, pyelonephritis should be suspected. If there is no fever or flank pain and large numbers of white blood cells are found in the urine with positive nitrites, it is more likely to be a lower urinary tract infection (i.e., cystitis). Cystitis is more common in adolescent females, whereas younger children are more likely to have pyelonephritis. In some instances, it is difficult to determine conclusively whether the infection has ascended the urinary tract and led to pyelonephritis. In either case, if the suspicion of infection is strong, empiric antibiotic treatment should be started after ensuring that an adequate specimen for urine culture has been obtained (catheterization, suprapubic aspiration, or clean-catch specimen). *Escherichia coli* and other enteric pathogens will be the most likely cause, and therefore a third-generation cephalosporin is often the best choice. Pyelonephritis should be treated with intravenous antibiotics, whereas cystitis may be treated orally with a third-generation cephalosporin, trimethoprim-sulfamethoxazole, or in older children, ciprofloxacin.

Hemorrhagic Cystitis

In the absence of a history of administration of medications that can cause hemorrhagic cystitis, hemorrhage in the urine associated with dysuria may be the result of renal calculi, hypercalciuria, or viral hemorrhagic cystitis. Adenovirus is a common cause of hemorrhagic cystitis and requires only supportive treatment, with resolution generally occurring within several days. However, if cyclophosphamide or another medication that can cause hemorrhagic cystitis has been administered, the child is frequently in significant pain and requires prompt attention. Consultation with a urologist will be necessary, and bladder irrigation should be initiated. A Foley catheter should be placed and normal saline irrigation begun. In some instances, administration of alum or silver nitrate into the bladder may be necessary. These steps should be undertaken only after consultation with a urologist.

Sexually Transmitted Infections

If the patient is an adolescent with dysuria, an STI is possible. Certainly, a history of previous similar infections or the presence of a vaginal or urethral discharge increases the likelihood of an STI. An adolescent female should undergo a pelvic examination, and appropriate cervical specimens for culture of gonococcus and *Chlamydia* should be obtained. A wet preparation should be performed with analysis for clue cells and *Trichomonas*. If there is cervical motion tenderness or adnexal tenderness on examination and/or significant purulent cervical discharge, treatment should be considered before confirmation of infection by culture. Treatment regimens for uncomplicated STI and those for pelvic inflammatory disease are presented in Tables 20-1 and 20-2, respectively. In males, a urethral swab can be performed to obtain specimens for culture of gonococcus and *Chlamydia*. Performing polymerase chain reaction (PCR) for gonococcus and *Chlamydia* on urine samples is an alternative to culture in both males and females. When the index of suspicion for an STI is high, treatment should be considered (Table 20-1).

TABLE 20–1 **Treatment of Uncomplicated Sexually Transmitted Infection in Adolescents**

Chlamydia trachomatis	Azithromycin, 1 g orally in a single dose *or* Doxycycline,* 100 mg orally twice daily for 7 days
Neisseria gonorrhoeae	Cefixime,† 400 mg orally in a single dose *or* Ciprofloxacin,‡ 500 mg orally in a single dose *or* Ofloxacin,‡ 400 mg orally in a single dose *or* Levofloxacin,‡ 250 mg orally in a single dose *or* Ceftriaxone, 125 mg intramuscularly in a single dose *plus* Treatment of *C. trachomatis* if indicated§

*Eight years of age or older.

†Cefixime is no longer produced in the United States; availability is limited.

‡Fluoroquinolones have not been recommended for persons younger than 18 years because they damage articular cartilage in juvenile animal models. However, in children treated with fluoroquinolones, no joint damage attributable to therapy has been observed. Quinolones should not be used to treat gonorrhea infections acquired in Asia or the Pacific Islands, including Hawaii.

§The Centers for Disease Control and Prevention recommend treating persons with a positive gonorrhea test result for both gonorrhea and chlamydia unless a negative result has been obtained with a sensitive chlamydia test.

From Kliegman RM, et al: Practical Strategies in Pediatric Diagnosis and Therapy, 2nd ed. Philadelphia, Elsevier, 2004, p 481. Adapted from the Centers for Disease Control and Prevention. Sexually transmitted diseases treatment guidelines 2002. MMWR Morb Mortal Wkly Rep 51:1-84, 200.

SCROTAL PAIN

PHONE CALL

Questions

1. How long has the pain been present?
2. Has there been any history of injury or trauma?
3. Is there any radiation of the pain?
4. Are there systemic or other symptoms?
5. Is there swelling?

The sudden onset of pain or pain after minor injury is suggestive of torsion of the testes or the appendix testis. Radiation of the pain may suggest inguinal hernia, and systemic symptoms such as fever and chills might indicate infection. Nausea and vomiting can be

TABLE 20–2 **Treatment of Pelvic Inflammatory Disease**

Parenteral Regimens (One of the Following)

Cefotetan, 2 g IV q12h, or cefoxitin, 2 g IV q6h, plus doxycycline, 100 mg
IV or PO q12h

or

Clindamycin, 900 mg IV q8h, plus gentamicin, loading dose (2 mg/kg
body weight) IV or IM followed by maintenance dose (1.5 mg/kg q8h)

Parenteral therapy may be discontinued 24 hours after clinical improvement
and continue

    Doxycycline, 100 mg PO bid, or clindamycin, 450 mg orally qid,
    continued for 14 days of total therapy

    For tubo-ovarian abscess, addition of either metronidazole, 500 mg
    PO bid, or clindamycin, 450 mg PO qid, to oral doxycycline
    provides better coverage against anaerobes

Outpatient Regimens (One of the Following)

Ofloxacin, 400 mg PO bid, or levofloxacin, 500 mg PO qd for 14 days with
or without metronidazole, 500 mg PO bid for 14 days

or

Ceftriaxone, 250 mg IM in a single dose, or cefoxitin, 2 g IM, with
probenecid, 1 g PO in a single dose once, or other parenteral third-
generation cephalosporin (e.g., ceftizoxime or cefotaxime) plus doxycycline, 100 mg PO bid for 14 days, with or without metronidazole,
500 mg PO bid for 14 days

bid, twice daily; IM, intramuscularly; IV, intravenously; PO, per os (orally); qd, every day;
qid, four times daily.

From Kliegman RM, et al: Practical Strategies in Pediatric Diagnosis and Therapy, 2nd ed.
Philadelphia, Elsevier, 2004, p 491. Adapted from the Centers for Disease Control and
Prevention. Sexually transmitted diseases treatment guidelines 2002. MMWR Morb
Mortal Wkly Rep 51:1-84, 200.

associated with testicular torsion, and dysuria may be seen with
urinary tract infection or epididymitis.

Orders

Ask the nurse to collect and save a urine sample if possible.

Inform RN

"Will arrive at the bedside in... minutes." Scrotal pain is an emergency and should be evaluated immediately.

ELEVATOR THOUGHTS

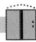

What causes scrotal pain?
    Testicular torsion (adolescent > prepubertal)
    Torsion of testicular appendage (prepubertal > adolescent)
    Trauma

Incarcerated inguinal hernia
Epididymitis (adolescents)
Orchitis (mumps)
Vasculitis (Henoch-Schönlein purpura)
Referred pain (nephrolithiasis, appendicitis)
Malignancy
Fournier's gangrene

MAJOR THREAT TO LIFE

Interruption of vascular flow to the testes with risk of subsequent infarction and loss of the testes is the major immediate threat. Testicular torsion results in the greatest risk for infarction, but severe trauma or vasculitis may rarely also place the patient at risk. Fournier's gangrene is unusual in children, but it is a life-threatening infection.

BEDSIDE

Quick-Look Test

Does the child appear well (comfortable), sick (distressed, agitated), or critical (lethargic, unresponsive)?
    A child with scrotal pain will generally appear very uncomfortable regardless of the cause. Those with torsion of the appendix testis will not be as uncomfortable as those with testicular torsion. In the rare event of Fournier's gangrene, the child may be in septic shock.

Airway and Vital Signs

The airway and vital signs should not be compromised, with the exception that tachycardia and mild hypertension may be present secondary to pain. If fever is noted, infection is obviously a consideration.

Selective Physical Examination

The examination will focus on the scrotum, its contents, and the inguinal canal, as well as the abdomen. The abdomen should be inspected and palpated for signs of an acute abdominal process with potential referred pain to the scrotum. Any scars should be noted because they will indicate a possible previous hernia or undescended testes. When examining the scrotum, note the position of the testis. A high-riding, swollen, exquisitely tender testis is suggestive of testicular torsion. The scrotum may be erythematous, and the cremasteric reflex should be absent. If a firm mass is palpated at the upper pole of the testis and the cremasteric reflex is present, torsion of the appendix testis is much more likely. In some instances, the "blue dot sign" may be seen in which the twisted appendix testis is visible through the skin. With epididymitis, the epididymis itself will be firm, tender, and swollen.

Attention should be directed to the inguinal area to look for evidence of hernia. Swelling and pain in the scrotum and inguinal canal, especially with additional signs indicative of potential bowel obstruction, may occur with an incarcerated inguinal hernia.

Selective History and Chart Review

If the patient is an adolescent, is there a history of STI or dysuria?
This will increase the likelihood of epididymitis.

Has there been intermittent pain in the scrotum in the past?
Such pain might reflect previous intermittent episodes of testicular torsion.

Are there rashes, abdominal pain, and other systemic features?
Vasculitides such as Henoch-Schönlein purpura and polyarteritis nodosa may cause scrotal pain and swelling secondary to vasculitis within the spermatic cord.

Management

It may be difficult to distinguish testicular torsion, torsion of the appendix testis, and other causes of scrotal pain by the history and physical findings alone. This is critical because testicular torsion is managed surgically and the other conditions may be managed nonoperatively. Imaging studies may help determine whether blood flow to the testis is reduced, as seen in testicular torsion. A color Doppler ultrasound is quick and often the most readily available imaging study. A radionuclide testicular flow scan can also be performed, but it requires more time and is often less convenient. When testicular torsion is a consideration, prompt consultation with a pediatric urologist is most helpful.

Testicular Torsion

Testicular torsion is a surgical emergency. If there is a reasonable likelihood of testicular torsion, the patient should be taken to the operating room for surgical exploration because time spent on imaging studies may be detrimental. Even if the torsion can be reduced manually by the pediatric urologist, surgical fixation is necessary to prevent recurrence.

Torsion of the Appendix Testis

Torsion of the appendix testis will eventually lead to infarction of the appendix with subsequent resolution of the pain and swelling. Bed rest plus analgesics for several days is usually sufficient. Imaging studies will most often reveal increased blood flow to the testis.

Incarcerated Hernia

If an incarcerated hernia is suspected, immediate pediatric surgical consultation is necessary, with surgical correction performed. Manual reduction of the hernia may be attempted before surgical repair.

Epididymitis

In prepubertal boys, epididymitis is most often secondary to an anatomic abnormality of the lower genitourinary tract and is usually caused by the same organisms that cause urinary tract infections. In these young boys, urinalysis with culture should be performed, appropriate antibiotics administered when indicated, and consultation with pediatric urology obtained. In adolescent boys, epididymitis is most often an STI, with gonococcus and *Chlamydia* being most common, and should be treated as described earlier in this chapter under "Sexually Transmitted Infections."

Fournier's Gangrene

Systemic symptoms of fever, chills, and potentially shock often accompany this severe necrotizing infection of the perineum. Multiple organisms, including staphylococcus, streptococcus, anaerobes, and gram-negative organisms, have been associated with Fournier's gangrene. Surgical débridement and broad-spectrum antibiotics should be instituted promptly.

VAGINAL BLEEDING

Vaginal bleeding is always abnormal in the absence of secondary sexual characteristics and in girls younger than 8 years. The exception is in a newborn, in whom small amounts of vaginal bleeding may occur as a result of withdrawal from circulating maternal estrogens. In adolescents, it may also be the result of irregular menstruation. Vaginal bleeding is rarely an emergency, but you may need to be prepared to evaluate this problem should it begin while you are on call.

PHONE CALL

Questions

1. How old is the child?
2. Has the child been menstruating previously?
3. Has there been any trauma?
4. What medications is the child receiving?
5. Is there bleeding at other sites?

The age and menarchal status of the child will affect your differential diagnosis, as will a history of trauma, medications, and the presence of bleeding at multiple sites.

Orders

A complete blood count (CBC) with differential, prothrombin time (PT), and partial thromboplastin time (PTT) should be ordered if not performed recently.

Inform RN

"Will arrive at the bedside in ... minutes." Unless the child is unstable or bleeding profusely, vaginal bleeding is rarely an emergency, and if other situations are a priority, the patient can be evaluated when time allows.

ELEVATOR THOUGHTS

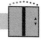

What causes vaginal bleeding?

Prepubertal child	Vaginal foreign body (toilet paper)
	Infectious vulvovaginitis
	Urethral prolapse
	Trauma
	Lichen sclerosus
	Pinworms
	Hemangioma
	Malignancy
	Precocious menarche
Pubertal child	Foreign body
	Trauma
	Malignancy
	Cervical polyp
	Coagulopathy
	Hemangioma
	Cervicitis
	Endometrial polyp
	Pelvic inflammatory disease

MAJOR THREAT TO LIFE

Massive bleeding with exsanguination is the primary threat to life.

BEDSIDE

Quick-Look Test

Does the child appear well (comfortable), sick (distressed, agitated), or critical (lethargic, unresponsive)?
    If the child is distressed or agitated, excessive bleeding, infection, or an uncomfortable foreign body should be considered.

Airway and Vital Signs

Fever, tachycardia, or hypotension should increase your suspicion of infection or massive hemorrhage.

Selective Physical Examination

The examination will focus on the external genitalia, and in adolescents, consideration will need to be given to performing a pelvic examination if there is considerable bleeding and the cause is not apparent after examining the external genitalia. In addition, the general examination should focus on the mucous membranes of the nasal and oral cavities and the skin in a search for other signs of hemorrhage that might be indicative of a systemic coagulopathy.

The labia should be examined for signs of trauma such as lacerations. Any discharge from the vagina and any lesions should be noted, such as hemangiomas or urethral prolapse. The presence of a foreign body should be obvious. The Tanner stage of the child should be documented. Lichen sclerosus of the vulva leads to thinning of the epidermis and has a characteristic appearance.

Selective History and Chart Review

Has the child had menarche?

If other signs of pubertal development are apparent, the current bleeding may represent menarche.

If the child has begun menstruating, what has the pattern of the menstrual periods been and when was the last one?

Soon after menarche, menstruation can be very irregular.

Is there a history of bleeding disorders in the family?

Coagulopathies, including von Willebrand's disease, may cause menorrhagia without necessarily causing bleeding at other sites.

Management

The cause of the vaginal bleeding may be obvious after your physical examination and selective history, particularly if a laceration, vaginal discharge, foreign body, or mass is evident. If signs of vaginal discharge are present, cultures should be obtained and appropriate antibiotics begun. If the cause is not easily discerned, further evaluation will be necessary, but it does not necessarily need to occur in the middle of the night. Checking the results of the CBC, PT, and PTT can help reassure you that the bleeding is not excessive, and the patient may require frequent evaluation to ensure that the bleeding does not worsen and that her vital signs do not suggest impending hypovolemia. As long as this is the case, further assessment, including evaluation for precocious puberty and potential consultation with a gynecologist or pediatric endocrinologist, can proceed in a less urgent manner. Remember, your goal while on call is to ensure that nothing will occur immediately to endanger the patient.

SUMMARY

Genitourinary problems are infrequent while on call and are rarely an emergency. However, a few life-threatening and organ-threatening processes can cause dysuria, scrotal pain, and vaginal bleeding and may need to be addressed while on call. Although it is always optimal to make a definitive diagnosis, when this is not possible, evaluating the patient frequently, providing supportive care, and remaining alert for potential life-threatening processes will allow you to keep your patient safe and comfortable while on call.

Headache

Wendy Z. Gavidia, MD

Headache is a frequent complaint of hospitalized children. It may be a symptom secondary to a life-threatening intracranial process, or it may be a relatively benign and self-limited complaint. The goal while on call is not necessarily to definitively diagnose the cause of the headache. Although a definitive diagnosis would be most helpful, the more immediate goal is to exclude conditions that require urgent attention and treatment. Once this is accomplished, headache can be managed symptomatically and expectantly while planning for further diagnostic evaluation when a clear cause cannot be immediately established.

PHONE CALL

Questions

1. How old is the child?
2. Why is the patient in the hospital?
3. How severe is the headache? Can the child rate the pain such as with a pain scale (Fig. 21-1)?
4. Was the onset sudden or gradual?
5. What are the vital signs?
6. Has the child had a headache like this before?
7. Is the headache positional (is it worse when lying down flat)?

Orders

If a recent set of vital signs have not been recorded, ask the nurse to obtain them, including temperature.

Inform RN

"Will arrive at the bedside in … minutes."

Increased intracranial pressure (ICP) is the most concerning possible explanation for headache and needs to be considered in all patients with this complaint. ICP headaches are associated with nausea, vomiting, mental status changes, and eventually vital sign abnormalities, such as bradycardia and hypertension. Recurrent or chronic headaches should be addressed within a reasonable time

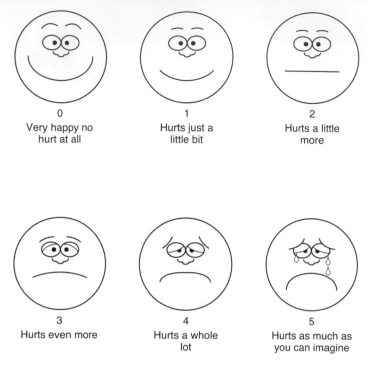

0
Very happy no
hurt at all

1
Hurts just a
little bit

2
Hurts a little
more

3
Hurts even more

4
Hurts a whole
lot

5
Hurts as much as
you can imagine

Figure 21–1 The Bieri faces scale. (Adapted from Bieri D, Reeve RA, Champion GB, et al: The faces pain scale for the self-assessment of the severity of pain experienced by children: Development, initial validation, and preliminary investigation for ratio scale properties. Pain 41:139-150, 1990.)

but do not warrant an immediate assessment if the vital signs are stable, the pain is not severe, and the child has no other symptoms.

ELEVATOR THOUGHTS

What causes headaches?

Many of the causes are the same as in adults, but the relative frequencies may be very different. For example, brain tumors are the most commonly diagnosed solid tumor of childhood, and many, especially posterior fossa tumors, are associated with characteristic headaches.

Headaches may be a symptom of a disorder outside the nervous system or may arise directly as a result of dysfunction within the nervous system. The pain-sensitive structures in the head are as follows:

Intracranial	Cerebral and dural arteries
	Large veins and venous sinuses
	Dura at the base of the brain
	Periosteum of the skull
Extracranial	Cervical roots
	Cranial nerves
	Extracranial arteries
	Muscles attached to the skull
	Periosteum/paranasal sinuses
	Eyes/ears
	Mouth/dental structures
	Skin or soft tissue over the skull

Acute Headache

1. Increased ICP. Headache results from compression and distortion of pain-sensitive dural and vascular structures surrounding the brain. It is worse after a few hours of being recumbent or asleep and decreases after a period of being awake and upright (positional headache). When more severe, it increases with coughing, straining, and bending over and may be associated with visual obscuration. Causes include:
   Brain tumor
   Subdural or epidural hematoma
   Malignant hypertension
   Pseudotumor cerebri
   Trauma (closed head injury)
2. Infectious. Meningismus occurs as a result of inflammation of pain-sensitive structures surrounding the brain. It is usually generalized, severe, throbbing, and associated with nuchal rigidity and photophobia. Causes include:
   Meningitis
   Encephalitis
   Sinusitis or mastoiditis
   Brain abscess
3. Vascular. Subarachnoid hemorrhage causes an explosive, sudden-onset, "worst headache of my life." Pain is followed by meningismus and later by headache secondary to increased ICP. Causes include:
   Intraparenchymal hemorrhage
   Vasculitis
   Migraine
   Arteriovenous malformation with bleeding
   Cerebral venous sinus thrombosis: seizures, increased ICP, altered mental status

4. Post-traumatic
    Concussion
    Subdural or epidural hematoma
    Cerebral contusion
5. Other
    Acute angle-closure glaucoma
    Alcohol or drug ingestion
    Low-pressure headache. Because of loss of cerebrospinal fluid (such as after a lumbar puncture [LP]), the brain's buoyancy is decreased such that the organ descends when the individual is in the upright position; as a result, traction is exerted on structures at the apex, and structures at the base are compressed. Pain is relieved by laying flat.
    Pituitary apoplexy. Acute headache referred to the temples/ears, meningismus, visual field changes, and raised ICP-type headache may be caused by pituitary apoplexy.

Chronic (Recurrent) Headache

Progressive

1. Vascular
    Migraine
    Cluster headaches
    Hypertension
    Subdural hematoma
2. Metabolic
    Hypoglycemia
3. Drugs
    Alcohol
    Nitrates
    Calcium channel blockers
    Nonsteroidal anti-inflammatory drugs (NSAIDs)
4. Increased ICP
    Tumor
    Pseudotumor
    Central nervous system (CNS) vasculitis
    Hydrocephalus
5. Infectious
    Abscess (intracranial, dental)

Nonprogressive

1. Psychogenic
    Tension headaches
    Stress
    Depression
    Anxiety

2. Other
   Temporomandibular joint disease
   Post-traumatic
   School avoidance/attention seeking

MAJOR THREAT TO LIFE

Headaches caused by increased ICP can result in the following major threats to life:

- Intracranial bleeding: subarachnoid, subdural, epidural hemorrhage
- Meningitis
- Herniation (transtentorial, cerebellar, central)
- Tumor
- Cerebral venous thrombosis

All of these conditions can progress rapidly and are associated with a poor outcome if unrecognized. Herniation is a significant cause of death secondary to cerebral edema after trauma, intraparenchymal bleeding, or hypoxic-ischemic encephalopathy (Fig. 21-2).

BEDSIDE

Quick-Look Test

Does the patient appear well (comfortable), sick (uncomfortable, distressed), or critical (about to die)?

Most patients with chronic or recurrent headaches are fairly comfortable. Those with migraines, meningitis, subarachnoid hemorrhage, or subdural or epidural hematomas generally appear ill.

Airway and Vital Signs

What is the temperature?

Fever in the setting of headache should prompt a search for infectious causes, including meningitis, abscess, encephalitis, and sinus disease.

What is the blood pressure?

Significant hypertension of any origin can cause headache.

What is the heart rate?

Cushing's triad of hypertension, bradycardia, and respiratory changes is a most ominous and generally very late finding that is accompanied by significant mental status change. Tachycardia would be expected in any child complaining of severe headache.

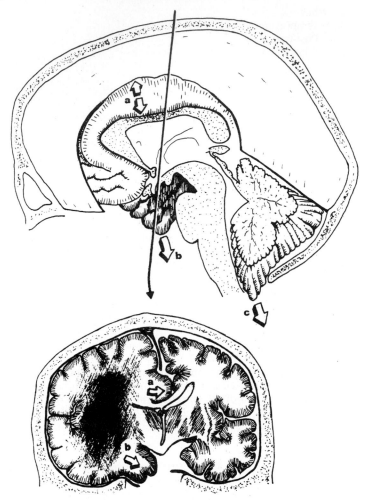

Figure 21–2 Central nervous system herniation. a, Cingulate herniation. b, Uncal herniation. c, Cerebellar herniation. (From Marshall SA, Ruedy J: On Call: Principles and Protocols, 4th ed. Philadelphia, Elsevier, 2004, p 122.)

Selective Physical Examination

HEENT   **Funduscopic examination is *ABSOLUTELY ESSENTIAL*** for detecting vascular changes, hemorrhages, and papilledema (Fig. 21-3) (loss of the optic nerve margin and lack of

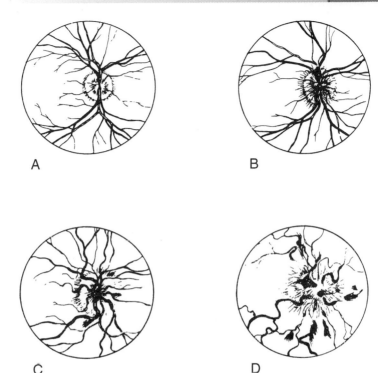

Figure 21–3 Disk changes seen in papilledema. **A**, Normal. **B**, Early papilledema. **C**, Moderate papilledema with early hemorrhage. **D**, Severe papilledema with extensive hemorrhage. (From Marshall SA, Ruedy J: On Call: Principles and Protocols, 4th ed. Philadelphia, Elsevier, 2004, p 123.)

	venous pulsations are specific signs of increased ICP); also check visual acuity, symmetry of pupils, photophobia, extraocular movements, ptosis, sinus tenderness, hemotympanum (basilar skull fracture), mastoid tenderness, depressed skull fractures, contusions, jaw pain, or restriction of movement
Neck	Nuchal rigidity, positive Kernig's or Brudzinski's sign (Fig. 21-4).
Neurologic	Cranial nerve examination; symmetry of reflexes, tone, and strength; cerebellar function, including balance and gait; mental status examination. *MAKE THE CHILD WALK IF AT ALL POSSIBLE!*

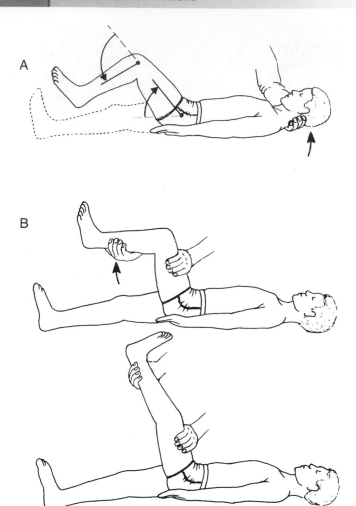

Figure 21–4 A, Brudzinski's sign. The test result is positive when the patient actively flexes his hips and knees in response to passive neck flexion by the examiner. **B**, Kernig's sign. The test result is positive when pain or resistance is elicited by passive knee extension from the 90-degree hip-knee flexion position. (From Marshall SA, Ruedy J: On Call: Principles and Protocols, 4th ed. Philadelphia, Elsevier, 2004, p 124.)

Management I

In a child with nuchal rigidity, altered mental status, or focal neurologic findings, order an immediate computed tomography (CT) scan of the head.

If meningitis is suspected, order an LP tray at the bedside and appropriate intravenous broad-spectrum antibiotics to be given as soon as the CT scan and LP are completed. The CT scan and LP should be completed within 1 hour. If there is to be any delay, give the antibiotics and complete the studies thereafter.

The necessity for a head CT scan is controversial in patients with a completely nonfocal neurologic examination, normal mental status, and no signs of increased ICP, including papilledema. One can proceed either by performing the LP and administering the antibiotics (if you feel comfortable that there is no increase in ICP) or by administering the antibiotics empirically and performing the LP after the head CT scan has been obtained (if increased ICP remains a concern).

In children with nuchal rigidity and signs of increased ICP, LP is absolutely contraindicated because of the risk of brain herniation. Meningitis, subdural empyema, and brain abscess can all produce increased ICP and be manifested as headache. Head CT helps distinguish among these conditions. In general, when evaluating for acute blood and ventricular size, CT of head without contrast is better than magnetic resonance imaging (MRI). If inflammation is suspected, CT of head with contrast helps. To evaluate the posterior fossa, order an MRI. When evaluating arteries, order MRI/magnetic resonance angiography (MRA). To evaluate the venous sinuses, order magnetic resonance venography (MRV). The empiric antibiotic coverage suggested for children and adolescents is cefotaxime, 50 mg/kg intravenously every 6 hours, along with vancomycin, 15 mg/kg every 6 hours. Vancomycin is a recent addition to the recommended empiric antibiotics because of the alarming increase in resistant *Streptococcus pneumoniae*. Higher doses of antibiotics are needed to allow for meningeal penetration. If abscess or subdural empyema is suspected, clindamycin or metronidazole is added to cover for anaerobes.

In addition to immediate antibiotic treatment, children with a brain abscess or subdural empyema require the expertise of a pediatric neurosurgeon. Moreover, it is prudent to anticipate a therapeutic plan for seizure control (see Chapter 29, Seizures). If any signs of altered mental status and/or increased ICP are present, therapy should begin immediately (see Chapter 7, Altered Mental Status).

Selective History and Chart Review

If the headache is a new complaint, have the child describe in detail what it feels like, where it hurts the most, and what makes it better or worse. Was there a warning or an aura? Are there associated symptoms? Did it start suddenly or gradually? Has the child ever had a headache like this before?

Characterize the onset, duration, frequency, and pattern of chronic headaches. Do they awaken the child from sleep or keep the child from falling asleep? Are the headaches present as soon as the child awakens in the morning? What time of day does the headache occur? Are there known precipitants, such as foods, change in sleep pattern, trauma, toxins, medications, or psychosocial stressors? Are there any associated symptoms such as an aura, tinnitus, visual changes, mental status changes, seizure activity, nausea, or vomiting?

The chart may contain additional information about past complaints of headache, as well as reports of a family headache history.

A medication history plus a history of head trauma over the last 6 to 8 weeks should be obtained. Headaches secondary to subdural hemorrhage may be delayed for days or even weeks, and therefore the patient and family may not associate the headache with a "distant" head injury.

Management II

Tension Headaches

Also known as stress headaches, muscle tension headaches are the most common headaches in childhood. Frequently described as "band-like," they are usually bilateral. Pain tends to be mild to moderate, and the duration is highly variable, from 2 to 72 hours. This type of headache is frequently related to undiagnosed refraction defects in school-aged children straining to see the blackboard. Chronic exposure to loud music or noise can also provoke this type of headache. Patients are generally treated conservatively with acetaminophen or ibuprofen and re-evaluated in the morning.

Migraine Headaches

Migraine headaches can be incapacitating regardless of the patient's age. Migraines may be preceded by an aura, which can consist of homonymous visual disturbances, unilateral weakness or sensory changes, aphasia or other language disturbances, or the "Alice in Wonderland" syndrome of spatial disorientation. Be aware that these symptoms are similar to those of ischemic stroke. Migraines are frequently unilateral but can be bilateral. Pain intensity is moderate to severe, and the duration is typically about 8 hours. Acute therapy should begin with acetaminophen or NSAIDs. Narcotic analgesics should be avoided if possible, but when necessary, codeine followed by meperidine can be used. The acute administration of vasoconstricting agents such as ergotamine or sumatriptan succinate (Imitrex) should be avoided in children younger than

10 years, if possible. β-Blockers are extensively used for migraine prophylaxis but are of little use as acute therapy.

Post-traumatic (Postconcussive) Headache

Given a history of trauma but no signs of intracranial edema or hemorrhage, postconcussive headaches can occur in the acute post-traumatic phase or at much later times. Mild analgesics such as acetaminophen or NSAIDs, which do not adversely affect the child's mental status or level of consciousness, should be administered. If the headache continues to worsen, consider a CT scan of the head to look for subdural or intraparenchymal blood.

Complicated Migraines

Basilar migraine is characterized by adolescent onset, occurrence in females more frequently than in males, and usually absence of a positive family history; it is frequently accompanied by visual disturbances, ataxia, vertigo, nausea, vomiting, loss of consciousness, and/or drop attacks. Cranial nerve deficits can be observed. In treatment, avoid sumatriptan because it will constrict vessels in an already ischemic area. Hemiplegic migraine must be distinguished from stroke. There is a slow progression of unilateral weakness and/or sensory changes usually preceding the headache. Symptoms may last hours to days, and in recurrent attacks the alternate side may be affected. Associated symptoms include aphasia, paresthesias, and rarely, seizures. Permanent deficits can result from repeated attacks. Ophthalmoplegic migraines generally have an age of onset of less than 10 years. Unilateral eye pain is followed by third nerve palsy, a dilated pupil, and downward and outward deviation of the eye. The fourth and sixth cranial nerves are frequently involved. Ophthalmoplegia resolves in 1 to 4 weeks. Permanent third nerve injury can result from multiple attacks.

Cluster Headaches

Cluster headaches are nonfamilial and tend to afflict males more than females. These headaches are rare before 10 years of age. The headache tends to be rather brief, 30 to 60 minutes, but is severe to excruciating. Often, there is unilateral nasal stuffiness and tearing attributed to histamine release, hence the term histamine cephalgia.

Brain Tumor Headaches

Although headaches can be an initial symptom of a brain tumor, in general, brain tumors are an uncommon cause of headache in children. Brain tumor headaches tend to be chronic and progressive, and their onset commonly has a positional component, with maximal pain in the early morning on first rising from bed. The vast majority of children with brain tumors have abnormal findings on neurologic or ophthalmologic examination. A meticulous history and neurologic examination detect most brain tumors, especially in the setting of chronic, progressive headache.

Hemorrhages and Effusions

Subdural, epidural, and subarachnoid hemorrhages can result in headache and are generally diagnosed by CT scan. Therapy may be surgical, with decompression required to avoid herniation. Prompt neurosurgical consultation is warranted. Chronic subdural effusions can occur after meningitis, as well as after trauma, especially child abuse.

Malignant Hypertension

Malignant hypertension is unusual in children. Prompt but careful reduction in blood pressure should be undertaken, as discussed in Chapter 24, Hypertension.

Hydrocephalus

Though more common in younger children than in adolescents, hydrocephalus, like brain tumors, tends to cause recurrent, progressive headache. Therapy requires neurosurgical consultation. Obtaining the opening pressure when performing an LP is very important and may suggest the diagnosis of pseudotumor cerebri if the ventricles are not dilated on CT scan. Pseudotumor is most often seen in obese, adolescent girls but is also associated with several systemic illnesses.

TABLE 21-1 **Differential Diagnosis of Headache**

Acute isolated headache	Meningitis
	Subarachnoid hemorrhage
	Systemic infection with fever
Acute recurrent headache	Brain tumor
	Vascular malformation
	Migraine
	Hypertension
	Sinusitis (rare in younger children)
Chronic progressive headache	Brain tumor
	Hydrocephalus
	Brain abscess
	Subdural hemorrhage
	Pseudotumor cerebri
Chronic nonprogressive headache	Depression
	Stress, tension headache
	Post-traumatic
	School avoidance or attention seeking

SUMMARY

Headache is not an uncommon complaint in hospitalized children. Most headaches are due to benign causes that require only analgesic therapy. The house officer on call must distinguish these mild headaches from those that are life threatening. Thus, headaches warrant prompt evaluation. It is important in the history to distinguish an isolated acute headache from a recurrent acute headache, as well as a pattern of chronic progressive versus chronic nonprogressive headaches. Table 21-1 can be helpful in organizing the differential diagnosis. Key physical examination findings include meningismus, funduscopic irregularities, and abnormal ambulation of the child.

Heart Rate and Rhythm Abnormalities

B. Joann Patterson, MD

The terms *dysrhythmia* and *arrhythmia* are often used interchangeably, but in fact these terms describe different abnormalities in rhythm. Dysrhythmia refers to an abnormal rhythm, the more common problem. Arrhythmia means the absence of rhythm, which is a more acute and urgent problem.

Fortunately, cardiac rhythm disturbances are relatively rare in children. This is both a blessing and a curse because the lack of experience results in most pediatric house officers feeling relatively ill prepared to both perform and adequately interpret an electrocardiogram (ECG).

It is best to think of rhythm disturbances in general categories first: too fast, too slow, regular, or irregular. Cardiac output is equal to *stroke volume* times *heart rate*, and rhythm has a profound effect on both factors in that equation. Loss of atrial and ventricular synchrony compromises ventricular filling and adversely affects stroke volume. Likewise, very high heart rates decrease ventricular filling time and, again, compromise stroke volume.

The task for a house officer confronted by a dysrhythmia is to find a cause, if possible, and to intervene immediately in order to preserve cardiac output before damage to vital organs occurs, including the brain, the kidney, the liver, and the heart itself. This means, however, assessing the condition of the patient, regardless of what is on the monitor, and treating the patient, **not** the monitor!

In pediatrics, tachydysrhythmias are far more common than bradydysrhythmias. Bradycardia is usually secondary to respiratory compromise and hypoxemia. Tachydysrhythmias can include any of the supraventricular tachycardias (SVTs) and, rarely, ventricular tachycardia (VT). Regardless of the cause, rhythm disturbances can be life threatening and must be evaluated without delay.

RAPID HEART RATES

PHONE CALL

Abnormal heart rhythms provoke an immediate reaction from the nursing staff. Questions should include the following:

1. How old is the patient?
2. Why is the patient in the hospital?
3. What is the heart rate?
4. Is the rhythm regular or irregular?
5. Is the QRS complex narrow or wide?
6. What are the patient's blood pressure and perfusion status?
7. Are there any associated symptoms (chest pain, palpitations, respiratory distress)?
8. What are the rest of the patient's vital signs (temperature, respiratory rate)?

Orders

1. If the child is hypotensive, start a bolus of normal saline or lactated Ringer's solution, 20 mL/kg over a 5- to 10-minute period.
2. Call for a stat 12-lead ECG and rhythm strip, if available. If they are not available, ask the nurse to attach the patient to a cardiorespiratory monitor immediately.
3. Obtain another blood pressure reading now.
4. Start the child on supplemental oxygen, 1 to 2 L/min by nasal cannula.
5. Inform the RN that you will arrive at the patient's bedside in ... minutes.

ELEVATOR THOUGHTS
(CAUSES OF RAPID HEART RATES)

Regular SVTs	Sinus tachycardia
	Reentrant SVT
	Atrial flutter
	Junctional ectopic tachycardia
Irregular SVTs	Multifocal atrial tachycardia
	Sinus tachycardia with premature atrial contractions (PACs)
	Sinus tachycardia with premature ventricular contractions (PVCs)
	Atrial flutter with variable block
	Atrial fibrillation
Ventricular tachycardia	

MAJOR THREAT TO LIFE

- Hypotension leading to shock
- Congestive heart failure leading to pulmonary compromise and hypoxia

As noted previously, keep in mind the following formulas:

Cardiac output (CO) = Heart rate (HR) × Stroke volume (SV)

Blood pressure (BP) =
Cardiac output (CO) × Systemic vascular resistance (SVR)

Once the heart rate becomes so high that ventricular filling is compromised, stroke volume and therefore cardiac output fall. The body tries to preserve blood pressure by increasing SVR through vasoconstriction, especially in the extremities, thereby resulting in compromised peripheral perfusion.

BEDSIDE

Quick-Look Test

Does the patient look well (comfortable), sick (uncomfortable or distressed), or critical (about to die)?
  Tachycardia is uncomfortable and may cause agitation and irritability in infants and toddlers. Older children describe palpitations, pounding of the heart or chest, or racing of the heart. A patient in shock may have mental status changes.

Airway and Vital Signs

What are the heart rate and rhythm, temperature, and blood pressure?
  Hypotension requires immediate action. Sinus tachycardia may be due to fever, or it may be secondary to hypotension from hypovolemia, septic shock, or medications. It rarely occurs at rates high enough to be a primary cause of hypotension. No more than a rhythm strip is usually necessary to recognize reentrant SVT, atrial fibrillation with a rapid ventricular response, or VT. You must be careful to verify that the rhythm strip determinations and ECG are performed at the standard paper speed of 25 mm/sec. This is the sweep speed for all monitors and is the standard for all ECG machines. However, monitors and ECG machines allow the operator to change the recording speed to 12.5 mm/sec, which slows the paper and makes the QRS complexes very narrow and crowded. Conversely, changing the paper speed to 50 mm/sec widens the complexes and appears to slow the rate. This speed can be used for tachycardias to try to determine whether P waves are present. Always be sure that the monitor and your assessment of the pulse rate coincide with one another.

Recognition of the rhythm disturbance is critical. The following are examples of regular and irregular tachydysrhythmias:

Rapid regular rhythms
- Sinus tachycardia (Fig. 22-1)
- SVT: atrial flutter (Fig. 22-2)
- SVT: atrioventricular (AV) nodal reentry SVT or Wolff-Parkinson-White orthodromic SVT (Fig. 22-3). Figure 22-4 shows the typical "delta" wave seen with Wolff-Parkinson-White syndrome when *not* in reentrant SVT
- SVT: ectopic atrial tachycardia (Fig. 22-5)
- VT (Fig. 22-6); Figure 22-7 shows the variant called torsades de pointes, seen with the long QT syndrome

Rapid irregular rhythms
- Atrial fibrillation (Fig. 22-8)
- Atrial flutter with variable block (Fig. 22-9)
- Multifocal atrial tachycardia (Fig. 22-10)
- Sinus tachycardia with PACs (Fig. 22-11)
- Sinus tachycardia with PVCs (Fig. 22-12)

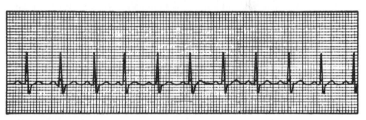

Figure 22–1 Rapid regular rhythms with sinus tachycardia. (From Marshall SA, Ruedy J: On Call: Principles and Protocols, 4th ed. Philadelphia, Elsevier, 2004, p 137.)

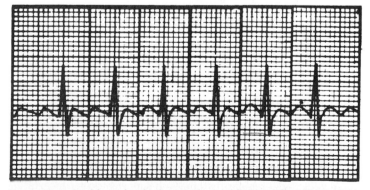

Figure 22–2 Rapid regular rhythms with atrial flutter. (From Marshall SA, Ruedy J: On Call: Principles and Protocols, 4th ed. Philadelphia, Elsevier, 2004, p 138.)

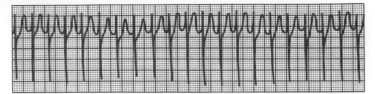

Figure 22–3 Rapid regular rhythms with supraventricular tachycardia and atrioventricular nodal reentry or Wolff-Parkinson-White tachycardia. (From Marshall SA, Ruedy J: On Call: Principles and Protocols, 4th ed. Philadelphia, Elsevier, 2004, p 138.)

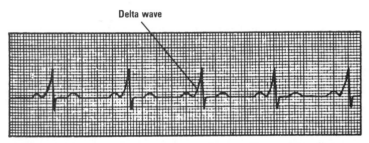

Figure 22–4 Wolff-Parkinson-White syndrome. This condition is characterized by a regular rhythm, a PR interval less than 0.12 second, a QRS complex longer than 0.11 second, and a delta wave (i.e., slurred beginning of the QRS). (From Marshall SA, Ruedy J: On Call: Principles and Protocols, 2nd ed. Philadelphia, WB Saunders Co, 1993, p 121.)

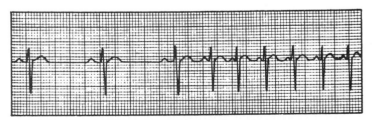

Figure 22–5 Rapid regular rhythms with supraventricular tachycardia (ectopic atrial tachycardia). (From Marshall SA, Ruedy J: On Call: Principles and Protocols, 4th ed. Philadelphia, Elsevier, 2004, p 138.)

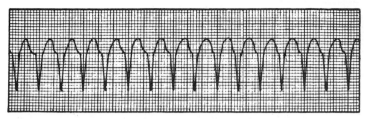

Figure 22–6 Rapid regular rhythms with ventricular tachycardia. (From Marshall SA, Ruedy J: On Call: Principles and Protocols, 4th ed. Philadelphia, Elsevier, 2004, p 135.)

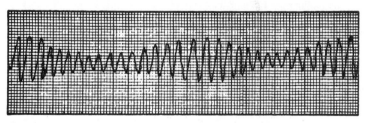

Figure 22–7 Torsades de pointes. (From Marshall SA, Ruedy J: On Call: Principles and Protocols, 4th ed. Philadelphia, Elsevier, 2004, p 149.)

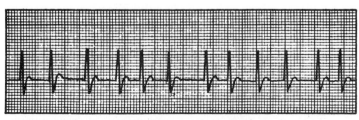

Figure 22–8 Rapid irregular rhythms with atrial fibrillation. (From Marshall SA, Ruedy J: On Call: Principles and Protocols, 4th ed. Philadelphia, Elsevier, 2004, p 136.)

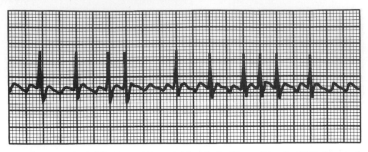

Figure 22–9 Atrial flutter with variable block. (From Marshall SA, Ruedy J: On Call: Principles and Protocols, 4th ed. Philadelphia, Elsevier, 2004, p 136.)

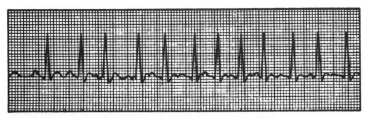

Figure 22–10 Rapid irregular rhythms with multifocal atrial tachycardia. (From Marshall SA, Ruedy J: On Call: Principles and Protocols, 4th ed. Philadelphia, Elsevier, 2004, p 137.)

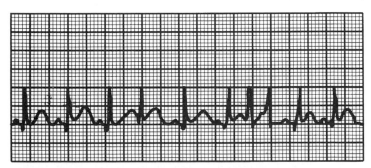

Figure 22–11 Rapid irregular rhythms with sinus tachycardia and premature atrial contractions. (From Marshall SA, Ruedy J: On Call: Principles and Protocols, 4th ed. Philadelphia, Elsevier, 2004, p 137.)

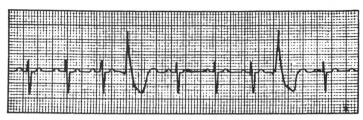

Figure 22–12 Rapid irregular rhythms with sinus tachycardia and premature ventricular contractions. (From Marshall SA, Ruedy J: On Call: Principles and Protocols, 4th ed. Philadelphia, Elsevier, 2004, p 137.)

Selective History and Chart Review

Look for causes of tachycardia. Fever causes sinus tachycardia, as do anemia, acute blood loss, pain, and sympathomimetic drugs (albuterol, pseudoephedrine, caffeine, and theophylline). Does the child have a history of heart disease and recent surgery or any history of syncope? These may indicate a cause or chronicity of disease.

Management I

Regardless of the cause of the tachycardia, ventricular filling must be improved by immediately increasing preload (with intravenous [IV] fluids, packed red blood cells, etc.). However, if the patient has significant cardiovascular compromise and atrial fibrillation with a rapid ventricular response, SVT, or VT, emergency direct-current electrocardioversion is indicated. Give the following instructions:

Page the senior resident and pediatric intensive care unit physician immediately, or call for the "code team."

Bring the cardiac arrest resuscitation cart to the patient's bedside and attach the ECG leads of the defibrillator to the child.

Make sure that the child is receiving oxygen by nasal cannula or mask and that airway management equipment is on hand.

Ensure that an adequate IV line is in place.

Select the appropriate energy (0.5 to 1.0 joule/kg) and *synchronize* to the patient's R wave (select the monitor lead with the most obvious R wave).

Clear everyone from contact with the patient and deliver the synchronized shock *while recording the ECG.*

If sinus rhythm is obtained, proceed with a fluid bolus and further stabilization.

Continue to follow the Pediatric Advanced Life Support (PALS) and/or Advanced Cardiac Life Support (ACLS) protocol for resuscitation.

Management of Hemodynamically Stable Reentrant Supraventricular Tachycardia

If the patient has no evidence of significant cardiovascular compromise, other methods may be used to convert the rhythm. For reentrant SVT, this may include vagal maneuvers such as applying ice to the face or eliciting a Valsalva maneuver. Alternatively, IV adenosine (0.1 mg/kg) given by *rapid push*, followed immediately by a large-volume flush, is effective in causing the same short-term AV nodal blockade achieved by vagal stimulation. If the initial dose is ineffective, the dose should be doubled, to a maximum of 12 mg. The most common reason for failure of adenosine is administration in an inadequate IV line or inadequate flush. The half-life of adenosine in the bloodstream is 6 to 10 seconds; therefore, an IV site above the diaphragm is preferable, with at least a 10-mL normal saline solution flush.

Refractory SVT can be treated with an esmolol infusion or with amiodarone. These drugs should not be started without cardiology or critical care input.

It is very important in infants and younger children that the calcium channel blocker verapamil be avoided for acute SVT because of its long duration and the possibility of persistent high-grade (life-threatening) AV block. Despite its utility in adults, verapamil has very limited indications in children.

Management of Atrial Fibrillation

Atrial fibrillation is a very rare rhythm in children with anatomically normal hearts. In children with congenital heart disease, atrial fibrillation can arise as a late complication of corrective surgery; it is also a complication of tricuspid regurgitation, pulmonary hypertension, and dilated cardiomyopathy. Atrial fibrillation becomes hemodynamically significant if the ventricular response rate is very high or when atrial systole is needed to augment filling of a noncompliant ventricle; both cases result in reduced ventricular filling. Because of variable ventricular response rates in children, atrial fibrillation is not usually tolerated as well as it can be in adults. Atrial fibrillation occasionally resolves spontaneously; more often, it requires direct-current cardioversion by the aforementioned technique.

Management of Hemodynamically Stable Ventricular Tachycardia

VT is a dangerous rhythm and must be treated immediately. IV amiodarone is an effective treatment of VT/ventricular fibrillation (VF); lidocaine is the alternative. Pediatric dosing of amiodarone is a rapid bolus of 5 mg/kg for pulseless VT/VF. For recurrent VT, 5 mg/kg intravenously infused over a period of 20 to 60 minutes (which may be repeated up to a maximum of 15 mg/kg/day) is recommended.

Synchronized cardioversion may also be used if medical therapy alone does not convert the patient to sinus rhythm.

Once the patient is converted to sinus rhythm, it is important to search for possible causes of the VT, such as myocardial injury or ischemia, hypoxia, electrolyte imbalance (hyperkalemia, hypokalemia, hypomagnesemia, hypocalcemia), cardiomyopathy (arrhythmogenic right ventricular dysplasia), and drugs, especially quinidine, procainamide, digoxin, disopyramide, tricyclic antidepressants, phenothiazines, sotalol, and amiodarone.

SLOW HEART RATES

PHONE CALL

Questions
1. How old is the patient?
2. Why is the patient in the hospital?
3. What is the heart rate?
4. What is the rhythm?
5. What is the blood pressure?
6. What medications is the child receiving?

Digoxin, β-blockers, and calcium channel blockers can prolong AV nodal conduction and result in bradycardia with a prolonged PR interval; they can also inhibit sinus node automaticity.

Orders
1. Call respiratory therapy immediately, administer 100% oxygen, and have a bag-valve-mask and intubation supplies at the bedside.
2. If the child is hypotensive, make sure that a secure IV line is in place and give 10 to 20 mL/kg of normal saline or lactated Ringer's solution by IV push. Place the patient in the Trendelenburg position (15 degrees head down) to achieve an "autotransfusion."
3. Bring the resuscitation "code" cart to the bedside and attach the patient to the defibrillator monitor.
4. Obtain an ECG rhythm strip immediately.
5. If the heart rate is less than 60 beats per minute (bpm) in an infant or 40 bpm in a child or adolescent, a dose of 0.1 mg/kg atropine should be prepared.

Inform RN

"Will arrive at the bedside in ... minutes." Bradycardia is an indication of imminent circulatory collapse and must be evaluated immediately.

ELEVATOR THOUGHTS (CAUSES OF SLOW HEART RATES)

Sinus bradycardia (Fig. 22-13)	**Drugs**
	Digoxin, β-blocker therapy, calcium channel blockers
	Cardiac
	Neurocardiogenic (vagal) bradycardia, sick sinus syndrome
	Other
	Hypothyroidism, increased intracranial pressure (ICP) (Cushing's triad), respiratory compromise (hypoxemia), anorexia nervosa
Second-degree AV block Mobitz type I (Wenckebach) (Fig. 22-14) Mobitz type II (Fig. 22-15)	**Drugs**
	Digoxin, β-blockers, calcium channel blockers
	Cardiac
	Sick sinus syndrome, acute myocardial infarction, blunt trauma
	Other
	Head trauma
Third-degree AV block (complete heart block) (Fig. 22-16)	**Drugs**
	Digoxin, β-blockers, calcium channel blockers
	Cardiac
	Sick sinus syndrome, acute myocardial infarction
Atrial fibrillation with slow ventricular response (Fig. 22-17)	**Drugs**
	Digoxin, β-blockers, calcium channel blockers
	Cardiac
	Sick sinus syndrome

Note: In the absence of respiratory compromise, bradycardia most often results from drugs or primary cardiac disease.

MAJOR THREAT TO LIFE

- Hypotension
- Asystole

Especially in infants, cardiac output is very dependent on heart rate; consequently, bradycardia significantly decreases cardiac output and thereby leads to end-organ dysfunction. Bradycardia secondary to myocardial infarction or contusion may deteriorate into a more ominous rhythm, such as VF or asystole.

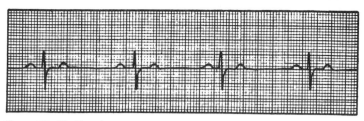

Figure 22–13 Slow heart rate with sinus bradycardia. (From Marshall SA, Ruedy J: On Call: Principles and Protocols, 4th ed. Philadelphia, Elsevier, 2004, p 150.)

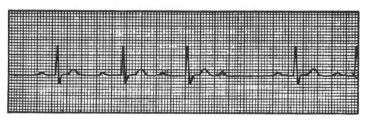

Figure 22–14 Slow heart rate with second-degree atrioventricular block (type I). (From Marshall SA, Ruedy J: On Call: Principles and Protocols, 4th ed. Philadelphia, Elsevier, 2004, p 151.)

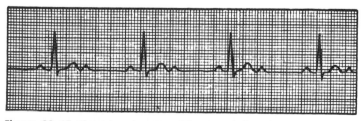

Figure 22–15 Slow heart rate with second-degree atrioventricular block (type II). (From Marshall SA, Ruedy J: On Call: Principles and Protocols, 4th ed. Philadelphia, Elsevier, 2004, p 151.)

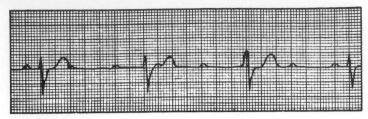

Figure 22–16 Slow heart rate with third-degree atrioventricular block. (From Marshall SA, Ruedy J: On Call: Principles and Protocols, 4th ed. Philadelphia, Elsevier, 2004, p 152.)

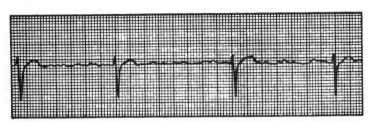

Figure 22–17 Atrial fibrillation with slow ventricular rate. (From Marshall SA, Ruedy J: On Call: Principles and Protocols, 4th ed. Philadelphia, Elsevier, 2004, p 152.)

BEDSIDE

Quick-Look Test

Does the patient appear well (comfortable), sick (uncomfortable or distressed), or critically ill (about to die)?

Unless the patient is very comfortable and has normal mental status, the "code" cart and other resuscitative measures should be close at hand. Make sure that the patient is attached to a monitor and that the sweep speed of the monitor is set at 25 mm/sec rather than 50 mm/sec, which falsely appears to be wide-complex bradycardia. Make sure that the monitor and the patient's pulse correlate with one another.

Airway and Vital Signs

First, be sure that the patient is ventilating adequately—address airway and breathing first of all.

What is the heart rate?

Analyze the rhythm strip and identify the rhythm. Profound bradycardia may require immediate intervention, including the administration of 0.1 mg/kg atropine via an IV or endotracheal tube if necessary.

What are the blood pressure and perfusion status?

Regardless of the rhythm, the lack of blood pressure means that cardiopulmonary resuscitation must be started, including chest compressions if necessary. *Remember:* Electromechanical dissociation gives a false sense of security because an electrical rhythm is seen despite inadequate contraction. Volume resuscitation is required and can be started by positioning the patient supine with the legs raised or by putting the head of the bed down 15 degrees.

Selective History and Chart Review

Look for a cause or for previous episodes of bradycardia. Remember that the most common causes of bradycardia are related to medications prescribed for the child, followed by medications prescribed for another family member.

Does the child have a past history of Kawasaki disease with coronary artery aneurysms? Has the child been in an area endemic for Lyme disease? Is there a family history of hyperlipidemia?

Was there associated syncope that might point to a vasovagal episode? Was the bradycardia associated with vagal maneuvers, such as straining, micturition, or Valsalva maneuvers?

Selective Physical Examination

Again, look for clues to the cause of the patient's bradycardia (if stable).

Vital signs	Bradypnea (hypothyroidism), hypothermia (hypothyroidism, exposure), hypertension (ominous in combination, indicating increased ICP, Cushing's triad)
HEENT	Coarse facial features, macroglossia; loss of the lateral third of the eyebrows (hypothyroidism); diabetic or hypertensive funduscopic changes, papilledema
Neck	Goiter, jugular venous distention
Cardiovascular	New S_3 or S_4, mitral regurgitation murmur (myocardial infarction with papillary muscle injury)
Abdomen	Hepatosplenomegaly
Extremities	Poor perfusion and/or peripheral pulses
Neurologic	Mental status changes, evidence of trauma, delayed return phase of deep tendon reflexes (hypothyroidism)

Management

Sinus Bradycardia

If the child is not hypotensive, no acute intervention is necessary. Search for a cause. If the child has been receiving digoxin, β-blockers, or calcium channel blockers, no further doses should be given until the heart rate normalizes.

Second-Degree Atrioventricular Block (Type I or Type II)

If the patient is hemodynamically stable, no acute intervention is required. Cardiotonic drugs should be withheld until the rhythm normalizes. Continuous monitoring is advisable. If the child is unstable, consider isoproterenol infusion.

Third-Degree Atrioventricular Block

If the child is hemodynamically stable, no acute intervention is required. If the child is unstable, begin resuscitative measures and consider using a transcutaneous pacemaker unit. This may sometimes be necessary in a newborn infant with congenital complete heart block secondary to maternal lupus erythematosus.

Atrial Fibrillation with Slow Ventricular Response

Again, intervention is indicated by symptoms, which are generally due to hypotension. Stop the administration of drugs such as digoxin, β-blockers, and calcium channel blockers. Be prepared to either externally pace the ventricle or insert a transvenous pacing wire (requires intensive care unit stay), if necessary.

REMEMBER

1. Discontinuation of digoxin, β-blockers, calcium channel blockers, or antiarrhythmic medications may allow the original rhythm disturbance or congestive heart failure to re-emerge.
2. Abrupt discontinuation of β-blockers may cause rebound hypertension, angina, or myocardial infarction. The drug should be reinstituted at a lower dose once the heart rate has normalized.
3. In the setting of acute digoxin ingestion with high blood levels, bradycardia, and second- or third-degree heart block, the digoxin-specific binding antibody Digibind must be given to reduce the toxic effects.

In order to identify a rhythm disturbance, you must be able to *perform* and *interpret* the ECG. You can't get the answer if you don't get the data!

Hematuria

Priya Pais, MD

Few patients have a complaint of "hematuria." Rather, patients with hematuria may describe "red urine," "brown urine," or "blood in my urine." Detection of blood in a child's urine usually alarms the patient, the parents, and the physician. The first step in evaluating these patients is determining whether the child really has hematuria. Frankly red or pink urine suggests macroscopic hematuria. Tea- or cola-colored urine may reflect hemoglobinuria, myoglobinuria, or excretion of organic dyes, such as those in beets and some confectionery dyes. An orange stain in a diaper is often mistaken for blood when it is more likely to be urate crystals.

Hematuria is a sign of injury to the lining of the lower genito-urinary tract, as in trauma or infection, or it may represent glomerular injury as a result of trauma, infection, or an autoimmune phenomenon.

PHONE CALL

Questions

1. How old is the patient?
2. Why is the patient in the hospital?
3. Is the child male or female? What is the child's age?
4. Are there any associated symptoms, such as frequency, urgency, fever, dysuria, oliguria, or polyuria?
5. If female, is the child menstruating?

Orders

Ask the nurse to obtain a sterile urine specimen for dipstick, microscopic analysis, culture, and Gram stain. In any child younger than 5 years, it should be a clean catheterized specimen only.

Repeat a full set of vital signs immediately.

Inform RN

"I will arrive at the bedside in … minutes." Hematuria requires evaluation but rarely is so urgent that other activities need to be abandoned at once. In the setting of a trauma patient, it deserves

prompt attention because significant traumatic kidney injury or
pelvic fracture can precipitate internal bleeding and shock.

ELEVATOR THOUGHTS

The differential diagnosis of hematuria (red blood cells in the urine)
includes the following:
    Infections
        Urinary tract infection
        Viral bladder infection
    Trauma
    Nephrolithiasis
    Glomerular
        Postinfectious glomerulonephritis
        Hemolytic-uremic syndrome
        Lupus
        IgA nephropathy
        Henoch-Schönlein purpura
    Anatomic
        Polycystic kidney disease
        Tumor
    Vascular
        Renal artery/vein thrombosis
        Miscellaneous
        Exercise induced
        Medications, e.g., cyclophosphamide
        Sickle cell trait
        Fictitious
        Menses

MAJOR THREAT TO LIFE

Blunt trauma to the flank, back, or abdomen of a child may result in
significant renal injury and not only hematuria but also intra-
abdominal or retroperitoneal bleeding leading to shock. The urine
of every trauma victim should be dip-tested for occult blood.
Hematuria in the setting of a known bleeding disorder should also
be considered a warning of potentially life-threatening coagulopathy.

BEDSIDE

Quick-Look Test

*Does the patient appear well (comfortable), sick (uncomfortable or
distressed), or critical (about to die)?*
    Pain may suggest trauma but, in the setting of dysuria, fever,
frequency, and pyuria, is more likely to indicate pyelonephritis.

Painless hematuria can be seen in patients with glomerulonephritis, as well as tumor.

Airway and Vital Signs

What are the temperature, heart rate, blood pressure, and respiratory signs?

Hypertension may suggest renal artery stenosis with high renin production or glomerulonephritis. Tachycardia may accompany pain. Respiratory distress can be seen with renal failure and fluid overload. Fever may indicate pyelonephritis.

Selective History and Chart Review

See Table 23-1.

Selective Physical Examination

HEENT	Carefully examine the fundi for signs associated with hypertension
Neck	Check for jugular venous distention and thyromegaly
Lungs	Rales and/or consolidation with hemoptysis suggests Goodpasture's syndrome or vasculitis
Cardiovascular	Tachycardia, hypertension, or an S_3 gallop rhythm can imply fluid overload
Abdomen	Flank pain, tenderness, fullness, masses, ascites
Genitourinary	Discharge, edema, erythema, trauma
Skin	Petechiae, purpura

TABLE 23–1 **History and Chart Review**

Question	Etiology (from History)
Dysuria/frequency/fever?	Urinary tract infection/urethritis
Abdominal or flank pain?	Stones/pyelonephritis/Henoch-Schönlein purpura
Trauma/exercise?	Direct trauma/exercise induced
Bleeding tendency?	Coagulopathy
Impetigo/streptococcal pharyngitis?	Postinfectious glomerulonephritis
Family history	
Kidney disease?	Alport's syndrome/polycystic kidneys
Deafness?	Alport's syndrome
Stones?	Nephrolithiasis
Other: medications/menses?	Medication induced/fictitious

Management I

In the short term, it is important to assess the patient's urine output and adjust fluid intake appropriately. Hematuria accompanied by oliguria requires fluid restriction to cover insensible losses only because of the possibility of renal failure with resultant electrolyte disturbances, hypertension, and fluid overload. Hypertension must be managed to avoid complications, and strict dietary protein and potassium restriction may be necessary (see Chapter 24, Hypertension). In severe cases, dialysis may be necessary because of uremia, fluid overload, or severe electrolyte disturbances.

Laboratory Data

It is important to determine what is causing coloration of the urine. The presence of red blood cells (hematuria), hemoglobin (hemoglobinuria), and myoglobin (myoglobinuria) colors the urine. Obviously, each has its own differential diagnosis and management strategy.

If the patient has true hematuria, a look at the rest of the elements of the urinalysis might provide some clues:

Finding	*Possible Diagnosis*
Proteinuria	Glomerular disease
White blood cells	Urinary tract infection
Crystals	Stones

At the same time that management initiatives are begun, diagnostic tests should be performed:

Lab Test	*Possible Diagnosis*
Creatinine/serum K$^+$	Kidney dysfunction
C3, C4 (low)	Postinfectious glomerulonephritis/lupus
Antistreptolysin-O, anti-DNAse B	Postinfectious glomerulonephritis
Urine calcium	Hypercalciuria
Urine culture	Urinary tract infection
Complete blood count	Hemolytic-uremic syndrome
IgA	IgA nephropathy
Antinuclear antibody	Lupus
Albumin/cholesterol	Nephrotic syndrome

Management II

The pediatric nephrologist should be called for several reasons:
- Red blood cell casts on microscopic examination (may need biopsy)
- Significant proteinuria (may need biopsy)
- Hypertension, edema
- Abnormal renal function
- Renal structural abnormality

SUMMARY

Hematuria, though rarely presenting a major threat to life, may occur in a variety of conditions associated with significant morbidity and, in some cases, death. As with many conditions, a diagnostic work-up should be performed simultaneously with empiric management.

Hypertension

Shenell Y. Miller, MD

Hypertension is a very common problem in adults, but in children it is relatively rare. The normal ranges for systolic and diastolic blood pressure differ at various ages, thus making the definition of "high blood pressure" variable. Nomograms have been developed by conducting blood pressure screening programs in very large populations of "normal" children. Persistent measurements above the 95th percentile have generally been used to define hypertension. It is important to remember that a single measurement recording a high blood pressure does not necessarily indicate hypertension.

Probably the most common "cause" of hypertension in children is the use of an inappropriate cuff size. If the cuff is too small, a spuriously high reading is obtained. The cuff width should be two thirds the length of the upper part of the arm and have a bladder that encircles the arm. Similarly, when obtaining a leg pressure, the cuff should cover two thirds the length of the thigh. A second common "cause" of high readings is agitation and movement during the blood pressure reading. Even in toddlers a blood pressure reading can usually be obtained without undue agitation if the child is approached slowly and patiently and reassured that the cuff will only squeeze his or her arm for a short time.

Approximately 80% to 90% of hypertension in children results from renal disease, but other treatable causes must also be considered in any evaluation for hypertension.

PHONE CALL

Questions

1. Why is the child hospitalized?
2. How high is the blood pressure and how was it obtained (manual cuff or Dynemap, arm or leg)?
3. Is this a new finding? What have previous blood pressure readings been?
4. Is the child having any other associated symptoms (chest pain, tachycardia, sweating, shortness of breath, nausea, vomiting, headache)?

5. **If the patient is female, could she be pregnant?**
6. **What medications has the child received?**

Orders

Ask the nurse to have a manual blood pressure cuff of the appropriate size at the patient's bedside.

If the child does not have an intravenous (IV) line, ask the nurse to have IV supplies ready at the bedside.

Inform RN

"Will arrive at the bedside in ... minutes." Situations requiring emergency evaluation include severely elevated blood pressure (in children, systolic pressure above 200 and/or diastolic pressure above 110 mm Hg), hypertension in a pregnant adolescent female, altered mental status, or pain of any kind.

ELEVATOR THOUGHTS

Major etiologic categories of hypertension include the following:
  Renal (glomerulonephritis, vasculitis, tumors, polycystic kidneys, renal scarring)
  Coarctation of the aorta (upper extremity pressure > lower extremity pressure)
  Increased intracranial pressure (ICP)
  Eclampsia
  Hyperthyroidism
  Drugs (sympathomimetic agents, corticosteroids, oral contraceptives)
  Hypercatechol states

Although rare, some life-threatening conditions in children may result in hypertension. Pre-eclampsia in a pregnant adolescent is accompanied by proteinuria and edema. Headache is frequently associated with the rise in blood pressure.

Catecholamine crisis may be precipitated by a number of conditions:
  Drug overdose
  Especially common with cocaine, phencyclidine (PCP), and amphetamines; overdose must be suspected regardless of age
  Drug interactions
  Monoamine oxidase (MAO) inhibitors and indirect-acting catechols (wine, cheese, ephedrine)
  Tricyclic antidepressants and direct-acting catechols (epinephrine, norepinephrine, pseudoephedrine)
  Pheochromocytoma
  Neoplasm overproducing catechols
  Burns

Transient hypertension develops in some patients with second- or third-degree burns because of high levels of circulating endogenous catecholamines, renin, and angiotensin II

Head trauma may result in increased ICP secondary to expanding subdural or epidural hematomas or cerebral edema. The need for the cerebral perfusion pressure to exceed ICP causes the release of endogenous catechols to preserve cerebral blood flow.

The consequences of hypertension include intraventricular hemorrhage in low-birth-weight premature infants. Cerebrovascular accidents are less common in full-term infants and older children but are still a possible complication of extreme hypertension. Hypertensive encephalopathy can include nausea, vomiting, headache, lethargy, confusion, visual disturbances, and seizures.

MAJOR THREAT TO LIFE

The major immediate threat to life is the rapid increase in blood pressure that can occur with eclampsia, drug ingestion, and head injuries, especially with extra-axial hemorrhage and hypertensive encephalopathy.

BEDSIDE

Quick-Look Test

Does the patient appear well (comfortable), sick (uncomfortable or distressed), or critical (about to die)?

A patient having seizures (eclampsia, drug ingestion, glomerulonephritis) or marked respiratory distress (critical coarctation of the aorta) requires immediate action to normalize the blood pressure. Patients with surprisingly high blood pressure can appear quite comfortable and in little or no distress.

Airway and Vital Signs

What is the blood pressure?

Check that the appropriate cuff size has been used and then proceed to take the blood pressure yourself from both arms and at least one leg. Coarctation of the aorta is a common source of upper extremity hypertension. The lower extremity blood pressure should always *equal or exceed* the upper extremity blood pressure. Comparison of upper and lower extremity blood pressure is the definitive diagnostic technique for coarctation of the aorta. It is important to remember that **coarctation of the aorta is the only cardiac cause of hypertension.**

What is the heart rate?

Bradycardia and hypertension in a patient not taking β-blockers may indicate increased ICP. When accompanied by irregular respirations, it is known as Cushing's triad. Tachycardia with hypertension is consistent with catecholamine-mediated changes and, if episodic, is suggestive of pheochromocytoma.

Is the patient in pain?
Pain is a very powerful stimulant for catecholamine release, regardless of the source. Patients hospitalized after trauma may have undiagnosed injuries, such as fractures or abdominal injuries, that can be overlooked, especially if the patient is unconscious on arrival and admission.

Selective History and Chart Review

What has the patient's blood pressure been up to this point?
Any previous recorded blood pressure readings are useful to put the patient's current pressure into perspective. Remember, however, that how and where the pressure was obtained are not usually recorded, thus making the previous results less reliable as a comparison. A normal leg pressure may be reassuring except in an infant or child with coarctation of the aorta, whose arm pressure may be significantly higher.

Is the child having any symptoms of complications because of the hypertension?
Chest pain
Respiratory distress (pulmonary edema, congestive heart failure [CHF])
Back pain (aortic dissection)
Headache, lethargy, mental status change (hypertensive encephalopathy)
Focal neurologic signs

Does the patient have a history of renal disease, especially reflux nephropathy, chronic or recurrent pyelonephritis, nephrotic syndrome, or any of the glomerulonephropathies?

Does the patient have a recent history of sore throat or upper respiratory symptoms?
Postinfectious glomerulonephritis is a common cause of sudden hypertension in children. Probably 80% to 90% of hypertension is a complication of infectious and/or inflammatory renal disease. Primary injury to the renal arteries can occur after umbilical artery cannulation in a newborn and results in altered renal perfusion and high renin production. Proximal tubular disease can result in poor sodium excretion and inappropriate loss of bicarbonate with poor urine acidification.

Selective Physical Examination

Does the patient have evidence of a hypertensive emergency?

HEENT   Assess the fundi for hypertensive changes (generalized or focal arteriolar narrowing, hemorrhages, exudates). Papilledema is

HEENT—Cont'd	an ominous and late finding and is the hallmark of malignant hypertension and hypertensive encephalopathy
Neck	Jugular venous distention may suggest heart failure; thyromegaly may indicate hyperthyroidism
Respiratory	Rales, pleural effusion (CHF)
Cardiovascular system	Increased precordial activity, loud S_2 (pulmonary hypertension), S_3 gallop (CHF), continuous murmur in the back (collaterals secondary to coarctation of the aorta), weak or absent femoral pulses, brachiofemoral delay, diffusely weak or absent pulses (Takayasu's arteritis)
Abdomen	Presence of bruits over the kidneys (renal artery stenosis), enlarged kidneys (ureteropelvic junction obstruction, renal vein thrombosis)
Neurologic	Confusion, lethargy, headache, vision disturbances, delirium, agitation, focal neurologic signs

Management

Remember, the object is to treat the patient, not a number. Hypertension must be viewed in the context of the entire patient. If the patient is asymptomatic, there is less urgency to normalize the blood pressure than if the child is encephalopathic. There is a very real risk of overshooting the mark during acute reduction of blood pressure in patients with long-standing hypertension and high levels of autoregulated cerebral blood flow. Do not treat a blood pressure reading! Treat the condition underlying it or associated with it.

True emergencies require special management. Such emergencies include eclampsia, intracranial hemorrhage, and hypertensive encephalopathy (Fig. 24-1).

It is important to involve your senior resident and an attending physician in such crisis situations and inform the pediatric intensive care unit (PICU) that your patient requires transfer to a higher level of care and monitoring. No matter how "comfortable" you may feel with managing hypertension, it is important to recognize the critical condition of these patients and the many complications inherent in their management.

Hypertensive Encephalopathy

Hypertensive encephalopathy is almost always accompanied by papilledema, retinal hemorrhages, and exudates. Focal neurologic signs, although unusual early on, suggest the presence of a stroke. It is important to remember that lowering the blood pressure precipitously can cause a stroke as well as syncope.

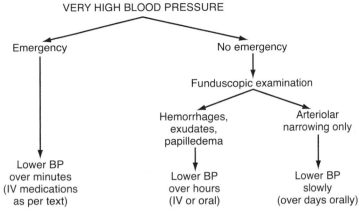

Figure 24–1 Approach to the management of very high blood pressure (BP).

1. Transfer the child to the PICU for electrocardiographic (ECG) and intra-arterial blood pressure monitoring.
2. While the transfer is being arranged, an initial dose of oral nifedipine can be administered and adequate IV access obtained.
3. If there is evidence of hypertensive encephalopathy, diazoxide (Hyperstat) is often used in adults. In children, however, IV nitroprusside is preferred because it can be titrated gradually. It is absolutely necessary to have intra-arterial monitoring to safely use such powerful afterload reduction. It is also necessary to administer IV fluid if the vasodilation that results overshoots the desired blood pressure.
4. Labetalol, a combination α- and β-blocking agent, may also be administered and can be particularly useful in a patient whose hypertension is mediated by overproduction of endogenous catecholamines or increased sympathetic tone. Bradycardia may result, and if the patient has a history of reactive airway disease, the respiratory findings must be monitored closely.
5. Once the blood pressure is under control by parenteral means, a suitable oral medication regimen must begin in order to discontinue the IV medications and allow the patient to leave the PICU.

Malignant Hypertension

Unless malignant hypertension is accompanied by other emergency conditions such as encephalopathy, control of blood pressure can be accomplished more gradually. Control of blood pressure must often be pursued while a search for the cause is ongoing. As you are gaining control of the blood pressure, begin to arrange the work-up to document renal perfusion and function (ultrasonography with Doppler flow study of the renal artery and vein, renal arteriography if necessary, dimercaptosuccinic acid [DMSA] renal scan with or without captopril challenge, blood urea nitrogen, creatinine, urinalysis, creatinine clearance, electrolytes, calcium, phosphate), serum and urine steroid metabolite levels, and serum renin and angiotensin II levels. Especially if renal disease is suspected, include streptococcal antibody (antistreptolysin-O [ASO], anti-DNAse B) and complement (C3 and C4) studies.

Pre-eclampsia and Eclampsia

A pregnant adolescent presents a variety of special problems and can be difficult to manage. Hypertension poses a risk to both the adolescent and her unborn fetus. If she is near term, the treatment of choice is magnesium sulfate ($MgSO_4$), a nonspecific smooth muscle relaxant, until delivery of the child can be arranged. Obviously, obstetric consultation is required and, frequently, transfer to a labor and delivery unit. $MgSO_4$ is administered intravenously as an infusion with an initial loading dose of 4 g intravenously over a 20-minute period (16 g of $MgSO_4$ in 1 L of 5% dextrose in water [D_5W]). The maintenance infusion is then 1 to 4 g/hr or more as required. Serum magnesium levels must be monitored every 4 hours, with target serum magnesium levels of 6 to 8 mmol/L.

Note that $MgSO_4$ does not lower blood pressure. Other medications, such as nitroprusside, labetalol, and hydralazine, are typically used to lower blood pressure. Diuretics are to be avoided because these patients are usually relatively volume depleted and have an activated renin-angiotensin system.

Intracranial Hemorrhage

Your index of suspicion should be high in the setting of a child with altered mental status, suspicion of child abuse, focal neurologic signs, or associated bradycardia. Subarachnoid bleeding and subdural or epidural hemorrhage can cause increased ICP and secondary hypertension. Intraparenchymal bleeding is a risk in children with known coagulopathies and requires close monitoring and a judicious approach.

Catecholamine Crisis

Pheochromocytoma presents the classic syndrome of pallor, palpitations, and diaphoresis associated with intermittent and alarmingly high blood pressure. Other circumstances that can mimic this syndrome include drug ingestion, especially cocaine and PCP. Food (cheese), drug (ephedrine), and drink (wine) interactions with MAO inhibitor antidepressant medications can result in similar findings, as can the interaction of tricyclic antidepressants with pseudoephedrine in over-the-counter cold preparations. MAO inhibitors are not widely used in children. Symptoms of catecholamine crisis should prompt immediate transfer to the PICU for close ECG and intra-arterial monitoring. Besides nitroprusside and labetalol, phentolamine mesylate, a powerful direct α-blocker, may be given to decrease systemic vascular resistance (afterload) and venous capacitance by directly relaxing smooth muscle. β-Blockade is especially important with cocaine and PCP ingestion because of the generalized increase in sympathetic nervous system activity that most children exhibit. When amphetamines have been taken, psychosis and hyperactivity may require the use of chlorpromazine (Thorazine) or haloperidol (Haldol) to control hallucinations and delirium.

SUMMARY

Hypertension is unusual in children and must be taken seriously. Be sure that the correct cuff size has been used and that the conditions for checking the blood pressure have been optimized. Take four-extremity blood pressure readings manually, and carefully record the results to rule out coarctation of the aorta. Acute hypertension implies an intracranial process, drug ingestion or interaction, or another source of catecholamine overproduction. Treat acute hypertension carefully and always in the context of the entire patient. Rapid normalization of blood pressure can itself precipitate problems.

Hypotension and Shock

Tannaz G. Hild, MD

Hypotension frequently prompts a call in the middle of the night. A variety of disease processes in pediatric patients follow a common pathway of hypotension, decreased tissue perfusion, acidosis, and shock. The house officer's task is to quickly assess the magnitude of the problem, intervene to prevent progression of shock, and discover the underlying problem that resulted in hemodynamic deterioration. This seems like a tall order, but remember that fundamentally the blood pressure must be adequate to perfuse the brain, the heart, and the kidneys. Accordingly, assessment of the child's mental status, pulses and perfusion, and urine output gives all the data necessary. Remember too that blood pressure is preserved by a variety of mechanisms and falls only as a late consequence; therefore, early recognition and intervention are essential.

PHONE CALL

Questions

1. How old is the patient?
2. Why is the patient in the hospital?
3. What is the blood pressure? What method of measurement was used and from what site on the body was the blood pressure taken?
4. What are the heart rate, temperature, and respiratory rate?
5. What is the child's mental status (agitated, somnolent, unresponsive)?

Orders

1. If the child does not have an intravenous (IV) line, the largest possible IV line should be started immediately. Normal saline or lactated Ringer's solution, 10 to 20 mL/kg, should be administered over a period of 5 to 10 minutes by IV push if necessary.
2. Oxygen should be administered.

3. If the child is not on a cardiorespiratory monitor, one should be obtained immediately. Request frequent repeat measurements of blood pressure (every 5 minutes).

4. If the child is febrile, acetaminophen or ibuprofen should be given if the patient is alert enough to take medication by mouth.

Inform RN

"Will arrive at the bedside immediately." There should be no delay in seeing a child with impending shock.

ELEVATOR THOUGHTS

Shock is caused by the following conditions:
Sepsis
Hypovolemia
Cardiogenic causes
Anaphylaxis
Adrenal insufficiency
Trauma
Toxins
Two formulas are useful when considering the cause of hypotension:

$$\text{Blood pressure (BP)} =$$
$$\text{Cardiac output (CO)} \times \text{Total systemic vascular resistance (SVR)}$$

$$\text{Cardiac output (CO)} = \text{Heart rate (HR)} \times \text{Stroke volume (SV)}$$

With these formulas in mind, one can see that hypotension results from a decrease in either cardiac output or SVR. Sepsis and anaphylaxis cause hypotension as a result of systemic vasodilatation (decreased SVR) and relative hypovolemia (because of capillary leak), both of which decrease cardiac output. Hypovolemia decreases cardiac filling and lowers stroke volume, thereby leading to tachycardia and ultimately resulting in decreased cardiac output and hypotension. Cardiogenic causes include decreased stroke volume because of decreased ejection fraction, as in dilated cardiomyopathies, dysrhythmias, and cardiac ischemia; decreased heart rate, as in heart block; restriction of cardiac filling (and therefore stroke volume), as in hypertrophic states, mitral stenosis, restrictive cardiomyopathy, and pericardial tamponade; and loss of systemic output via left-to-right shunts when pulmonary vascular resistance is less than SVR.

The most common cause of decreased cardiac output is lack of intravascular volume. This can be caused by external losses, as seen with vomiting and diarrhea, or by internal losses from third spacing, as seen with intestinal obstruction or after major abdominal surgery.

MAJOR THREAT TO LIFE

Shock is the major threat to life. Hypotension becomes life threatening when there is evidence of inadequate end-organ perfusion. Making the diagnosis of shock or impending circulatory collapse is not usually difficult, but treating shock and its underlying cause can be a challenge. The duty of the house officer is to prevent end-organ damage and to find and correct the cause of hemodynamic compromise.

BEDSIDE

Quick-Look Test

Does the patient look well (comfortable), sick (uncomfortable or distressed), or critical (about to die)?

A child who is hypotensive but not in shock appears quite well. However, as soon as perfusion of vital organs is compromised, the patient appears quite ill. The blood pressure may be normal in a child in shock, so attention to end-organ function is of utmost importance.

Airway and Vital Signs

Is the airway clear?

If the child's mental status is compromised, the ability to protect the airway may be impaired. Airway support should be readily at hand for any patient in shock.

Is the child ventilating adequately?

Children in shock are often tachypneic (to blow off accumulated CO_2), grunting (to provide positive end-expiratory pressure and prevent atelectasis), and retracting (to maximize tidal volume). Assess the respiratory rate, aeration, breath sounds, and chest movement. If the work of breathing is excessive, intubation and ventilatory support are indicated.

Assess the Circulation

1. Mild hypotension may be manifested as postural dizziness. Assess for postural hypotension by checking the pulse and blood pressure in the supine position and again after standing for 3 minutes. A postural rise in heart rate of more than 15 beats per minute, a fall in systolic blood pressure of more than 15 mm Hg, or any decrease in diastolic blood pressure indicates hypovolemia.
2. What is the heart rate? Sinus tachycardia is the first response to stress, hypovolemia, sepsis, and decreased myocardial function in infants and children. Nonsinus tachydysrhythmias can

lead to circulatory collapse and shock, and therefore at least an electrocardiographic rhythm strip should be checked to rule out a supraventricular tachydysrhythmia (see Chapter 22, Heart Rate and Rhythm Abnormalities). Bradycardia in the setting of shock is an ominous, life-threatening sign of circulatory collapse. If bradycardia is present, make sure that the patient is not in heart block and therefore unable to respond to his or her own catecholamine signals (Fig. 25-1). Vagal stimuli can produce profound bradycardia and even asystole in young patients. Episodes are usually short lived and respond promptly to laying the patient supine with the legs elevated or even in the Trendelenburg position. Prolonged bradycardia should respond to IV atropine (0.02 mg/kg).

Children who are receiving β-blockers or calcium channel blockers or who have ingested such medications accidentally are not able to respond normally to their intrinsic catecholamine signals. Likewise, children with sick sinus syndrome may not respond to β_1-chronotropic stimulation and do not compensate with tachycardia in response to stress.

3. Is the child in shock? This should take less than 30 seconds to determine, and shock, if present, requires immediate action regardless of the underlying cause.

Vital signs	Repeat immediately (include urine output)
Cardiovascular	Heart rate, blood pressure, pulse pressure, pulse quality, capillary refill (normal, <2 seconds)
Neurologic	Mental status

Shock is a clinical diagnosis. No single sign or test establishes the diagnosis. The constellation of low systolic blood pressure for age, cool clammy extremities, poor capillary refill, acrocyanosis, altered mental status (confusion, delirium, lethargy, coma), and decreased urine output (number of wet diapers in infants) indicates progressive circulatory compromise.

4. Is the child febrile? Obviously, fever frequently means sepsis, and prompt administration of antibiotics may be indicated. Fever also results in peripheral vasodilatation, which decreases SVR and causes decreased cardiac output. A neonate may not have significant fever and may indeed be hypothermic. Sepsis is always in the differential diagnosis of shock in children.

Selective Physical Examination

Determine the severity of the hypotension by assessing volume status and end-organ function. Cardiogenic shock may be manifested as volume overload, but in general, most shock states have evidence of hypovolemia.

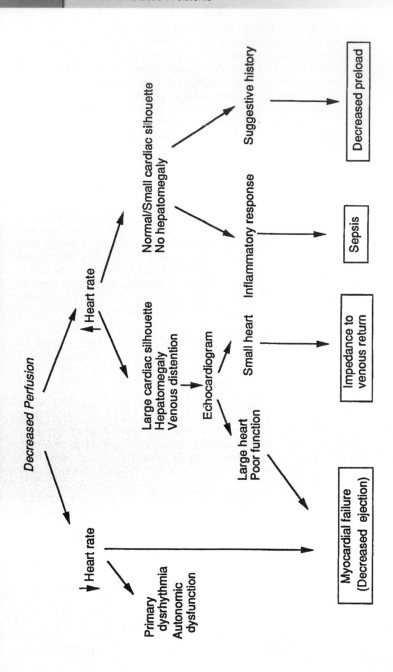

Vital signs	Repeat and document regularly
HEENT	Pupils (narcosis), mucous membranes, tears, fontanelle, periorbital edema, lip edema
Neck	Jugular venous distention (congestive heart failure [CHF], tamponade), deviation of the trachea (tension pneumothorax)
Respiratory	Grunting, retracting, stridor, or wheezing (anaphylaxis); rales (CHF)
Cardiovascular	Displaced point of maximal impulse (dilated cardiomyopathy), distant heart sounds (pericardial effusion, myocarditis), gallop rhythm, holosystolic regurgitant murmurs (ventricular septal defect, mitral or tricuspid regurgitation), loud S_2 (pulmonary hypertension), weak femoral pulses and/or brachiofemoral delay (coarctation of the aorta). Also assess perfusion, skin temperature, and color
Abdomen	Hepatosplenomegaly, ascites, distention and/or tenderness (ischemia or perforation)
Extremities	Presacral and/or ankle edema (CHF); cold, clammy hands and feet; poor capillary refill
Neurologic	Mental status
Skin	Urticaria (anaphylaxis), skin turgor, burns or wounds, anasarca (capillary leak secondary to sepsis), petechiae or purpura (sepsis and disseminated intravascular coagulopathy)

Figure 25–1 Algorithm for discerning the cause of decreased perfusion. Although the heart rate is usually increased in response to poor systemic perfusion, the presence of bradycardia should provoke a search for a primary dysrhythmia (e.g., heart block) or autonomic dysfunction (e.g., spinal cord trauma) or raise concern that there is severe myocardial failure. Alternatively, when the heart rate is increased, one should attempt to determine whether signs of systemic venous engorgement are present. When the heart silhouette is enlarged and there is venous distention, it is important to distinguish whether the heart is well filled and suffering from poor inotropic function or there is impedance to venous return (e.g., cardiac tamponade or tension pneumothorax). In these circumstances, an echocardiogram is an invaluable tool. When there is tachycardia with no sign of venous distention, inadequate perfusion can be caused by decreased preload and insufficient cardiac filling (e.g., hemorrhage or dehydration) or by diminished effective circulation, as in sepsis (with diffuse inflammation, venodilatation, and maldistribution of blood flow). It is also important to recognize that many of the problems that cause decreased perfusion can do so by more than one mechanism. Sepsis is a good example of a process that can diminish preload and produce myocardial failure simultaneously. (From Behrman RE: Nelson Textbook of Pediatrics, 15th ed. Philadelphia, WB Saunders, 1995, p 248.)

Selective History and Chart Review

Anaphylaxis has a preceding, inciting event, such as food, drug, or radiologic dye exposure, with an abrupt onset and rapidly progressive course. Angioedema and urticaria are present, as well as wheezing with or without stridor. A neonate with sepsis may have been exposed to an older child with a specific infectious illness. Children with known immunologic compromise, such as human immunodeficiency virus (HIV) infection, sickle cell disease, asplenia, or neoplasms, may be more susceptible to septic shock. In addition to sepsis or distributive shock, cardiogenic shock may develop in children with known cardiac disorders. A history of significant steroid therapy for autoimmune illnesses or cystic fibrosis increases susceptibility to infection. Rapid withdrawal of steroids may precipitate adrenal crisis and subsequent shock. Recent surgery can result in hemorrhage and hypovolemia. Spinal trauma may lead to neurogenic shock (disturbance in vasomotor tone). Children with dehydration secondary to diarrhea need to be assessed carefully. Just because the patient was admitted does not mean that the diarrhea is gone. Children in diapers need to be carefully assessed for intake and output. Watery diarrhea can be confused with urine output because modern diapers absorb extremely well. Make sure that the documented urine output is really urine and not watery stool.

Management

What immediate measures need to be taken to restore circulatory function and prevent progression of shock and end-organ hypoperfusion?

Normalize intravascular volume. The heart needs preload to function high on the Frank-Starling curve and maximize ejection fraction and therefore stroke volume. Even in some forms of cardiogenic shock, volume expansion is indicated initially. (Children with dilated or hypertrophic cardiomyopathy require high filling volume and pressure to compensate for low ejection fraction and high end-diastolic volume or for poor diastolic compliance with high end-diastolic pressure.)

Volume expansion should start by positioning the patient supine with the legs raised 15 degrees or in the 15-degree head-down Trendelenburg position. In infants, volume replacement should be in the form of 5% albumin if possible; 10 to 20 mL/kg should be administered over a 5- to 10-minute period by IV push if necessary. Reassess volume status and end-organ function (mental status, heart rate, urine output, perfusion) after each intervention.

Anaphylactic Shock

If the patient is in anaphylactic shock, treat rapidly as follows:
1. A 10- to 20-mL/kg fluid bolus
2. Epinephrine, 0.01 mg/kg as a 1:1000 solution intravenously immediately (subcutaneously only if necessary)

3. Diphenhydramine, 1 mg/kg intravenously
4. Methylprednisolone sodium succinate, 1 to 2 mg/kg intravenously now and every 6 hours

Treat signs of hypovolemia and simultaneously assess the magnitude of end-organ damage by obtaining an arterial blood gas reading.

Cardiogenic Shock

Although much less common in pediatric patients, cardiogenic shock can occur because of intrinsic cardiac disease (including structural lesions and dysrhythmias), injury to cardiac muscle (myocardial infarction, trauma, myocarditis), and extrinsic processes such as sepsis. Promptly obtaining a 12-lead electrocardiogram and chest radiograph greatly assists the house officer in assessing the cause and gravity of cardiac failure. It is critical that the house staff determine whether the child is preload dependent to maximize cardiac output, as mentioned earlier. Other clues should exist to suggest CHF, including jugular venous distention, hepatosplenomegaly, a history of congenital heart disease, and differential pulses. Other conditions, however, can be manifested similarly and result in hypotension and shock.

Acute Pericardial Tamponade

Tamponade physiology results in poor cardiac filling, which compromises stroke volume, elevates right-sided pressure, and causes jugular venous distention and tachycardia (Beck's triad: arterial hypotension, jugular venous distention, and soft or distant heart sounds). Tamponade can be seen in postoperative cardiac patients, children with viral pericarditis, and patients with blunt chest trauma; after cardiac catheterization; and with inflammatory conditions such as systemic juvenile rheumatoid arthritis and systemic lupus erythematosus. Suspect tamponade in patients who appear well hydrated, nonvasodilated, and poorly perfused. They may have a narrow pulse pressure and a pulsus paradoxus of greater than 10 mm Hg during relaxed respirations (Fig. 25-2).

Tension Pneumothorax

A rather rare entity, tension pneumothorax precipitates circulatory collapse by inhibiting cardiac filling and therefore stroke volume because of high intrathoracic pressure, which decreases venous return to the heart. The result is jugular venous distention, severe dyspnea, unilateral hyperresonance, tracheal deviation *away from* the affected side, and unequal breath sounds. Trauma is the most common cause, but spontaneous pneumothorax can progress to tension pneumothorax as well. Tension pneumothorax is a life-threatening emergency, and there may not be time to wait for a radiograph. Call the senior resident immediately, administer oxygen, and prepare an 18- to 20-gauge needle on a three-way stopcock with a 20-mL syringe. Scrub the second intercostal space of the affected side with

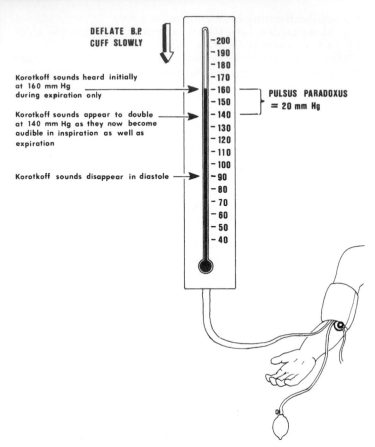

Figure 25–2 Determination of pulsus paradoxus. B.P., blood pressure. (From Marshall SA, Ruedy J: On Call: Principles and Protocols, 4th ed. Philadelphia, Elsevier, 2004, p 266.)

povidone-iodine (Betadine) quickly, and insert the needle at the midclavicular line in a slightly lateral direction, aspirating as you go. When air is aspirated, fill the syringe and flush it out with the stopcock, and repeat until air is no longer freely aspirated. This should rapidly improve the patient's clinical condition. **Tension pneumothorax is a true medical emergency and requires prompt, definitive action**.

Pulmonary Embolism

Though rather unusual, pulmonary embolization can occur in children, especially in adolescents, and is a cause of sudden, severe hypotension and circulatory collapse. Because of the acute obstruction to pulmonary blood flow, left atrial filling decreases, which causes compromise in left ventricular filling, decreased stroke volume, acute tachycardia, tachypnea, and chest pain. Cardiac output can rapidly decrease and lead to shock. Preexisting coagulopathy, immobility secondary to trauma or burns, birth control pills, and indwelling central venous catheters may predispose young patients to pulmonary embolization. Fat emboli are a well-known serious consequence of long bone fractures, especially of the femur. Embolization and subsequent infarction may also result in the acute chest syndrome of hemoglobin SS disease.

The pathophysiologic consequences of these diverse processes are essentially the same: ventilation-perfusion mismatch, hypoxemia with or without hypercapnia, increased pulmonary vascular resistance, decreased left heart filling, and decreased cardiac output. Secondary decreased perfusion and tissue hypoxemia result in acidemia, which worsens the ventilation-perfusion mismatch (intrapulmonary shunt), and an elevation in pulmonary vascular resistance.

Acute therapy for pulmonary embolism is largely supportive and includes oxygen with positive pressure ventilation if necessary, volume and inotropic support as needed, and close monitoring of arterial blood gases for gas exchange and acid-base status. The diagnosis may be suggested by the history and chest radiograph. Definitive diagnosis requires chest computed tomography, pulmonary perfusion scanning, ventilation scintiphotographic studies, and/or pulmonary angiography. Anticoagulant therapy (maintaining the activated partial thromboplastin time at 1.5 to 2 times control) and/or thrombolytic therapy requires monitoring in the intensive care unit. Patients with sickle cell disease require at least partial exchange transfusion to lower their percentage of hemoglobin SS.

Hypovolemia

In infants and children, fluid losses from diarrhea, vomiting, excessive sweating, acute blood loss, chronic gastrointestinal bleeding, polyuria, and third-space losses (capillary leak syndromes, including sepsis and systemic inflammatory response syndrome [SIRS]) all can result in hypovolemia and shock. A number of medications can lead to relative or actual hypovolemia, including diuretics, β-blockers, calcium channel blockers, acetylcholinesterase inhibitors, and other antihypertensive medications. Normal compensatory mechanisms for hypovolemia include increased sympathetic tone with resultant tachycardia, increased myocardial contractility, and peripheral vasoconstriction. Increased myocardial work and oxygen consumption are the price paid for this compensation. Therefore, the first goal of therapy is to reduce myocardial work by fluid resuscitation.

Practicality, availability, and the type of fluid losses that the child has suffered should guide the choice of fluid for resuscitation. Normal saline and lactated Ringer's solution are readily available

TABLE 25–1 **Intravenous Fluids Available for Pediatric Volume Resuscitation**

Crystalloids	Colloids
0.9% sodium chloride Lactated Ringer's solution Hypertonic saline (3%)	5% human serum albumin in 0.9% sodium chloride 25% human serum albumin in 0.9% sodium chloride 6% hydroxyethyl starch in 0.9% sodium chloride 10% dextran 40 in 5% dextrose in water Fresh frozen plasma Whole blood

From Behrman RE, Kliegman R: Nelson Essentials of Pediatrics, 2nd ed. Philadelphia, WB Saunders, 1994, p 118.

and economical; however, crystalloid solutions have a greater propensity for leaking the tissues, and thus colloid solutions are sometimes indicated, as in infants and patients with obvious capillary leak syndromes (Table 25-1). Likewise, a multiple trauma patient may require whole blood during resuscitation, frequently without the luxury of cross-matching. Children in severe hypovolemic shock may require a fluid bolus of 60 to 80 mL/kg within the first 1 to 2 hours. However, the risk of fluid overload must be continually reassessed.

Volume expansion may not be enough to sustain cardiac output and perfusion. In this case inotropic and/or vasodilator support is indicated. Table 25-2 lists the inotropic agents used. Dopamine is generally given first.

The use of inotropic and vasodilator therapy generally requires transfer to an intensive care unit for appropriate, usually invasive monitoring. It is important to remember that **inotropic support is not a replacement for volume resuscitation**.

TABLE 25–2 **Catecholamines Used for Cardiopulmonary Resuscitation**

	Direct Pressor	Positive Inotrope	Positive Chronotrope	Indirect Pressor	Vasodilator
Dopamine	++	+	+/–	++	++*
Dobutamine	++	+/–	–	–	+
Epinephrine	+++	+++	+++	–	–
Isoproterenol	+++	+++	–	–	+++
Norepinephrine	+++	+++	+++	–	–

*Primarily splanchnic and renal in low doses (3 to 5 μg/kg/min).
From Behrman RE, Kliegman R: Nelson Essentials of Pediatrics, 2nd ed. Philadelphia, WB Saunders, 1994, p 119.

Sepsis

Any kind of infection can result in circulatory collapse and shock. Again, the use of inotropic support should not precede volume resuscitation. Obtaining at least a sample of blood for culture immediately before administration of broad-spectrum antibiotics may be crucial in determining the length of administration and the dose of antibiotics. Sepsis is often accompanied by a SIRS-like capillary leak that allows proteinaceous fluid to leach into tissues, including the lungs, with the subsequent development of adult respiratory distress syndrome.

Adrenal Crisis

Adrenal insufficiency is characterized by hyponatremia, hyperkalemia, acidosis, hypoglycemia, and hypotension or shock. It may occur in combination with other causes of shock (e.g., meningococcemia and secondary adrenal infarction, sepsis in a steroid-dependent patient). In addition to fluid resuscitation, if adrenal crisis is suspected, prompt treatment with IV hydrocortisone, 1 to 2 mg/kg, can result in dramatic improvement. Continuation of IV hydrocortisone, 25 to 250 mg/day divided two or three times daily, is usually necessary. Hydrocortisone is preferred to other IV steroid preparations because of its mineralocorticoid effect.

REMEMBER

1. Shock is a clinical diagnosis characterized by inadequate end-organ perfusion and subsequent dysfunction. One must assess its severity by noting the child's mental status (brain), pertusion, heart rate and blood pressure (heart), and urine output (kidney). Blood pressure may be normal and the child may still be in shock. Compensatory mechanisms (tachycardia, vasoconstriction) will maintain blood pressure, but end-organ perfusion will be inadequate.
2. Although the skin is not generally considered a "vital" organ, it can provide valuable information regarding volume status and tissue perfusion. Do not be misled or falsely reassured by a well-perfused patient who has other manifestations of shock. So-called warm shock is no less threatening and frequently precedes circulatory collapse. (Be alert for a patient with tachycardia, wide pulse pressure, and warm extremities.)
3. Hypovolemia is the most common cause of shock in infants and children, with sepsis following close behind.
4. Accurate assessment and prompt intervention are required in the diagnosis and treatment of hypotension and shock in children.

Lines, Tubes, and Drains

Richard W. Hendershot, MD

Nearly every child admitted to the hospital requires an intravenous (IV) line, a catheter, a tube, or a drain of some sort. These devices are necessary but may also be a source of problems. Not only is their placement sometimes difficult, but also, once in place, a line or a tube may clog, leak, or stop functioning.

This chapter discusses the placement of a few of these devices, as well as the approach to some of the problems that may arise while you are on call. IV and intraosseous line placement, as well as femoral and arterial line placement, is discussed in Appendix A. Chest tube placement is discussed in Chapter 10, Chest Pain. Techniques of central line placement (subclavian and internal jugular lines) are beyond the scope of this book and are not discussed. This chapter is divided into the following sections:

Nasogastric (NG) and enteral feeding tubes
    Placement
    Blocked NG tube and enteral feeding tube
    Dislodged NG tube and enteral feeding tube
Urethral catheters
    Placement
    Blocked urethral catheter
    Gross hematuria
Umbilical catheters
    Placement
    Blocked umbilical arterial or venous catheter
Central lines
    Bleeding at the entry site
    Blocked central line
Chest tubes
    Persistent bubbling in the drainage container
    Bleeding at the entry site
    Drainage of blood
    Loss of fluctuation of the underwater seal
Dyspnea
Subcutaneous emphysema

NASOGASTRIC AND ENTERAL FEEDING TUBES

Placement of a Nasogastric Tube

NG tubes may be necessary for a number of reasons. A vomiting child may require drainage of gastric contents, gastric lavage may be necessary after an acute toxic ingestion, or a tube may be needed for enteral feeding. Placement of an NG tube is a relatively simple procedure, but as with other procedures in children, it may often be challenging. Small tubes (5 to 10 French [Fr]) may be used in neonates. Larger tubes (12 to 16 Fr) are necessary in older children. Generally, larger tubes are required if the goal is to empty gastric contents than if the tube is being placed for enteral feeding.

1. Make sure that you have help to restrain an uncooperative child. Sedation should not ordinarily be necessary unless the child is especially combative or insufficient help is available to provide restraint.
2. Measure the approximate length of tube required by holding the tube against the child's head and looping it back along the side of the ear and then down along the neck and the thorax until you have extended the tubing inferiorly past the lower ribs. Mark the location where the tube is adjacent to the child's nares so that you know how far to insert it.
3. Lubricate the end of the tube and the child's external nares with petroleum jelly.
4. Asking an older child to drink a cup of water or juice while the tube is inserted often makes the process easier. Drinking also closes the epiglottis, thus ensuring that the tube does not pass into the trachea.
5. Quickly and smoothly insert the end of the tube into the nares and direct it toward the child's occiput. Remember that the passage through the nasal turbinates is nearly perpendicular to the esophagus; therefore, the tube should not be angled too far superiorly or inferiorly.
6. The tube should be advanced in a smooth, continuous motion. Once it is through the nasal passages, resistance should be minimal and the tube should advance easily down the posterior of the pharynx, into the esophagus, and then into the stomach. Tilting the head forward slightly opens the esophagus wider, thus making it less likely for the tube to pass into the trachea. If excessive coughing or choking occurs, do not attempt to pass the tube farther; instead, withdraw it and start over.
7. When the tube is advanced to the point where your marking reaches the external nares, stop advancing and secure the tube in place with tape.

8. The location of the tube within the stomach can be checked by pushing air through the tube with a 20-mL syringe and listening over the stomach with a stethoscope for the sound of air escaping from the distal end of the tube. Alternatively, aspirating the tube with the same syringe may bring up gastric fluid, thereby confirming proper positioning. If there is any doubt regarding location, a radiograph can be obtained to confirm the position.

Blocked Nasogastric Tube or Enteral Feeding Tube

PHONE CALL

Questions

1. How long has the tube been blocked?
2. What type of tube is it?
3. Is the tube dislodged?
4. What are the vital signs and status of the patient?

Orders

Ask the nurse to place several 20- and 50-mL syringes, normal saline solution, and an emesis basin at the bedside.

Inform RN

"Will arrive at the bedside in … minutes." A blocked feeding tube is not an immediate concern but should be evaluated as soon as possible in an infant and within several hours in an older child. A blocked drainage tube is a greater problem and requires prompt evaluation to avoid complications from the accumulation of gastric fluid or gas.

ELEVATOR THOUGHTS

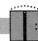

What causes blocked NG or enteral feeding tubes?
1. Debris within the lumen of the tube
2. Blood within the tube
3. Failure to irrigate the tube

MAJOR THREAT TO LIFE

- Aspiration: If the NG tube is blocked and does not empty the stomach, gastric contents may rise around the tube and can then be aspirated into the lungs and lead to pneumonia.

BEDSIDE

Quick-Look Test

Does the patient look well (comfortable), sick (uncomfortable or distressed), or critical (about to die)?
If aspiration has occurred, the patient may look quite ill.

Airway and Vital Signs

What is the respiratory rate? The airway and vital signs should not be affected by a blocked tube unless aspiration has occurred or the blocked tube has led to nausea and vomiting.

Management

1. Irrigate the tube with 5 to 10 mL of normal saline solution for an infant, 20 mL for an older child, and 25 to 50 mL for an adolescent. As you irrigate, listen with a stethoscope over the stomach to ensure proper placement of the tube.
2. If irrigation is unsuccessful, remove the tube and replace it.

Dislodged Nasogastric Tube and Enteral Feeding Tube

PHONE CALL

Questions

1. How long has the tube been dislodged?
2. What type of tube is it?
3. What are the vital signs and the status of the patient?

Orders

You should make sure that the nurse knows to give nothing further (feeding, medication) through the tube until you have a chance to evaluate the patient.

Inform RN

"Will arrive at the bedside in ... minutes." As with blocked tubes, infants with dislodged tubes should be evaluated as soon as possible.

ELEVATOR THOUGHTS

What causes an NG or feeding tube to become dislodged?
1. Failure to secure the tube
2. Uncooperative child (normal for infants and young children)

MAJOR THREAT TO LIFE

- Aspiration: If the tube is dislodged and gastric contents are not being drained, these contents may be aspirated. Alternatively, if the tube is being used for feeding, the feeding formula may be instilled into the lungs rather than the gastrointestinal tract.

BEDSIDE

Quick-Look Test

Does the patient look well (comfortable), sick (uncomfortable or distressed), or critical (about to die)?
    Aspiration may cause the patient to appear ill.

Airway and Vital Signs

If the airway or vital signs are compromised, you should suspect that aspiration has occurred.

Management

1. Inspect the tube. The markings may allow you to estimate the positioning of the tube.
2. Aspirate the tube to determine whether you can obtain gastric fluid. Alternatively, instill a small amount (10 to 20 mL) of air into the tube and listen with a stethoscope over the stomach for the rush of air to confirm positioning.
3. If the tube is an enteral feeding tube (e.g., a jejunal tube), it needs to be removed and replaced. It should not be pushed farther down if it has become dislodged.

URETHRAL CATHETERS

Placement

Urethral catheters are used to obtain sterile urine specimens and are also placed to allow more accurate determination of urine output in those who are critically ill. In infants, feeding tubes are often used for this purpose, whereas in older children, standard Foley catheters may be used. Sterile technique should be ensured when placing a urethral catheter. As with other procedures in pediatric patients, having an experienced "holder" to distract and gently restrain the child during the procedure can be a tremendous help.

1. Position the child supine. Cleanse the urethral opening thoroughly with a povidone-iodine (Betadine) solution.
2. Lubricate the end of the catheter with petroleum jelly and insert it into the urethral opening; advance the tube with gentle, steady pressure.

3. Once urine flow is visualized in the tube, stop advancing the catheter if this is a one-time catheterization to obtain a sterile urine specimen. If the catheter is to remain in place, advance the catheter a little farther to ensure that the end is within the bladder.

4. If a Foley catheter is being used, inflate the balloon on the end of the catheter and exert gentle traction to make sure that the balloon is against the bladder trigone.

5. Secure the catheter to the medial aspect of the thigh with tape. Leave a generous portion of the catheter tubing between the tape and the urethral opening to allow some "give" as the child moves the leg.

Blocked Urethral Catheter

PHONE CALL

Questions

1. How long has the catheter been blocked?
2. What are the vital signs?
3. Is the child complaining of suprapubic or abdominal pain?

Orders

Ask the nurse to try flushing the catheter with 10 mL of normal saline solution if this has not been done already.

Inform RN

"Will arrive at the bedside in ... minutes." If the child is uncomfortable, you should evaluate the child immediately.

ELEVATOR THOUGHTS

What causes blocked urethral catheters?
1. Urinary sediment
2. Blood clots
3. Kinked or compressed catheter
4. Displaced catheter

MAJOR THREAT TO LIFE

- Bladder rupture
- Progressive renal insufficiency
- Urosepsis

Bladder rupture may occur if the bladder is unable to drain an increasing volume of urine. Pain may be expected to precede rupture; therefore, an uncomfortable child is worrisome. However, some children may be incapable of sensing a distended bladder (e.g., those with spinal cord lesions and comatose or sedated children).

Renal failure may occur secondary to hydronephrosis from chronic urinary tract obstruction. Urinary stasis also increases the risk for infection of the urinary tract, which may potentially progress to sepsis.

BEDSIDE

Quick-Look Test

Does the child look well (comfortable), sick (uncomfortable or distressed), or critical (about to die)?

Most patients look well unless the bladder has been distended enough to cause pain.

Airway and Vital Signs

Unless pain or infection is present, the vital signs are not usually affected by a blocked urethral catheter.

Management

1. Palpate the suprapubic area for fullness suggestive of bladder distention.
2. Carefully inspect the catheter and drainage tubing for kinks, compression, or an obvious blockage in the external portion of the tube.
3. Aspirate and irrigate the catheter as follows:
   a. Using sterile technique, disconnect the catheter from the drainage tubing.
   b. With a syringe, aspirate the catheter to dislodge and extract any sediment or blood clot that may be obstructing the lumen.
   c. If aspiration does not reveal anything, flush the catheter with 10 to 20 mL of normal saline solution.
   d. If aspiration and flushing fail to relieve the obstruction, remove the catheter and insert a new one. **Remember to re-evaluate the need for a urethral catheter before inserting a new one**.

Gross Hematuria

PHONE CALL

Questions

1. Why does the child have a urethral catheter?
2. What are the vital signs?
3. Has the patient received heparin, warfarin, or cyclophosphamide?

Orders

None

Inform RN

"Will arrive at the bedside in ... minutes." Gross hematuria should be evaluated immediately.

ELEVATOR THOUGHTS

What causes gross hematuria in a child with a urinary catheter?

Urethral trauma (either from displacement or during insertion)	
Coagulopathies	Factor deficiencies
	Disseminated intravascular coagulopathy (DIC)
	Thrombocytopenia
Drugs	Anticoagulants
	Thrombolytic agents
	Cyclophosphamide
Other causes	Massive hemolysis
	Cystitis (e.g., adenovirus)
	Renal stones
	Glomerulonephritis

MAJOR THREAT TO LIFE

- Hemorrhagic shock: Although gross hematuria is frightening to the child (and often the physician as well), it is rare for the child to bleed enough to result in shock.

BEDSIDE

Quick-Look Test

Does the child look well (comfortable), sick (uncomfortable or distressed), or critical (about to die)?

The child may be frightened but does not appear sick or critical unless an associated cause is present.

Airway and Vital Signs

Tachycardia and/or hypotension may be indicative of hypovolemia or impending shock.

Selective History and Chart Review

Has the child received any medication that may cause hematuria?
> Anticoagulants, streptokinase, urokinase, and cyclophosphamide, among others, may cause hematuria.

Do abnormal laboratory findings suggest a coagulopathy or hemolysis?
> Prolongation of the prothrombin time (PT) or partial thromboplastin time (PTT), thrombocytopenia, or anemia with a high reticulocyte count and high indirect bilirubin level may be clues to the cause of the hematuria. Reviewing the peripheral smear for evidence of DIC or a microangiopathy may be helpful.

Is there a history of urethral trauma?
> Recent surgery, difficulty inserting or removing a urethral catheter, or an obstructed catheter suggests the possibility of trauma.

Management

1. If the cause is a coagulopathy, management should address correction of the specific problem (see Chapter 33, Anemia, Thrombocytopenia, and Coagulation Abnormalities).
2. If drugs are suspected to be the cause, review the need for the medication and discontinue administration if at all possible.
3. If trauma is the suspected cause, a period of observation with frequent monitoring of the vital signs and degree of hematuria allows time for the bleeding to subside. Consultation with a urologist should be considered if the bleeding does not diminish or the vital signs are compromised.

UMBILICAL CATHETERS

Umbilical Arterial Catheter Placement

An umbilical arterial catheter (UAC) is placed in a critically ill newborn to monitor blood pressure and arterial blood gases. It may also be used to obtain blood samples, although this is not an indication for placement. For infants under 1500 g body weight, a 3.5-Fr catheter may be used. For larger infants, a 5-Fr catheter should be appropriate. The tip of the catheter, once in place, should rest in the aorta at the approximate level of the diaphragm (high UAC, at the level of the sixth to ninth thoracic vertebra on a posterolateral chest radiograph) or at the bifurcation of the aorta (low UAC, at the level of the second to fourth lumbar vertebra on an abdominal radiograph). If the catheter is inserted to a point between these two sites, it may obstruct one or more of the major aortic branches (celiac axis, superior mesenteric artery, renal arteries, inferior mesenteric artery). Placement should proceed as follows:

1. Place the infant supine on a warming table.

2. Estimate the length of catheter to be inserted in the following way:
   a. Measure the length of the infant.
   b. For a high UAC, the length inserted is one third the length of the infant.
   c. For a low UAC, the length inserted is one sixth the length of the infant.
   d. Note the marking on the catheter that corresponds to the appropriate length. This mark is positioned at the umbilical stump once the catheter is in place.
3. Restrain the infant's legs by extending a diaper or small blanket across the thighs and securing it to the warming table with tape so that that the infant is not able to raise the legs.
4. Tie a heavy string or umbilical cord tape around the umbilical stump just proximal to where the infant's skin meets the soft tissue of the cord and make certain that it is tight enough to prevent blood from oozing out of the umbilical arteries.
5. Sterile technique should be used to place the catheter. Apply povidone-iodine to the entire umbilical stump and the cord distally to the point where the cord is clamped. Drape the infant's abdomen so that only the stump and cord are exposed.
6. Prepare the catheter for insertion by attaching a 10-mL syringe filled with a heparinized solution and a three-way stopcock to the end. Fill the entire length of the catheter with the solution, and then turn the stopcock to the catheter off.
7. Using a scalpel, cut the cord transversely approximately 1 cm above the stump and remove the distally clamped cord. This exposes the two umbilical arteries and umbilical vein in cross section so that they can be visualized clearly. Leaving some of the cord itself allows you to shave some off at a later time if placement is difficult and the distal umbilical arteries become frayed.
8. Grasp the wall of the cord with a hemostat in one hand and pull up gently so that the cord is vertical and perpendicular to the abdomen. (Alternatively, ask a colleague to do this for you. This procedure is easier if two people work on it.) With curved forceps in the other hand, insert one tip of the forceps into the lumen of one of the umbilical arteries. These arteries are constricted; therefore, the lumen may initially be difficult to visualize. Gently move the tip of the forceps in a circular fashion to gradually dilate the lumen of the artery. Patience is the key to success here, and rushing to dilate the artery may result in fraying and destruction of the distal end of the artery and make it impossible to insert the catheter (Fig. 26-1).
9. Once the lumen is slightly dilated, both tips of the closed forceps may be inserted and the artery dilated further by gently opening the forceps to stretch the walls of the artery. As this is being done, also gradually insert the tips of the

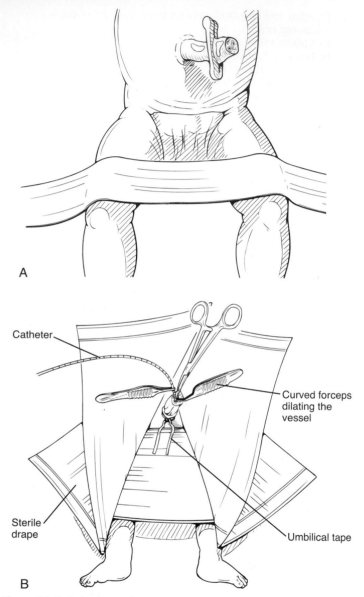

A

Catheter

Curved forceps
dilating the
vessel

Sterile
drape

Umbilical tape

B

Figure 26–1 A, Position of the infant for umbilical vessel catheterization.
B, Procedure for inserting an umbilical catheter.

forceps deeper and deeper into the lumen to dilate as far proximally as possible.

10. When the distal portion of the artery has been dilated enough to accommodate the umbilical catheter, grasp the catheter near the tip with forceps. While holding the lumen of the umbilical artery open with the forceps (again, this is much easier if two people work together), insert the catheter tip into the artery and gradually feed the catheter into the vessel with the forceps. Stop when you have reached the estimated length (the marking that you previously noted is positioned where the catheter enters the lumen of the vessel) that places the tip at either a high level (aortic bifurcation) or a low level (diaphragm).

11. With successful catheterization, pulsating blood is usually visible in the catheter. Opening the stopcock and aspirating on the syringe should result in blood being easily drawn into the catheter.

12. While feeding the catheter into the umbilical artery, obstruction may be encountered at the point where the vessels turn at the umbilical wall or because of vasospasm. When obstruction occurs, steady, gentle pressure on the catheter while pulling up on the umbilical stump often allows the catheter to pass. If it does not pass, a false tract external to the lumen of the vessel may have been created, and it may be necessary to withdraw the catheter and try again. If after several attempts the catheter still cannot be passed, it may be necessary to attempt insertion in the other umbilical artery. Alternatively, shaving the cord again with the scalpel may expose the artery proximal to the false tract and allow you to attempt insertion again.

13. Placement of the catheter should always be confirmed with a radiograph. If the sterility of the field and the catheter is maintained during radiography, the catheter may be advanced if necessary. Once positioning is confirmed, the catheter should be secured to the cord with a suture and then taped in place.

14. It is common for pallor or cyanosis to appear in a lower extremity after placement of a UAC. This occurs secondary to vasospasm in response to the catheter and is often relieved by warming the opposite leg. Warmth increases blood flow to the affected extremity as a result of reflex vasodilatation.

Umbilical Venous Catheter Placement

Umbilical venous catheters are placed for IV access and for monitoring central venous pressure. The umbilical vein is a readily available site for IV access in a critically ill newborn. Placement of a venous catheter is identical to that for an arterial catheter except that it is generally easier and less time consuming. The umbilical vein is thin walled and does not usually require dilatation. Once identified, the lumen is typically easily opened, and the catheter tip may pass freely with gentle pressure. Umbilical venous catheters should be placed so that the tip lies within the inferior vena cava just above the diaphragm. The length to be inserted can be estimated by multiplying the length of the infant by one sixth, similar to a low UAC. As with a UAC, proper positioning should be confirmed with a radiograph and the catheter secured with a suture and tape.

Blocked Umbilical Arterial or Venous Catheter

PHONE CALL

Questions

1. How long has the line been blocked?
2. What are the vital signs? Hypertension or narrowing of the recorded pulse pressure may be a sign of a thrombus at the tip of the arterial catheter.

Orders

None

Inform RN

"Will arrive at the bedside in ... minutes." A blocked umbilical catheter should be evaluated immediately.

ELEVATOR THOUGHTS

What causes an umbilical catheter to be blocked?
1. Thrombus at the catheter tip
2. Kinked or compressed tubing

MAJOR THREAT TO LIFE

- Gangrene of an extremity secondary to thrombosis of an arterial line.
- Pulmonary or cerebral embolism (through a patent foramen ovale) secondary to thrombosis of a venous line.

BEDSIDE

Quick-Look Test

If the infant appears ill, suspect a complication such as embolization or distal gangrene.

Airway and Vital Signs

As noted earlier, hypertension or a narrowed recorded blood pressure may be an indication of a thrombus at the tip of an arterial catheter.

Management

Inspect the external portion of the catheter for kinks or compression. **Unless there is an obvious kink or compression that can be relieved, the line must be removed.** After pulling the line, inspect the tip for a thrombus. Re-evaluate the need for the catheter to be replaced before replacing it.

CENTRAL LINES

Bleeding at the Entry Site

PHONE CALL

Questions

1. What are the vital signs?
2. What was the reason for admission?

Orders

Ask the nurse to have a dressing set, sterile gloves, and povidone-iodine at the child's bedside.

Inform RN

"Will arrive at the bedside in ... minutes." Bleeding at the central line site needs to be evaluated immediately.

ELEVATOR THOUGHTS

What causes bleeding at the entry site?
1. Bleeding from skin capillaries
2. Coagulation disorders
   a. Drugs (heparin, warfarin, nonsteroidal anti-inflammatory drugs, thrombolytic agents)
   b. Coagulopathy (thrombocytopenia, factor deficiency, DIC, microangiopathy)

MAJOR THREAT TO LIFE

- Upper airway obstruction
- Hemorrhagic shock

Bleeding into the soft tissues of the neck may compromise the airway. Massive bleeding at the entry site is required to cause shock.

BEDSIDE

Quick-Look Test

Does the child appear well (comfortable), sick (uncomfortable or distressed), or critical (about to die)?

The child should appear well unless airway compromise or shock has occurred.

Airway and Vital Signs

Check the airway and the respiratory rate carefully for signs of airway obstruction.

Selective Physical Examination and Management

1. Remove the dressing and try to localize the bleeding.
2. If you cannot localize the site, clean the area where the line enters the skin and reinspect.
3. If possible, elevate the site above the heart as tolerated.
4. Apply continuous, firm pressure to the site for 20 minutes (Fig. 26-2).
5. Reinspect. If the bleeding has stopped, clean the area and secure the line with an occlusive dressing. If bleeding persists, continue to apply pressure for another 20 minutes. If the bleeding has still not stopped, a coagulation defect should be suspected, and blood should be sent for a stat platelet count, PT, and PTT. Refer to Chapter 33, Anemia, Thrombocytopenia, and Coagulation Abnormalities, for further evaluation and management of coagulopathies. Review the child's medications for anticoagulants and drugs that may affect platelet function.
6. Consider removal of the line if the bleeding is excessive and resistant to the aforementioned measures.

Blocked Central Line

PHONE CALL

Questions

1. How long has the line been blocked?
2. What are the vital signs?

Orders

Ask the RN for a dressing set, sterile gloves, povidone-iodine, a 5-mL syringe, and a 21-gauge needle to be placed at the child's bedside. You may need to remove the sterile dressing that is in place.

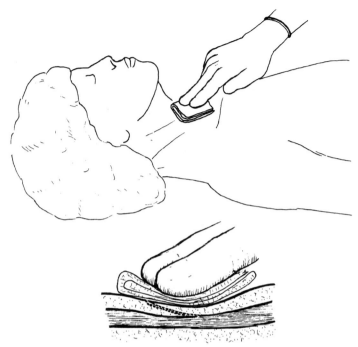

Figure 26–2 Continuous firm local pressure for 20 minutes is required to stop oozing of blood from the central line entry site. (From Marshall SA, Ruedy J: On Call: Principles and Protocols, 4th ed. Philadelphia, Elsevier, 2004, p 204.)

Inform RN

"Will arrive at the bedside in ... minutes." The child needs to be seen immediately.

ELEVATOR THOUGHTS

What causes a central line to become blocked?
1. Kinked or compressed tubing (Fig. 26-3A)
2. Thrombus at the catheter tip (Fig. 26-3B)

MAJOR THREAT TO LIFE

- Loss of access to allow appropriate central venous pressure monitoring and to deliver medications.

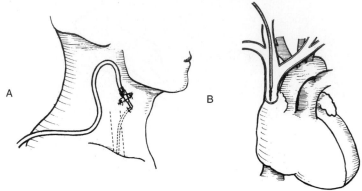

Figure 26–3 Causes of blocked central lines. **A,** Kinked tubing.
B, Thrombus at the catheter tip. (From Marshall SA, Ruedy J: On Call:
Principles and Protocols, 4th ed. Philadelphia, Elsevier, 2004,
p 200.)

BEDSIDE

Quick-Look Test

*Does the child appear well (comfortable), sick (uncomfortable or
distressed), or critical (about to die)?*

A blocked central line should not cause the child to appear ill.
If the child does appear ill, search for an alternative explanation.

Airway and Vital Signs

The airway and vital signs are not affected by a blocked central line
unless the line carries a vasoactive substance, such as dopamine,
dobutamine, or epinephrine.

Selective Physical Examination and Management

1. Inspect the line. Is there obvious kinking or compression? If
   so, remove the dressing, straighten the line, and see whether
   fluid now flows through the line. If flow is restored, secure
   the line with an occlusive dressing after cleaning the site.
2. If there is no flow with the line wide open, proceed as follows:
   a. Turn the IV line off.
   b. Place the child in the Trendelenburg position (head
      down). During the expiration phase of respiration, dis-
      connect the central line from the IV tubing. Quickly
      attach a 5-mL syringe to the central line and cap the IV
      tubing with a sterile 21-gauge capped needle to keep the

tip of the tubing sterile. The syringe must be attached quickly to the central line to avoid an air embolus, which may occur if air is sucked into the line from the negative intrathoracic pressure generated during inspiration.

    c. Draw back gently on the syringe. This may dislodge a small thrombus and restore flow to the line.

    d. Draw back 3 mL of blood, if possible. Again, during the expiratory phase of respiration, remove the capped needle from the IV tubing and the syringe from the central line and reattach the tubing to the central line. Turn the IV line on again and check for flow.

    e. Blocked central lines should never be flushed because flushing may dislodge a clot on the tip of the catheter and produce a pulmonary embolus.

3. If the preceding measures are unsuccessful, determine the necessity for the central line. If the central line is essential, a new central line needs to be placed at a different site. A new central line should not be reinserted over a guidewire at the same site because this may also disrupt a clot and result in a pulmonary embolus.

CHEST TUBES

Chest tubes are placed to evacuate air (pneumothorax), fluid (pleural effusion), pus (empyema), or blood (hemothorax) from the pleural space (Fig. 26-4). They are always connected to an underwater seal and may be set up for straight drainage (no suction) or suction. Common drainage setups are depicted in Figure 26-5, and common problems with chest tubes are shown in Figure 26-6.

Persistent Bubbling in the Drainage Container (Air Leak)

PHONE CALL

Questions

    1. Why was the chest tube placed?
    2. What are the vital signs?
    3. Is the child in respiratory distress?

Orders

None

Inform RN

"Will arrive at the bedside in … minutes." The patient needs to be seen as soon as possible and immediately if in respiratory distress.

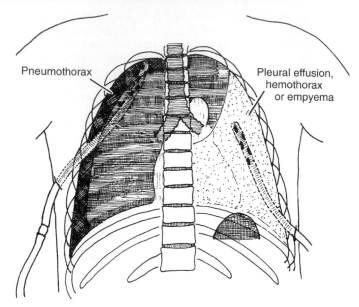

Figure 26–4 Chest tubes are inserted to drain air (pneumothorax), blood (hemothorax), fluid (pleural effusion), and pus (empyema). (From Marshall SA, Ruedy J: On Call: Principles and Protocols, 4th ed. Philadelphia, Elsevier, 2004, p 208.)

ELEVATOR THOUGHTS

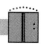

What causes persistent bubbling in the drainage container?
1. Loose tubing connection
2. Air leaking into the pleural space around the chest tube at the insertion site
3. Traumatic tracheobronchial injury (in children with traumatic pneumothorax, there may be additional injuries)
4. Persistent leak into the pleural space from the bronchoalveolar tree
   a. Postsurgical
   b. Ruptured bleb (e.g., asthma, cystic fibrosis)
5. Externalization of a proximal side hole on the chest tube (usually evident on a chest radiograph)

MAJOR THREAT TO LIFE

- Hypoxia: The major threat to life is the underlying intrathoracic process producing the air leak. As long as air is bubbling

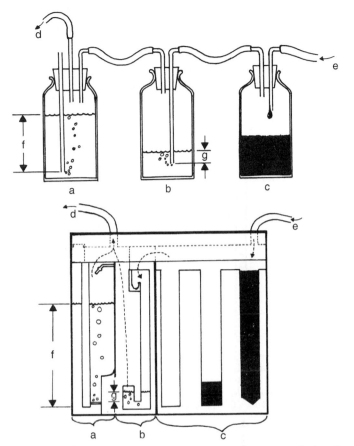

Figure 26–5 Chest tube apparatuses. **A**, Suction control chamber. **B**, Underwater seal. **C**, Collection chamber. **D**, To suction. **E**, From patient. **F**, Height equals amount of suction in cm H_2O. **G**, Height equals underwater seal in cm H_2O. (From Marshall SA, Ruedy J: On Call: Principles and Protocols, 4th ed. Philadelphia, Elsevier, 2004, p 209.)

through the collection chamber, the leak is being evacuated and air should not be accumulating in the intrapleural space (except in the rare coincidence in which the tube fails to drain the pleural space because of obstruction and an external loose connection accounts for the persistent bubbling).

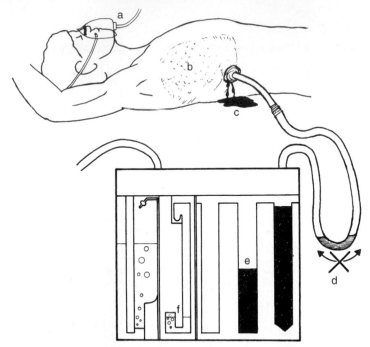

Figure 26–6 Common chest tube problems. **A**, Shortness of breath. **B**, Subcutaneous emphysema. **C**, Bleeding at the entry site. **D**, Loss of fluctuation. **E**, Excessive drainage. **F**, Persistent bubbling. (From Marshall SA, Ruedy J: On Call: Principles and Protocols, 4th ed. Philadelphia, Elsevier, 2004, p 210.)

BEDSIDE

Quick-Look Test

Does the child appear well (comfortable), sick (uncomfortable or distressed), or critical (about to die)?

A larger pneumothorax may be developing in a child who appears ill. Quickly evaluate the need for an additional chest tube in an ill-appearing child by listening over the lung fields and, if necessary (and if there is time), obtaining a stat portable chest radiograph.

Airway and Vital Signs

If all connections are tight and the chest tube dressing is airtight, a persistent air leak means that the patient has a pneumothorax. As long as air continues to bubble through the collection chamber, the air should drain from the pleural space and not alter the vital signs or compromise the airway.

Selective History and Chart Review

Why was the chest tube placed?

If the tube was placed for pneumothorax, the collection chamber should be bubbling unless the lung is fully expanded and the leak into the pleural space has sealed.

If the tube was placed to drain fluid (effusion, empyema, or blood) without suction, a new onset of bubbling indicates loose connections external to the chest, air leaking into the pleural space from around the insertion site, or the development of a pneumothorax.

Selective Physical Examination and Management

If the air leak is small, bubbling may be intermittent and appear only when intrapleural pressure increases (e.g., with coughing).

1. Inspect the tubing connections and ensure that all seals are airtight.
2. Remove the dressing at the entry site, listen for the sound of air being sucked into the chest, and observe the area around the site. If the incision for the tube is inadequately closed to form a seal around the tube, placing several sutures to seal the opening may be necessary. If this stops the bubbling, reapply the sterile dressing after cleaning the site.
3. If the tubing and entry site appear airtight, obtain a chest radiograph to confirm proper chest tube placement. The tube holes should be within the chest, and the tip of the tube should be clearly away from the mediastinal and subclavicular structures. Comparing this film with the previous film taken after insertion of the chest tube allows you to determine whether the pneumothorax has increased in size. If the pneumothorax is larger or the lung has not re-expanded, the single chest tube may not be adequate to evacuate the air leak. You may need to consider placing a second chest tube. This should be discussed with your senior resident and the patient's attending physician. Surgical consultation may also be necessary if the air leak occurred secondary to trauma or surgery.

Bleeding at the Chest Tube Entry Site

PHONE CALL

Questions

1. Why was the chest tube placed?
2. What are the vital signs?
3. Is the child in respiratory distress?

Orders

Ask the RN for sterile gloves, a dressing set, and povidone-iodine at the bedside. You need to remove the sterile dressing around the chest tube site.

Inform RN

"Will arrive at the bedside in ... minutes." You need to see the child immediately.

ELEVATOR THOUGHTS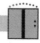

What causes bleeding around the chest tube entry site?
1. Inadequate pressure dressing
2. Inadequate closure of the incision
3. Coagulation disorders
4. Trauma to subcostal arteries and veins during tube placement
5. Blocked chest tube in a child with hemothorax

MAJOR THREAT TO LIFE

- Hemorrhagic shock: Usually the bleeding is not rapid. Blood loss would need to be substantial to result in shock.

BEDSIDE

Quick-Look Test

Does the child appear well (comfortable), sick (uncomfortable or distressed), or critical (about to die)?
    Only if a large amount of blood has been lost does the child appear ill.

Airway and Vital Signs

The airway and vital signs are stable unless significant bleeding has occurred.

Selective History and Chart Review

Why was the chest tube placed?
    If it was placed for hemothorax, the main concern is inadequate evacuation of blood from the pleural space.

Selective Physical Examination and Management

1. Remove the dressing and inspect the incision. Several sutures may stop the bleeding if the incision is inadequately closed. If the incision is adequately closed, reapply a pressure dressing at the site.

2. If bleeding continues, try milking the chest tube to relieve obstruction by blood clots or other debris.
3. If bleeding persists in a patient with hemothorax, consider placing a larger chest tube.
4. In those without hemothorax, apply firm pressure by hand over the site for 20 minutes. Repeat this step if necessary. If the bleeding still continues, further evaluation for a coagulopathy may be indicated. Remember to check the list of medications for any that may cause clotting abnormalities.

Drainage of Blood

PHONE CALL

Questions

1. **Why was the chest tube placed?**
2. **What are the vital signs?**
3. **Is the child in respiratory distress?**

Orders

None

Inform RN

"Will arrive at the bedside in ... minutes." You need to see the child immediately.

ELEVATOR THOUGHTS

What causes blood to drain from the chest tube?
    Intrathoracic bleeding

MAJOR THREAT TO LIFE

• Hemorrhagic shock

BEDSIDE

Quick-Look Test

Does the child appear well (comfortable), sick (uncomfortable or distressed), or critical (about to die)?
    Only if a large amount of blood has been lost does the child appear ill.

Airway and Vital Signs

Check the blood pressure and heart rate carefully for signs of hypovolemia.

Selective Chart Review and Management

What medications has the child received?
   Check the list for any that may lead to a clotting defect.

How much blood has been lost?
   If the amount of blood loss is small, you may continue to carefully monitor the loss and ask to be informed if the amount lost exceeds 10 mL/hr in an infant or 25 mL/hr in an older child. Increase the frequency of vital sign observations so that the heart rate and blood pressure can be monitored. In addition,
1. Order a chest radiograph to evaluate for potential sources of intrathoracic bleeding.
2. Send blood for typing and cross-matching for 4 adult units of packed red blood cells. Also ask for hemoglobin, hematocrit, platelet count, PT, and PTT measurements.
3. Consult cardiothoracic surgery. If the bleeding persists or is excessive, surgical exploration may be necessary to localize and stop the bleeding.

Loss of Fluctuation of the Underwater Seal

PHONE CALL

Questions

1. Why was the chest tube placed?
2. What are the vital signs?
3. Is the child in respiratory distress?

Orders

None

Inform RN

"Will arrive at the bedside in ... minutes." You need to evaluate the child immediately.

ELEVATOR THOUGHTS

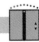

What causes loss of fluctuation of the underwater seal?
1. Kink in the chest tube
2. Obstructed chest tube
3. Misplaced chest tube

The underwater seal is a one-way, low-resistance valve. During expiration, intrapleural pressure increases and forces air or fluid from the pleural space through the chest tube and underwater seal (Fig. 26-7). Loss of fluctuation means that the tube is not functioning to evacuate air or fluid from the intrapleural space.

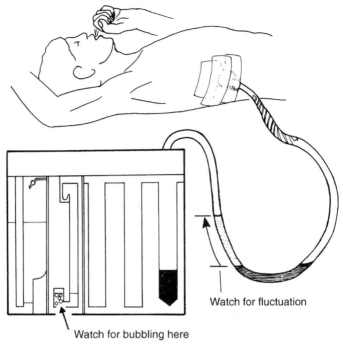

Watch for fluctuation

Watch for bubbling here

Figure 26–7 Loss of fluctuation of the underwater seal. Ask the patient to cough, and observe for any fluctuation or bubbling. (From Marshall SA, Ruedy J: On Call: Principles and Protocols, 4th ed. Philadelphia, Elsevier, 2004, p 212.)

MAJOR THREAT TO LIFE

- Tension pneumothorax: A malfunctioning chest tube may inadequately drain a pneumothorax and lead to tension pneumothorax (Figs. 26-8 and 26-9).

BEDSIDE

Quick-Look Test

Does the child appear well (comfortable), sick (uncomfortable or distressed), or critical (about to die)?

An ill-appearing child may have a tension pneumothorax.

Airway and Vital Signs

Hypotension and tachypnea may indicate a tension pneumothorax.

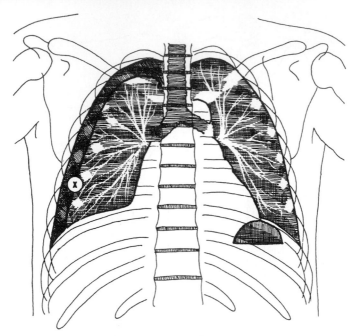

Figure 26–8 Pneumothorax. *x*, Edge of visceral pleura or lung. (From Marshall SA, Ruedy J: On Call: Principles and Protocols, 4th ed. Philadelphia, Elsevier, 2004, p 218.)

Selective History and Chart Review

Why was the chest tube placed?
How long ago did it stop fluctuating?
What and how much has been drained in the last 24 hours?

Selective Physical Examination and Management

1. Inspect the underwater seal. Is there any fluctuation? Ask the child to cough, and watch for fluctuation.
2. Inspect the tube for kinks or compression. You may need to remove the dressing at the insertion site. If a kink is found, reinspect for fluctuation after straightening or repositioning the tube.
3. Try milking the chest tube. Milking may dislodge an obstruction within the lumen of the tube.
4. Obtain a portable stat chest radiograph to determine the position of the tube. Reposition the tube if it appears to be close to structures that may be causing an obstruction.
5. If the tube is still not fluctuating, re-evaluate the need for the chest tube and consider placing a new one.

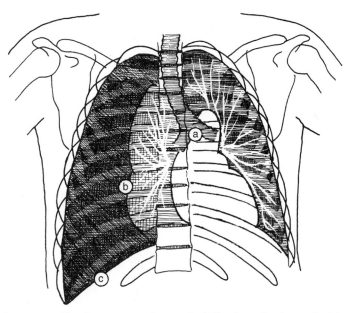

Figure 26–9 Tension pneumothorax. **A**, Shifted mediastinum. **B**, Edge of collapsed lung. **C**, Low flattened diaphragm. (From Marshall SA, Ruedy J: On Call: Principles and Protocols, 4th ed. Philadelphia, Elsevier, 2004, p 219.)

Dyspnea

PHONE CALL

Questions

1. Why was the chest tube placed?
2. What are the vital signs?

Orders

Ask the nurse for a dressing set, gloves, several sizes of angio-catheters, and povidone-iodine at the bedside. You may need the angiocatheters to evacuate a tension pneumothorax. Ask the nurse to call for an immediate portable chest radiograph.

Inform RN

"Will arrive at the bedside in ... minutes." You need to see the child immediately.

ELEVATOR THOUGHTS

What causes dyspnea in a patient with a chest tube?
1. Tension pneumothorax
2. Expanding pneumothorax
3. Subcutaneous emphysema (see later)
4. Expanding pleural effusion or hemothorax
5. Re-expansion pulmonary edema (after rapid evacuation of the pleural space)
6. Other causes unrelated to the chest tube (see Chapter 28, Respiratory Distress)

MAJOR THREAT TO LIFE

- Hypoxia

BEDSIDE

Quick-Look Test

Children with dyspnea usually appear ill.

Airway and Vital Signs

1. Inspect for any subcutaneous emphysema that may be obstructing the upper airway.
2. Tachypnea suggests hypoxia, pain, or anxiety.
3. Hypotension, pulsus paradoxus, and/or tachycardia may indicate a tension pneumothorax.

Selective Physical Examination

Does the patient have a tension pneumothorax?

HEENT	Deviation of the trachea away from the side of the pneumothorax
Chest	Unilateral hyperresonance and absence of breath sounds
Cardiovascular	Jugular venous distention
Chest tube	Is there bubbling in the collection chamber? Absence of bubbling suggests malfunctioning of the chest tube

Management

1. If subcutaneous emphysema has resulted in significant upper airway obstruction, the child may need to be intubated. Call your senior resident and the intensive care unit (ICU) immediately.

2. If you suspect tension pneumothorax, it needs to be evacuated (see Chapter 10, Chest Pain).
3. If you suspect an enlarging pneumothorax, look for a correctable cause (blocked or compressed tubing, inadequate suction on the chest tube, or dislodged chest tube). A chest radiograph helps determine whether the tube is properly positioned.
4. If the chest tube appears to be functioning and no tension pneumothorax or expanding pneumothorax is present, management should be directed at other causes of dyspnea unrelated to the chest tube (see Chapter 28, Respiratory Distress).

Subcutaneous Emphysema

PHONE CALL

Questions

1. Why was the chest tube placed?
2. What are the vital signs?
3. Is the child in respiratory distress?

Orders

Ask the nurse for a dressing set, gloves, and povidone-iodine at the bedside. You need to remove the sterile dressing around the insertion site.

Inform RN

"Will arrive at the bedside in ... minutes." You need to see the child immediately.

ELEVATOR THOUGHTS

What causes subcutaneous emphysema in a patient with a chest tube?
1. Inadequate size of tube
2. Inadequate suction
3. Chest tube aperture in the chest wall
4. Chest tube in the chest wall or abdominal cavity
5. Minor subcutaneous emphysema localized to the insertion site (not uncommon)

MAJOR THREAT TO LIFE

• Upper airway obstruction: Subcutaneous emphysema may extend into the soft tissues of the neck and compress the airway.

BEDSIDE

Quick-Look Test

Does the child appear well (comfortable), sick (uncomfortable or distressed), or critical (about to die)?

If upper airway obstruction is present, the child appears ill.

Airway and Vital Signs

1. Inspect and palpate the neck to feel for the crepitus of subcutaneous emphysema. It feels and may sound like "crunching" as you palpate.
2. Check the respiratory rate, blood pressure, and heart rate. Subcutaneous emphysema may be associated with a concurrent tension pneumothorax.

Selective Physical Examination and Management

1. If the airway is nearly obstructed (stridor, tachypnea), call your senior resident and the ICU and arrange to intubate the child.
2. Examine the size of the chest tube. If the tube is too small, air may escape from the pleural space into the chest wall. A new tube may be necessary.
3. Is the suction connected? A tube left only to straight drainage may be inadequate to evacuate a large pneumothorax.
4. Remove the dressing and inspect the insertion site and the chest tube. None of the holes in the tube should be visible. They should all be within the pleural space. If the tube has become misplaced and the holes now lie outside the chest wall, a new tube needs to be inserted. **Do not push an extruded tube back into the pleural space**. You may risk infecting the pleural cavity.

27

Rashes

Christopher J. Schwake, MD

Rashes can develop for a wide variety of reasons in a hospitalized child—some very serious and others quite benign. When you are called by the nurse to evaluate a rash in the middle of the night, remember that your goal is not necessarily to arrive at a specific diagnosis or explanation. Instead, excluding illnesses that might be harmful to the child, keeping the child comfortable, and reassuring the patient and family that you have done so may be more reasonable goals.

PHONE CALL

Questions

1. How long has the patient had the rash?
2. Is urticaria (hives) present?
3. Is the child wheezing or in any respiratory distress?
4. What are the vital signs?
5. What medications has the child received in the last 12 hours?
6. Does the child have any known allergies?
7. What is the child's admitting diagnosis?

Orders

If the rash is associated with signs of allergy or anaphylaxis (wheezing, stridor, dysphagia, shortness of breath, periorbital edema, lip swelling, or hypotension), order the following without delay:

1. Place the largest possible intravenous (IV) line immediately and start a normal saline bolus.
2. Have respiratory therapy place airway support materials at the bedside, including suction, a laryngoscopy tray, oxygen, and an Ambu bag.
3. Epinephrine, 0.01 mg/kg (0.1 mL/kg of a 1:10,000 solution for IV administration or 0.01 mL/kg of a 1:1,000 solution for subcutaneous administration). **Do not confuse these doses and routes of administration!**

4. IV diphenhydramine (Benadryl), 1 mg/kg
5. IV methylprednisolone, 2 mg/kg

If there are no signs of an acute allergic reaction, instruct the nurse to not put anything on the rash until you have examined the patient.

Inform RN

"Will arrive at the bedside in … minutes." Evidence of anaphylaxis or acute allergy requires immediate evaluation. A new onset of purpura or petechiae, particularly in a child with fever, also requires immediate evaluation.

ELEVATOR THOUGHTS

A wide variety of medications can cause skin eruptions, and such rashes are among the most common that you will be asked to evaluate. The lesions may be urticarial (rare but most alarming), macular, papular, erythematous, vesicular, bullous, petechial, or purpuric. Most drug rashes are widely distributed over the body. Some have typical distribution patterns that help identify their origin. Remember that rashes are dynamic processes, and changes are bound to occur with time. What the nurse observed may not be what you see 2 or 3 hours later. The more common rashes and some of their causes are listed here.

Urticaria (Rare but Potentially Life Threatening)

Histamine-mediated allergic reactions: IV contrast material, antibiotics, opiates, anesthetic agents, vasoactive agents
Drug reactions with an unknown mechanism: aspirin, nonsteroidal anti-inflammatory drugs
Food allergies: shellfish, nuts, tomatoes
Hereditary angioedema
Physical agents: detergents, perfumes, cold, heat, pressure
Idiopathic

Erythematous, Maculopapular (Morbilliform) Rashes

Measles (rubeola)
Rubella
Roseola
Kawasaki disease
Juvenile rheumatoid arthritis
Drug reaction
Antibiotics (reaction can be delayed as long as 2 to 3 weeks with ampicillin)
Antihistamines
Antidepressants

Diuretics
Sedatives
Because some drug rashes have a late onset, the medication history should include all medications taken in the last 4 weeks.

Vesicobullous Rashes

Varicella-zoster (primary, chickenpox; or secondary, herpes zoster)
Erythema multiforme (many viruses and drugs)
Stevens-Johnson syndrome
Drug reaction
Toxic epidermal necrolysis: Lyell's syndrome (sulfonamide, allopurinol)
Antibiotics (sulfonamides, dapsone)
Anti-inflammatory agents (penicillamine)
Sedatives (barbiturates)
Stevens-Johnson syndrome is a particularly life-threatening variant of erythema multiforme characterized by involvement of at least two mucous membranes, especially the oral mucosa and eye.

Petechiae or Purpura

Vasculitis (palpable purpura)
Sepsis or disseminated intravascular coagulopathy (DIC) (meningococcemia, *Haemophilus influenzae* sepsis, cytomegalovirus)
Drug reaction
Antibiotics (sulfonamides, chloramphenicol)
Diuretics
Anti-inflammatory agents (salicylates, indomethacin, phenylbutazone)
Thrombocytopenia

Exfoliative Dermatitis (Erythroderma)

Scarlet fever
Toxic shock syndrome
Drug reaction
Antibiotics (streptomycin)
Anti-inflammatory agents (gold, phenylbutazone)
Antiepileptics (carbamazepine, phenytoin)
Continued administration of the drug can lead to a generalized, dusky red, dry rash with profound exfoliation and scaling.

Fixed Drug Reaction

Antibiotics (sulfonamides, metronidazole)
Anti-inflammatory drugs (phenylbutazone)
Analgesics (phenacetin)
Sedatives (barbiturates, chlordiazepoxide)
Laxatives (phenolphthalein)

Certain drugs may produce a skin lesion in a specific area. Repeated administration of the drug reproduces the skin lesion in the same location. The lesions are usually dusky red patches over the trunk and limbs.

MAJOR THREAT TO LIFE

- Anaphylactic shock
- Septic shock with DIC
- Stevens-Johnson syndrome

Urticarial eruptions indicate histamine release and may be a prodrome to systemic histamine effects, including hypotension and shock. In hospitalized children, drugs and IV contrast materials are the most common causes of anaphylactic reactions.

Sepsis and septic shock can evolve rapidly. The rashes associated with certain conditions, such as meningococcemia and toxic shock syndrome, may develop during the early part of the hospitalization.

Stevens-Johnson syndrome presents a major risk of significant dehydration as a result of oral mucosal involvement, as well as a major threat of permanent visual impairment from uveitis or corneal scarring.

BEDSIDE

Quick-Look Test

Does the child appear well (comfortable), sick (uncomfortable or distressed), or critical (about to die)?

A patient in impending anaphylaxis appears anxious and hyperalert, usually with progressive respiratory distress.

Airway and Vital Signs

What is the blood pressure?

Hypotension is an ominous sign and requires immediate and aggressive intervention (see Chapter 25, Hypotension and Shock).

What is the temperature?

Almost all skin rashes become more apparent when the child is febrile because there is greater perfusion of the skin.

Selective Physical Examination

Is there evidence of impending anaphylaxis, sepsis or DIC, or Stevens-Johnson syndrome?

HEENT	Pharyngeal, periorbital, or facial edema; conjunctivitis or uveitis; oral mucosal lesions
Respiratory	Stridor, wheezing

Skin   Urticarial rash, erythema multiforme rash,
                        purpura, petechiae

What is the location of the rash? Is the rash generalized, acral (hands and feet), or localized?
   Remember that to evaluate a child for a rash, you must examine the entire child, including the buttocks (a common site for drug eruptions) and the genital region, as well as the scalp.

What is the color of the rash?
   Erythematous, pale, brown, purplish, pink

Describe the primary lesions (Fig. 27-1):
   Macules: flat, with or without a distinct margin (noticeable from the surrounding skin because of the color difference)
   Patch: a large macule
   Papule: solid, elevated, less than 1 cm

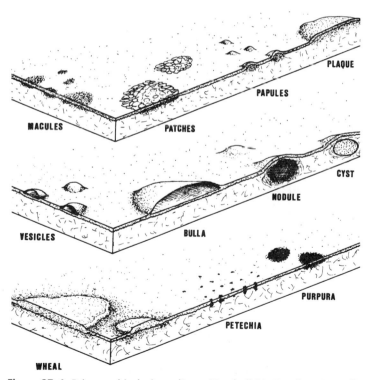

Figure 27–1 Primary skin lesions. (From Marshall SA, Ruedy J: On Call: Principles and Protocols, 4th ed. Philadelphia, Elsevier, 2004, p 291.)

Plaque: solid, elevated, greater than 1 cm

Vesicle: fluid filled, elevated, well circumscribed, less than 1 cm

Pustule: vesicle containing purulent fluid

Bulla: fluid filled, elevated, well circumscribed, greater than 1 cm

Nodule: deep-seated mass, indistinct borders, size less than 0.5 cm in both width and depth

Cyst: nodules filled with expressible fluid or semisolid material

Wheal (hives): urticaria; pruritic, well-circumscribed, flat-topped, firm elevation (papule, plaque, or dermal edema) with or without central pallor and with irregular borders

Petechiae: red or purple, nonblanching macules less than 3 mm

Purpura: red or purple, nonblanching macule or papule greater than 3 mm

Describe the secondary lesions (Fig. 27-2):

Scales: dry, thin plates of thickened keratin layers (white color differentiates scales from crusts)

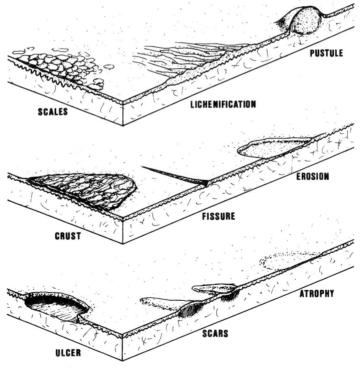

Figure 27–2 Secondary skin lesions. (From Marshall SA, Ruedy J: On Call: Principles and Protocols, 4th ed. Philadelphia, Elsevier, 2004, p 292.)

Crust: dried yellow exudate of plasma (results from broken vesicles, bullae, or pustules)

Lichenification: dry, leathery thickening; shiny surface with accentuation of skin markings

Fissure: linear, epidermal tear

Erosion: wide, epidermal fissure; moist and well circumscribed

Ulcer: erosion into the dermis

Scar: flat, raised (keloid), or depressed area of fibrosis

Atrophy: depression secondary to thinning of the skin

What is the configuration of the rash?

Annular: circular, well circumscribed

Linear: in lines

Grouped: clusters (e.g., vesicular lesions of herpes zoster or herpes simplex)

Selective History and Chart Review

How long has the rash been present?

Is it pruritic?

How has it been treated?

Is it a new or recurrent problem?

Which medications was the child receiving before onset of the rash?

Management

1. If the rash is suspected to be a manifestation of an allergy of any kind, it is usually pruritic and should respond to diphenhydramine (Benadryl).
2. If the rash is associated with urticaria and is secondary to a drug reaction, administration of the drug should be withheld until the diagnosis can be confirmed in the morning.
3. If the rash is nonurticarial and thought to be secondary to a drug reaction and the drug is essential to treatment of the child's underlying illness, administration of the drug should be continued with close monitoring of the patient's condition as long as there is no sign of respiratory compromise or abnormalities in blood pressure and other vital signs.
4. When the rash is not a drug reaction and the diagnosis is clear, the standard recommended treatment of that disorder should be instituted.
5. If the diagnosis of the rash is unclear, describe the lesions thoroughly in your note and to your senior resident. If the rash does not cause undue discomfort, no therapy is necessary until a specific diagnosis is made in the morning. Exceptions include the following:

    Petechial rash, which can indicate disorders of platelet number or function.

    Purpuric rash, which can indicate DIC and sepsis and requires checking a blood culture, prothrombin time, activated partial thromboplastin time, and platelet count, as well as prompt administration of antibiotics.

Vesicular rash secondary to varicella or herpes zoster, which requires immediate isolation of the patient from any potentially immunocompromised children. If the child is immunocompromised, urgent treatment with intravenous acyclovir is indicated to prevent dissemination of the infection to the central nervous system.

REMEMBER

Your ability to describe the rash is critical to establishing its cause and significance. This will help you think carefully about the possible explanations and appropriate management when you have been called to make a "rash decision."

28

Respiratory Distress

Keri A. Wheeler, MD

After fever, respiratory distress is probably the most common complaint that an on-call pediatric house officer is asked to assess. To adequately evaluate a child in respiratory distress, it is necessary to consider the respiratory rate in the context of the age of the child. Neonates typically breathe 35 to 50 times per minute, older infants and toddlers 30 to 40 times per minute, elementary school–aged children 20 to 30 times per minute, and preadolescents and adolescents 12 to 20 times per minute.

Besides the rate, it is important to observe the quality of the breathing, including depth, use of accessory muscles (retractions), grunting, and nasal flaring. Is there stridor with inspiration? Are the breath sounds equal at auscultation? Are there abnormal breath sounds, such as wheezes, rales, rhonchi, tubular breath sounds, egophony, and muffled or absent breath sounds? The specific characteristics of the breathing pattern combined with the physical findings and selective laboratory and radiographic tests (when necessary) will allow you to determine the probable cause of the respiratory distress.

PHONE CALL

Questions

1. How old is the patient?
2. Why is the patient in the hospital?
3. How long has the patient been in respiratory distress?
4. Was the onset sudden or gradual?
5. Does the child appear cyanotic?
6. What are the vital signs?
7. Is the child retracting, flaring, wheezing, or coughing?
8. Are oxygen and a pulse oximeter present in the room?

Orders

1. Have the nurse provide oxygen by nasal cannula or Venturi mask and obtain a pulse oximeter measurement immediately. Start with 1 to 2 L/min by cannula or 30% to 40% by mask.
2. Set up materials to obtain an arterial blood gas measurement or call the lab to draw blood for arterial blood gas studies.
3. If the child has been admitted for reactive airway disease and/or asthma, have the nurse set up an appropriate dose of a nebulized bronchodilator.
4. Inform the nurse that you are on your way. **Respiratory distress deserves immediate evaluation!**

ELEVATOR THOUGHTS

Respiratory distress may be a manifestation of several very different pathologic processes. Distress can include depressed respirations, as well as tachypnea.

Pulmonary processes	Pneumonia, bronchospasm, pulmonary hemorrhage, or interstitial lung disease
Airway processes	Croup, foreign body aspiration, retropharyngeal abscess, laryngeal edema or spasm, epiglottitis, tracheitis, laryngotracheal malacia, vascular ring, esophageal masses, or duplication cysts
Cardiac processes	Congestive heart failure (left-to-right shunt lesions, left ventricular failure), cardiac tamponade, or pulmonary embolism
Space-occupying lesions	Pleural effusion, empyema, pneumothorax, diaphragmatic hernia, massive ascites, or severe scoliosis. Abdominal distention can cause respiratory compromise, especially in infants, who rely on diaphragmatic breathing, or in children with restrictive lung disease (i.e., severe scoliosis)
Neurologic processes	Opiate overdose, increased intracranial pressure, anxiety, or chest wall and/or diaphragmatic weakness

MAJOR THREAT TO LIFE

Hypoxia resulting in inadequate tissue oxygenation is the most worrisome consequence of any process that results in respiratory distress. In addition, respiratory failure is the most common precipitant of cardiac arrest in children. It is therefore essential that clinicians who care for children recognize the manifestations of respiratory disease and be familiar with the principles of its treatment.

BEDSIDE

Quick-Look Test

Does the child appear well (comfortable), sick (uncomfortable or distressed), or critical (about to die)?

This simple observation is the critical first step in assessing this potentially life-threatening situation. An infant or child having difficulty breathing usually does not appear well. A child in distress should be placed on a cardiorespiratory monitor immediately. Oxygen should be administered and airway support supplies, including suctioning and intubation equipment, brought to the bedside. The pediatric intensive care unit (PICU) should be informed and consulted immediately.

Airway and Vital Signs

Is the upper airway clear, and can the patient protect his or her airway? Does the child have a gag reflex?

An obtunded patient in respiratory distress requires intubation. Upper airway obstruction may make intubation difficult or impossible, such as in a patient with oral or facial trauma, foreign body aspiration, or severe epiglottitis. A surgical airway may thus be necessary via emergency cricothyroidotomy.

What is the respiratory rate and pattern?

Rates less than 20 breaths per minute in most young children reflect central respiratory depression, such as with opiates, barbiturates, or alcohol. Tachypnea suggests hypoxia, hypercapnia, acidemia, pain, and/or anxiety. Retractions and nasal flaring indicate the use of accessory muscles of respiration because of inadequate tidal volume or airway obstruction. Thoracoabdominal dissociation is a worrisome finding. The chest and abdomen should rise and fall together and not paradoxically.

What is the heart rate?

Increased sympathetic tone secondary to respiratory distress results in sinus tachycardia. Hypercapnia causing acidosis will also cause tachycardia. Inappropriate bradycardia may herald impending cardiorespiratory collapse. Supraventricular tachycardia or nonsinus bradycardia may result in congestive heart failure and subsequent respiratory distress.

What is the temperature?

Fever is accompanied by tachypnea. Obviously, fever suggests infection, and respiratory distress may be due to airway, pleural, or parenchymal lung infection.

What is the blood pressure?

Hypotension in the setting of respiratory distress suggests shock, acidosis, and possible cardiac compromise as a result of tension pneumothorax. In children, pulsus paradoxus, or when inspiration causes a drop in systolic blood pressure of more than the usual 4 to 10 mm Hg, is rarely noted, but it may occur in the setting of respiratory distress and hypotension (pericardial effusion), as well as with obstructive airway disease as a reflection of the degree of airflow obstruction. Pulsus paradoxus is an inspiratory fall in systolic blood pressure greater than 10 mm Hg. To determine whether pulsus paradoxus is present, inflate the blood pressure cuff 20 to 30 mm Hg above the palpable blood pressure. Deflate the cuff slowly. Initially, Korotkoff sounds are heard only on expiration. At some point during cuff deflation, Korotkoff sounds appear on inspiration as well and give the impression of a doubling of the heart rate. The number of millimeters of mercury between the initial appearance of the Korotkoff sounds and their appearance throughout the respiratory cycle represents the degree of pulsus paradoxus (Fig. 28-1).

Hypertension can occur as a result of increased sympathetic tone from respiratory distress or significant hypercapnia and acidosis.

Selective Physical Examination

Is the patient cyanotic?

Vital signs	Repeat now, including pulse oximetry
HEENT	Nasal flaring, cyanotic mucous membranes, oropharyngeal foreign body
Neck	Midline trachea, stridor
Respiratory	Breath sound quality, symmetry, wheezing, rales, rhonchi, decreased breath sounds, dullness to percussion, ability to phonate, retractions, grunting
Neurologic	Mental status, ability to defend the airway (gag reflex)

Cyanosis is often not obvious unless the oxygen saturation is well below 90%. Especially in darkly pigmented children, oxygen saturation may be very difficult to assess visually. The absence of cyanosis should not falsely reassure the examiner. Significant pathologic conditions and inadequate ventilation may still be present.

Management

What immediate measures need to be taken to correct hypoxia?

Administer adequate oxygen. How much oxygen and by what route depend on the age of the child and the amount of distress. Infants may require an oxygen hood or tent because they do not keep a cannula or mask in place easily. Older children may do very well with either a nasal cannula or mask. The amount of oxygen should be just enough to normalize the oxygen saturation and/or Po_2. Remember, pulse oximetry does not give any information about the effectiveness of ventilation, such as Pco_2, pH, base excess or deficit, or the alveolar-arterial (A-a) O_2 gradient.

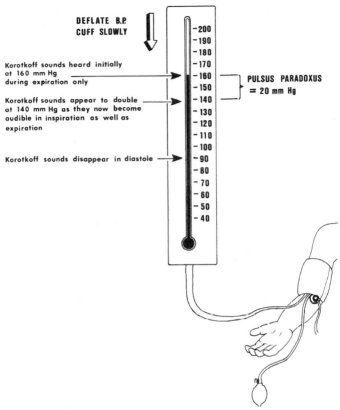

DEFLATE B.P.
CUFF SLOWLY

Korotkoff sounds heard initially
at 160 mm Hg
during expiration only

Korotkoff sounds appear to double
at 140 mm Hg as they now become
audible in inspiration as well as
expiration

Korotkoff sounds disappear in diastole

PULSUS PARADOXUS
= 20 mm Hg

-200
-190
-180
-170
-160
-150
-140
-130
-120
-110
-100
-90
-80
-70
-60
-50
-40

Figure 28–1 Determination of pulsus paradoxus. (From Marshall SA, Ruedy J: On Call: Principles and Protocols, 4th ed. Philadelphia, Elsevier, 2004, p 266.)

What harm can your treatment cause?

Oxygen is not without side effects. Giving 100% oxygen for a prolonged time can lead to atelectasis because the inert gases that are not absorbed help keep the alveoli inflated. With 100% oxygen these inert gases are washed out of the alveoli, and collapse can occur as the oxygen is absorbed. Oxygen also has direct toxic effects on the lungs, especially in neonates and infants.

The use of oxygen in adult patients with chronic obstructive airway disease is always done with caution because with chronic carbon dioxide retention, the drive for respiration becomes hypoxia, not hypercapnia. Therefore, in patients with chronic, poorly controlled asthma and in patients with cystic fibrosis, it is advisable to not exceed 30% oxygen without checking arterial blood gases carefully.

Is the child dyspneic with effective air movement or with poor air movement?

Children with alveolar disease have distress and hypoxia despite good air movement. This includes children with pneumonia and congestive heart failure. Children with airway disease have diminished air exchange for a variety of reasons.

Management depends on the underlying cause of the respiratory distress. Management of four general categories of respiratory distress is discussed here: pulmonary processes, airway processes, cardiac processes, and space-occupying processes. Management of asthma and respiratory failure is also included.

Pulmonary Processes

SELECTIVE HISTORY

Is there a history of fever, cough, or upper respiratory infection?
Is the child immunocompromised?
Does the child have a history of pneumonia, aspiration, or reactive airway disease?

SELECTIVE PHYSICAL EXAMINATION

Are the breath sounds heard equally in all areas of the chest?
Can areas of consolidation be identified by auscultation or percussion?
Are rhonchi, rales, or wheezing heard?
In older children, is egophony or whisper pectoriloquy appreciated?

CHEST RADIOGRAPHIC FINDINGS

Interpretation of chest radiographic findings is critical in a patient with respiratory distress. Pulmonary processes vary in their radiographic appearance and include lobar consolidation (bacterial pneumonia), streaky interstitial markings (bronchiolitis), patchy bilateral alveolar infiltrates (*Mycoplasma*), and pleural effusion. Trust your physical examination. Remember that a volume-depleted child with pneumonia may not manifest a full-blown infiltrate until rehydrated. Early in the course of pneumonia, the chest radiograph may also be unimpressive.

LABORATORY EVALUATION

Especially in infants and small children, one should obtain blood for culture. A complete blood count should be performed, as well as an arterial blood gas determination, for any child in significant distress. A chest radiograph must be ordered for children with severe respiratory distress to assist in determining the cause of the distress. A patient in distress should not be sent to the radiology department; instead, a portable radiograph should be obtained. Sampling sputum is impractical in small children, but in older children sputum should be obtained for Gram stain and culture. Always include tuberculosis (TB) in the differential diagnosis and consider performing a TB skin test with suitable controls if TB is a possibility. In an immunocompromised child one must consider *Pneumocystis carinii* pneumonia and other opportunistic pathogens. Sputum elicited or obtained via bronchoalveolar lavage should be examined with silver stain and immunofluorescence. In infants with bronchiolitis, nasal swabs should be obtained for immunofluorescent assay for respiratory syncytial virus, influenza, parainfluenza, and adenovirus.

TREATMENT
General Measures
* Oxygen

Specific Measures
ANTIBIOTICS. The choice of antibiotic therapy in neonates includes ampicillin and either gentamicin or cefotaxime to cover both gram-positive (*Streptococcus pneumoniae*) and gram-negative (*Escherichia coli, Haemophilus influenzae*) organisms, as well as *Listeria monocytogenes*. In older children, second- and third-generation cephalosporins are commonly used. Erythromycin is necessary for *Mycoplasma pneumoniae*. If aspiration is suspected, gram-negative coverage is very important. Hospital-acquired pneumonia may be caused by *Pseudomonas, Enterobacter,* or *Acinetobacter* species, as well as *Serratia,* especially in the cystic fibrosis population.

P. carinii requires intravenous pentamidine or trimethoprim-sulfamethoxazole (Bactrim). Steroids should be considered for *Pneumocystis* pneumonia.

BRONCHODILATORS. A mainstay of therapy for reactive airway disease, bronchodilators may have some utility in treating lobar bacterial pneumonia but are controversial in bronchiolitis. Nebulizer treatments combined with bronchial hygiene therapy may help loosen inspissated secretions and mucous plugs. Remember that bronchodilators are β_2-agonists but have β_1-activity and result in tachycardia, jitteriness, and sometimes agitation. Albuterol in particular also affects extracellular potassium transport.

STEROIDS. Another mainstay in the treatment of reactive airway disease, steroids have limited application in patients with pneumonia. Children with cystic fibrosis or immunocompromised children suspected of having *Pneumocystis* pneumonia may be considered for steroids.

ANTITUBERCULOSIS REGIMENS. TB must be treated with at least a two-drug regimen and often requires three- or four-drug combinations. Rifampin, isoniazid, ethambutol, pyrazinamide, and streptomycin are recommended in various combinations for extended periods.

Airway Processes

SELECTIVE HISTORY
Is there any history of a sudden choking or coughing spell preceding the respiratory distress?
Has the child's voice changed?
Can the child phonate?

Is there dysphagia or drooling?

Was the onset of respiratory distress sudden?

Was it associated with sudden high fever, chemical or noxious gas inhalation, or neck trauma?

SELECTIVE PHYSICAL EXAMINATION

Can the child swallow?

Is the child drooling?

Does the child hold his or her head in a particular position or assume a "tripod position"?

Is there evidence of a foreign body in the oropharynx?

Is the neck swollen or mobile, and does the child have any cervical adenopathy?

What is the appearance of the pharynx? (*Caution*: If acute suppurative epiglottitis is suspected, examination of the pharynx should occur in the operating room with an anesthesiologist and otolaryngologist present.)

Is the trachea in the midline?

Can the child phonate?

AIRWAY FILMS

A lateral neck film helps evaluate the integrity of the airway from the nasopharynx to the midtrachea. Significant tonsillar or adenoid enlargement, retropharyngeal abscess or cellulitis, epiglottitis, tracheal pseudomembrane, and foreign bodies may be seen. An anteroposterior airway film may show subglottic steepling in parainfluenza (croup), deviation of the trachea, foreign bodies, or external compression of the trachea.

LABORATORY EVALUATION

Febrile infants and children must be handled carefully if epiglottitis is suspected. Laboratory studies should include a complete blood count, blood culture, and possibly an arterial blood gas determination but should be postponed until the airway has been visualized and secured. Because not all foreign bodies are radiopaque, otolaryngology and/or general surgical consultation should be obtained for possible rigid bronchoscopy.

TREATMENT

Disturb a child with suspected epiglottitis as little as possible, and expedite transfer to the operating room for visualization. In other children, give humidified oxygen and consider nebulized epinephrine with or without steroids for subglottic edema if indicated clinically. For suppurative paratracheal processes, broad-spectrum antibiotics should be initiated promptly. Abscesses of the tonsils and retropharynx should be surgically drained as well.

Cardiac Processes

Congestive heart failure in infants and children is most often the result of left-to-right shunts as a consequence of congenital heart disease. Because of pulmonary overcirculation, pulmonary edema develops and respiratory distress gradually ensues.

SELECTIVE HISTORY

Is there a known cardiac defect?
In infants, what is the child's feeding pattern?
How has the child been growing?
Does the child become dyspneic, diaphoretic, and tired with feedings?
What medications does the child take?
Was the onset of symptoms abrupt and associated with pleuritic chest pain?

SELECTIVE PHYSICAL EXAMINATION

General	Assess the child's volume status. Is there fluid overload?
HEENT	Dysmorphic features (high association with congenital heart disease)
Neck	Jugular venous distention (rarely seen in infants and young children)
Chest	Symmetry, precordial activity
Respiratory	Rales, crackles at the bases, pleuritic pain, effusion
Cardiovascular	Location of the point of maximal intensity; abnormal impulses (right ventricular heave, thrills); tachycardia; S_1; S_2, including splitting; S_3; murmurs (systolic and diastolic); clicks, rubs, or gallops; brachial and femoral pulses
Abdomen	Hepatosplenomegaly, hepatojugular reflex, ascites
Extremities	Peripheral edema, thrombophlebitis

The most common congenital defect is a ventricular septal defect, which usually results in a left-to-right shunt. Other lesions can cause pulmonary edema, including patent ductus arteriosus, any of the left-sided obstructive lesions (coarctation, aortic stenosis, mitral stenosis), cardiomyopathies (dilated, hypertrophic, or restrictive), and some dysrhythmias.

CHEST RADIOGRAPHIC FINDINGS

Cardiomegaly (Fig. 28-2)
Increased pulmonary vascular markings
Right-sided aortic arch
Kerley's B lines
Pleural effusion
Pulmonary embolism findings (Fig. 28-3)

LABORATORY EVALUATION

A 12- to 15-lead electrocardiogram should be obtained. If the child is desaturated, a hyperoxia test should be performed (see Chapter 13, Cyanosis). Definitive diagnosis may require cardiology consultation

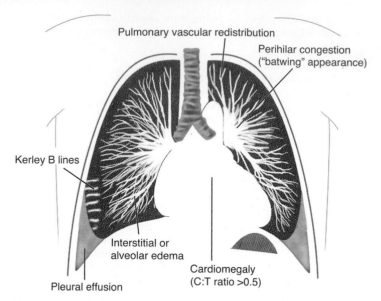

Figure 28–2 Chest radiographic features of congestive heart failure. C:T ratio, cardiac diameter to thoracic diameter. (From Marshall SA, Ruedy J: On Call: Principles and Protocols, 4th ed. Philadelphia, Elsevier, 2004, p 270.)

and an echocardiogram. Serum electrolytes, blood urea nitrogen, and creatinine should be checked to assess hydration status and renal function. If pulmonary embolism is suspected, an arterial blood gas determination is essential. A ventilation-perfusion (V/Q) scan or high-resolution computed tomography (CT) scan is necessary.

TREATMENT

General Measures
- Oxygen
- Elevate the head of the bed 30 degrees

Specific Measures. Frequently, the first response to a child with apparent cardiogenic respiratory distress is to give intravenous or intramuscular furosemide (Lasix). Although this may be indicated in infants and children with left-to-right shunt lesions, it could be disastrous in a child with cardiomyopathy who depends on a high end-diastolic volume or atrial filling pressure to maximize ventricular volume and maintain cardiac output. Therefore, it is imperative to define the child's physiologic features and obtain the cardiac

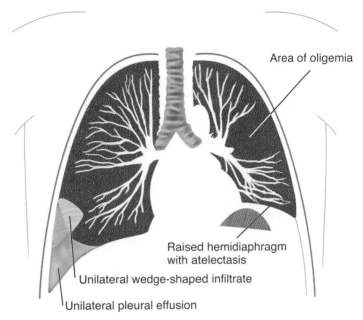

Area of oligemia

Raised hemidiaphragm
with atelectasis

Unilateral wedge-shaped infiltrate

Unilateral pleural effusion

Figure 28–3 Variable chest radiographic features of pulmonary embolism. (From Marshall SA, Ruedy J: On Call: Principles and Protocols, 4th ed. Philadelphia, Elsevier, 2004, p 274.)

diagnosis underlying the respiratory compromise before empirically treating with a diuretic.

If the child has known cardiac disease and is receiving diuretic therapy, an intravenous dose can be administered to augment diuresis. If a dilated cardiomyopathy is the problem, inotropic support is necessary, and diuretics may initially be contraindicated. Mitral regurgitation may be helped by reduction of systemic afterload.

Pericardial tamponade is a life-threatening emergency that is frequently manifested as respiratory distress with left chest and shoulder pain and coughing. Orthopnea is marked. Drainage of the pericardium, ideally via a catheter placed under echocardiographic guidance, is necessary.

In a crisis one may acutely decompress the pericardium as follows. First, the area of the xyphoid is prepared in sterile fashion. The skin and subcutaneous tissues should be anesthetized with 1% lidocaine. A No. 18 or 20 angiocatheter can then be placed on a three-way stopcock and attached to a 20-mL syringe. The angiocatheter is inserted lateral to the xyphoid, aiming for the left shoulder and aspirating as it is inserted. Watch the electrocardiographic monitor for signs of ectopy. If straw-colored fluid or thin bloody fluid is obtained, the catheter should be threaded fully and the needle withdrawn. The stopcock can then be attached directly to the catheter and the fluid aspirated. If blood is obtained again, check for ventricular ectopy and for pulsatile flow. If you suspect that you have entered the right ventricle, remove the apparatus and be prepared to give volume replacement. Obviously, placement of sharp objects very close to a beating heart is to be done carefully.

If pulmonary embolism is suspected, anticoagulation therapy must be started immediately. Be certain that the child has no contraindications to anticoagulant therapy, such as a history of a coagulopathy, previous stroke, peptic ulcer disease, or bleeding disorder. A baseline complete blood count, activated partial thromboplastin time (aPTT), prothrombin time, and platelet count must be obtained. Heparin is the mainstay of initial therapy and should be started with a 100-U/kg bolus, followed by an infusion of 15 to 25 U/kg/hr. The aPTT must be monitored closely and the heparin infusion adjusted to maintain the aPTT at 1.5 to 2 times baseline. Thrombolytic therapy is much higher risk and requires transfer to the PICU and consultation with both cardiology and cardiovascular surgery specialists.

Space-Occupying Processes

SELECTIVE HISTORY
  Does the patient complain of pleuritic pain?
  Was the onset gradual or sudden?
  Is the patient febrile?
  Has the patient ever had symptoms like this before?
  In a newborn, could this be a congenital diaphragmatic hernia?

SELECTIVE PHYSICAL EXAMINATION
  Is the trachea in the midline?
  Do both sides of the chest move together?
  Is there obvious splinting?
  Is there evidence of massive ascites or other abdominal processes
    that are limiting diaphragmatic excursion?
  Is there a pleural rub?
  Are the breath sounds equal right and left?
  Is the abdomen scaphoid?

CHEST RADIOGRAPHIC FINDINGS
  Pleural effusion
  Empyema
  Pneumothorax
  Intrathoracic masses, including the mediastinum
  Severe scoliosis

Massive ascites
Diaphragmatic hernia

LABORATORY EVALUATION

Thoracentesis may be indicated for diagnosis, as well as therapy. Arterial blood gases should be monitored in children with severe distress. Pleural and/or mediastinal masses require chest CT scanning and/or magnetic resonance imaging once the child's airway and breathing are secure. Pneumothoraces frequently require evacuation; at the least, the area should be prepared in sterile fashion and anesthetized. A pleural tap for a pneumothorax should be performed in the second intercostal space at the midclavicular line and the needle or catheter directed a bit laterally. Thoracostomy tube placement requires deeper anesthesia to the pleura (see Chapter 26, Lines, Tubes, and Drains).

Special Section on Asthma

Asthma is one of the most common admitting diagnoses in pediatrics. As a result, there is often a tendency to become complacent regarding the risk for decompensation in these children. Remember, asthma can cause respiratory distress very quickly.

SELECTIVE HISTORY

Did the child's condition suddenly become worse?
Has the child ever required intubation?
Are there any obvious precipitating factors?
Is this an anaphylactic reaction?
What are the child's current medications?

SELECTIVE PHYSICAL EXAMINATION

Is there evidence of acute airway obstruction?

Vital signs	Pulsus paradoxus
HEENT	Cyanosis
Neck	Midline trachea, jugular venous distention
Respiratory	Retractions, flaring, prolonged expiration, abnormal inspiratory-expiratory ratio, hyperinflation, wheezing, aeration, consolidation

CHEST RADIOGRAPHIC FINDINGS

Hyperinflation
Pneumothorax or pneumomediastinum
Flattened diaphragm
Atelectasis, infiltrates

LABORATORY EVALUATION

Arterial blood gases are very important in the assessment of an asthmatic patient who has deteriorated acutely. Pulse oximetry studies may be falsely reassuring when the patient's Pco_2 has begun to rise, which is indicative of impending respiratory failure.

TREATMENT

General Measures

- Oxygen
- Intravenous hydration

Specific Measures. The initial response should be nebulizer treatments with β-agonists (albuterol, 2.5 to 5 mg in 3 mL of normal saline solution) as often as necessary or even continuously. The anticholinergic agent ipratropium bromide, 0.5 mL in 3 mL of normal saline solution, may also be given via nebulizer in conjunction with albuterol. Side effects from either are obviously greater with an increased frequency of treatments.

Intravenous steroids should be given immediately (2 mg/kg methylprednisolone). Steroids should be continued every 4 hours initially at a dose of 1 mg/kg methylprednisolone.

In patients who remain in significant distress, xanthines, such as aminophylline or theophylline, can be used. An initial bolus of 6 mg/kg should be followed by a continuous infusion of 1.0 mg/kg/hr. Serum levels should be monitored closely until a steady state is achieved. Higher levels may cause nausea, vomiting, tachycardia, chest pains, headache, and irritability. Be careful when also giving erythromycin, cimetidine, β-blockers, allopurinol, and other drugs that may potentiate xanthine drug effects or affect serum levels.

Additional treatment may include intubation and mechanical ventilation, intravenous ketamine, and magnesium sulfate. Consultation with the critical care staff and transfer to the PICU will be necessary at the point that these measures are considered.

WARNING SIGNS IN ASTHMA

1. Sudden acute deterioration may signal the development of pneumothorax.
2. A rising P_{CO_2} in the face of maximal therapy portends respiratory failure. Arterial blood gases must be monitored closely.
3. The disappearance of wheezing is not always a good sign. Lack of wheezing may reflect lack of air exchange and indicate respiratory failure.
4. A sleepy patient with asthma is a worrisome patient. Because sedatives are contraindicated and both β-agonists and xanthines are stimulants, most patients will be hyperalert or agitated.
5. Rarely, there is a triad of asthma, nasal polyps, and aspirin hypersensitivity. Avoid aspirin and nonsteroidal anti-inflammatory drugs whenever possible in patients with asthma because fatal anaphylactoid reactions have been described.

Respiratory Failure

Any of the aforementioned conditions may lead to respiratory failure. Bradypnea (<20 breaths per minute), thoracoabdominal dissociation,

CO_2 retention, profound hypoxemia, and profound respiratory acidosis all imply respiratory failure.

1. Ensure that the patient has not received or is not receiving any respiratory depressant, especially narcotics, barbiturates, and benzodiazepines. Do not hesitate to give naloxone hydrochloride (Narcan), 0.2 to 2.0 mg intravenously, if opiates are suspected.

2. Notify the PICU early of a patient in distress. Direct therapy to the underlying causes of the respiratory problem, and assist ventilation and oxygenation as indicated. Acute respiratory acidosis frequently requires mechanical ventilatory support until the underlying cause is addressed.

REMEMBER

1. Abdominal problems may cause significant respiratory distress and compromise.

2. Do not be worried about your inexperience with endotracheal intubation. Unless there is severe upper airway obstruction, most patients can be effectively ventilated for an extended time with a bag-valve-mask unit until help and more hands arrive.

3. Even though respiratory distress is a very common cause of calls in the middle of the night, **it is essential to monitor patients frequently to make sure that they are responding appropriately to your treatment so that you can make changes in treatment as indicated.**

Seizures

James J. Nocton, MD

When a seizure unexpectedly develops, the sudden and often dramatic nature of the event has a tendency to create a sense of crisis among parents, other family members, nurses, and house officers. Everyone will feel a need to "do something" and to do it quickly to stop the seizure. The first order of business when you are called is to remain calm and recognize that although a seizure needs to be addressed immediately, the urgency to "do something" should not lead you to act reflexively or irrationally. There is time to organize your thoughts and develop a plan for further evaluation and treatment that is best for the patient. Remember, almost all seizures are paroxysmal events with abrupt onset, are variable in length but usually brief (minutes), and are generally self-limited. Careful attention to the airway, breathing, and circulation (ABCs) is often all that is initially necessary because this will maintain cerebral blood flow and oxygenation while you consider the need for further treatment or diagnostic tests.

PHONE CALL

Questions

1. Is the child still seizing?
2. What was witnessed? Ask the nurse to describe what happened. Was it generalized or focal, tonic-clonic, or just tonic? (Was the event actually a seizure and not merely a startle response or myoclonus?)
3. What was the patient's level of consciousness?
4. Was the event associated with apnea, cyanosis, or loss of bladder or bowel control?
5. What is the child's admitting diagnosis?
6. Is the child febrile?

Orders

1. Ask the nurse to see that the child is positioned on his or her side.

2. Ask the nurse to maintain seizure precautions, including suctioning and oxygen supplies at the bedside, padded bedrails, a properly sized oral airway at the bedside, and intravenous (IV) lorazepam readily available.
3. If the child does not have an IV line in place, ask the nurse to have the supplies at the bedside.
4. Ask the nurse to obtain a full set of vital signs immediately.
5. Check a Dextrostix.

Inform RN

"Will arrive at the bedside in ... minutes." Seizures require immediate evaluation.

ELEVATOR THOUGHTS

Did the child have a seizure?
    Remember that several conditions can mimic seizures, including breath-holding spells, syncope, chorea, narcolepsy, benign myoclonus, night terrors, and pseudoseizures. Your first task will be to determine the likelihood that the child experienced a seizure. You should be able to do this after your telephone discussion with the nurse.

What causes seizures?
    There are several types of seizures (Table 29-1) and an even longer list of potential causes (Table 29-2).

MAJOR THREAT TO LIFE

• Aspiration
• Hypoxemia
The majority of seizures will have stopped by the time you arrive at the child's bedside. Advise the nurse to try to position the child on his or her side to discourage airway obstruction or aspiration during the postictal state. Patients are rarely apneic during a seizure. Children can usually withstand status epilepticus for up to 30 minutes with no subsequent neurologic damage. The procedures to follow if the seizure has stopped are discussed subsequently, as are those for status epilepticus.

BEDSIDE

If the Seizure Has Stopped

Quick-Look Test

Does the patient appear well (comfortable), sick (uncomfortable or distressed), or critical (about to die)?

TABLE 29–1 **Classification of Epileptic Seizures and Some Epileptic Syndromes**

Clinical Seizure Type	Epileptic Syndrome
Partial Seizures	
Simple partial (consciousness not impaired) Motor signs	Benign focal epilepsy Juvenile myoclonic epilepsy
Special sensory (visual, auditory, olfactory, gustatory, vertiginous, or somatosensory) Autonomic Psychic (déjà vu, fear, and others)	West's syndrome Lennox-Gastaut syndrome Acquired epileptic aphasia Benign neonatal convulsions
Complex partial (consciousness impaired) Impaired consciousness at onset Development of impaired consciousness	
Generalized Seizures	
Absence Typical Atypical Tonic-clonic Atonic Myoclonic Tonic Clonic	
Unclassified	
Neonatal	

From Behrman RE, Kliegman R (eds): Nelson Essentials of Pediatrics, 2nd ed. Philadelphia, WB Saunders, 1994, p 681.

Most children have a period of postictal unresponsiveness after a generalized tonic-clonic seizure. Prolonged depression of mental status is ominous and requires prompt evaluation with head computed tomography (CT) or magnetic resonance imaging (MRI). A child in shock must be stabilized while addressing the seizure.

Airway and Vital Signs

In what position is the child lying?

The patient should be positioned in the left lateral decubitus position to prevent aspiration of vomited gastric contents (Fig. 29-1). If the child is unresponsive but adequately ventilating, it is prudent to insert an oral airway. (An awake child does not tolerate an airway, so be prepared to remove it as the child awakens.) Oxygen should be given via nasal prongs or face mask. Have the nurse obtain a repeat set of vital signs, again with a pulse oximeter saturation.

TABLE 29–2 Etiology of Seizures

Perinatal Conditions
Cerebral malformation
Intrauterine infection
Hypoxia-ischemia*
Trauma
Hemorrhage*

Infections
Encephalitis*
Meningitis*
Brain abscess

Metabolic Conditions
Hypoglycemia*
Hypocalcemia
Hypomagnesemia
Hyponatremia
Hypernatremia
Storage diseases
Reye's syndrome
Degenerative disorders
Porphyria
Pyridoxine dependency (deficiency)

Poisoning
Lead
Drugs
Drug withdrawal

Neurocutaneous Syndromes
Tuberous sclerosis
Neurofibromatosis
Sturge-Weber syndrome
Klippel-Trenaunay-Weber syndrome
Linear sebaceous nevus
Incontinentia pigmenti

Systemic Disorders
Vasculitis (central nervous system or systemic)
Systemic lupus erythematosus
Hypertensive encephalopathy
Renal failure
Hepatic encephalopathy

Other
Trauma*
Tumor
Febrile*
Idiopathic*
Familial

*Common.
From Behrman RE, Kliegman R (eds): Nelson Essentials of Pediatrics, 2nd ed. Philadelphia, WB Saunders, 1994, p 681.

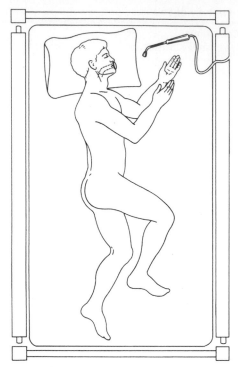

Figure 29–1 Positioning of the patient to prevent aspiration of gastric contents. (From Marshall SA, Ruedy J: On Call: Principles and Protocols, 4th ed. Philadelphia, Elsevier, 2004, p 254.)

What is the Dextrostix result?

Hypoglycemia may be rapidly treated, and raising the serum glucose level may prevent further hypoglycemic seizures.

Management I

Once you have established that the event was likely to be a seizure, establish IV access, and draw blood for the following studies: electrolytes, glucose, magnesium, calcium, blood urea nitrogen, creatinine, and serum levels of any anticonvulsant medications that the child may be taking. A toxicology screen and a serum lead level should also be considered. A complete blood count should be obtained, as well as a blood culture if the child is younger than 4 years and has a significant fever. A venous pH determination should be made after any prolonged seizure, and an arterial blood gas determination should be considered and obtained if any respiratory compromise is evident. If encephalitis or meningitis is a consideration because of the presence of fever or other signs and symptoms, a lumbar puncture with cerebrospinal fluid analysis and culture will be necessary.

Selective Physical Examination I

Mental status	Assess the response to verbal, tactile, and painful stimuli. Altered level of consciousness is discussed in Chapter 7, Altered Mental Status
Airway	Check body position, airway patency, and quality of breath sounds

Selective History and Chart Review

Was the event witnessed? Ask witnesses about the characteristics and duration of the seizure.

Was it generalized tonic-clonic or focal?

Did the seizure start focally or was it generalized?

Did the child suffer any injury as a result of the seizure (head trauma, tongue or lip trauma, bruises or lacerations on the extremities)?

Is the child normally receiving anticonvulsants or any other medications that might lower the child's seizure threshold?

What were the child's most recent laboratory results? Quickly review the child's chart before a more complete physical examination.

Selective Physical Examination II

Mental status	Assess whether the child has lost consciousness. Does the child respond to verbal, tactile, or painful stimuli? Is the child in a postictal state?
HEENT	Test the cranial nerves; again assure yourself that the child can defend his or her airway (gag reflex), and check the airway position (Fig. 29-2). Look for a potential source of infection in febrile patients (e.g., otitis, sinusitis). Any children who have had a seizure must have their fundi examined thoroughly, with dilation of the pupils if necessary, especially in infants (to look for retinal hemorrhages, as well as evidence of papilledema)
Neck	Nuchal rigidity
Lungs	Signs of aspiration (crackles, decreased breath sounds)
Neurologic	Complete neurologic examination within the limits of the child's level of consciousness, including reflexes, motor and sensory function, cerebellar function, visual fields, and short- and long-term memory

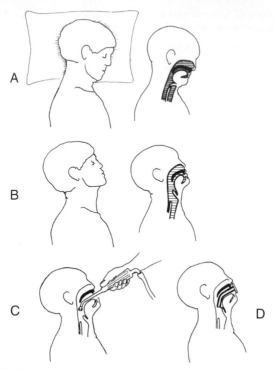

Figure 29–2 Airway management: correct positioning of the head, correct suctioning, and correct insertion of an oral airway. **A,** Neck flexion closes the airway. **B,** Neck extension to the sniffing position opens the airway. **C,** Suctioning. **D,** Placement of the airway. (From Marshall SA, Ruedy J: On Call: Principles and Protocols, 4th ed. Philadelphia, Elsevier, 2004, p 255.)

Miscellaneous	Check for oral and/or scalp lacerations, passive range of joint mobility, bruising, and other signs of injury incurred during the seizure

Management II

Given the history, one should establish a preliminary or provisional differential diagnosis. Remember that seizures are a symptom, not a diagnosis, and therefore there must be an underlying condition that is manifested by the seizure. **Your job is to find and treat the underlying condition**. In children, even hospitalized children, fever is a common underlying cause of seizures. It is thought that the rapidity with which the temperature rises precipitates the seizure activity. It may be difficult, however, to determine whether a febrile child with a seizure has simply had a "febrile seizure" or has had a seizure secondary to meningitis, encephalitis, or brain abscess. When this distinction cannot be made, it is necessary to perform a lumbar puncture to rule out meningitis. CT or MRI may be necessary before lumbar puncture to rule out cerebral edema and increased intracranial pressure.

Any child with an abnormal neurologic examination after a seizure should also have an imaging procedure (CT or MRI) performed to rule out tumor, edema, or other space-occupying lesions (arteriovenous malformation, abscess) as a cause of the seizure.

Remember also that there can be complications secondary to seizures, such as aspiration and trauma, especially to the head. Seizure precautions should be ordered immediately whenever an inpatient suffers a seizure.

In a hospitalized child who has a first-time seizure, it is usually prudent to maintain IV access but to withhold anticonvulsant therapy if the seizure is not prolonged and some readily identifiable underlying cause is apparent. Exceptions include a patient with a known seizure disorder who has a subtherapeutic serum anticonvulsant level. This, in fact, is the most common cause of in-hospital seizures in children. Other patients who warrant anticonvulsant therapy are victims of head injuries, children with central nervous system tumors, and those with known cerebrovascular accidents. Remember that benzodiazepines, such as diazepam (Valium) and lorazepam (Ativan), are useful in stopping status epilepticus but have no role in preventing recurrent events. The choice of anticonvulsant depends in part on the type of seizure and the age of the child. Anticonvulsant therapy should be discussed with a child neurologist (Table 29-3)

If the Child Is Still Seizing

Don't panic! Most seizures resolve spontaneously and last no more than several minutes. (This, of course, is an eternity to the child's parents and often the nurses.) Therefore, busy yourself with evaluating the child's ABCs. The child needs the evaluation, and it calms the parents to see that "something" is being done.

Quick-Look Test

Does the child appear well (comfortable), sick (uncomfortable or distressed), or critical (about to die)?
A generalized tonic-clonic seizure is a disconcerting event to witness. However, one should be reassured that a child who is seizing has both a heart rate and a blood pressure. Still, remember your limitations (a seizure *is* a medical emergency), and have a nurse page your senior resident immediately. You should not deal with a seizure alone if you do not absolutely have to do so. If there is clonic activity of the extremities, gently hold the extremity to see whether you can suppress the activity. If so, it is not seizure activity.

TABLE 29–3 Common Anticonvulsant Drugs

Drug	Seizure Type	Oral Dose	Loading Dose (IV)	Therapeutic Serum Level (µg/mL)	Side Effects and Toxicity
Carbamazepine (Tegretol)	Generalized tonic-clonic Partial	Begin 10 mg/kg/24 hr tid Increase to 20-30 mg/kg/24 hr tid	—	8-12	Dizziness, drowsiness, diplopia, liver dysfunction, anemia, neutropenia, SIADH, blood dyscrasias rare, hepatotoxic effects
*Clobazam (Frisium)	Adjunctive therapy when seizures poorly controlled	0.25-1 mg/kg/24 hr bid or tid	—	—	Dizziness, fatigue, weight gain, ataxia, behavioral problems
Clonazepam (Rivotril)	Absence Myoclonic Infantile spasms Partial Lennox-Gastaut Akinetic	Children <30 kg: Begin 0.05 mg/kg/24 hr Increase by 0.05 mg/kg/wk Maximum, 0.2 mg/kg/24 hr bid or tid Children >30 kg: 1.5 mg/kg/24 hr tid Not to exceed 20 mg/24 hr	—	>0.013	Drowsiness, irritability, agitation, behavioral abnormalities, depression, excessive salivation
Ethosuximide (Zarontin)	Absence May increase tonic-clonic seizures	Begin 20 mg/kg/24 hr Increase to maximum of 40 mg/kg/24 hr or 1.5 g/24 hr, whichever is less	—	40-100	Abdominal discomfort, rash, liver dysfunction, leukopenia

Gabapentin (Neurontin)	Adjunctive therapy when seizures poorly controlled	Children: 20-50 mg/kg/24 hr tid Adolescents: 900-3600 mg/24 hr tid	—	Not necessary to monitor	Somnolence, dizziness, ataxia, headache, tremor, vomiting, nystagmus, fatigue, weight gain
Lamotrigine (Lamictal)	Adjunctive therapy when seizures poorly controlled Broad-spectrum anticonvulsant activity in various seizure types, including complex partial, absence, myoclonic, clonic, tonic-clonic, and Lennox-Gastaut	Individualized based on age and additional anticonvulsants	—		Rash, dizziness, ataxia, somnolence, diplopia, headache, nausea, vomiting
*Nitrazepam (Mogadon)	Absence Myoclonic Infantile spasms	Begin 0.2 mg/kg/24 hr Increase slowly to 1 mg/kg/24 hr tid	—		Similar to clonazepam, hallucinations

Continued

TABLE 29–3 Common Anticonvulsant Drugs—Cont'd

Drug	Seizure Type	Oral Dose	Loading Dose (IV)	Therapeutic Serum Level (μg/mL)	Side Effects and Toxicity
Phenobarbital	Generalized tonic-clonic Partial Status epilepticus	3-5 mg/kg/24 hr bid	20 mg/kg 20-30 mg/kg in neonates	15-40	Hyperactivity, irritability, short attention span, temper tantrums, altered sleep pattern, Stevens-Johnson syndrome, depression of cognitive function
Phenytoin (Dilantin)	Generalized tonic-clonic Partial Status epilepticus	3-9 mg/kg/24 hr bid	20 mg/kg	10-20	Hirsutism, gum hypertrophy, ataxia, rash, Stevens-Johnson syndrome, nystagmus, nausea, vomiting, drowsiness, coarsening facial features, blood dyscrasias
Primidone (Mysoline)	Generalized tonic-clonic Partial	Children <8 yr: 10-25 mg/kg/24 hr tid or qid Children >8 yr: usual maintenance dose, 750-1500 mg/24 hr tid or qid	—	5-12	Aggressive behavior, personality changes, similar to phenobarbital

Drug	Indications	Dose	Comments	Therapeutic Level	Side Effects
Topiramate (Topamax)	Adjunctive therapy for poorly controlled seizures Refractory complex partial seizures	1-9 mg/kg/24 hr bid	—	—	Fatigue, cognitive depression
Tiagabine (Gabitril)	Adjunctive therapy for complex partial seizures	Average dose, 6 mg tid	—	—	Asthenia, dizziness, poor attention span, nervousness, tremor
Valproic acid (Depakene, Epival)	Generalized tonic-clonic Absence Myoclonic Partial Akinetic	Begin 10 mg/kg/24 hr Increase by 5-10 mg/kg/wk Usual dose, 30-60 mg/kg/24 hr tid or qid	Intravenous preparation now available Studies in children under way	50-100	Nausea, vomiting, anorexia, amenorrhea, sedation, tremor, weight gain, alopecia, hepatotoxicity
*Vigabatrin (Sabril)	Infantile spasms Adjunctive therapy for poorly controlled seizures	Begin 30 mg/kg/24 hr once daily or bid Maintenance dose, 30-100 mg/kg/24 hr once daily or bid	—	—	Hyperactivity, agitation, excitement, somnolence, weight gain Note: Reports of visual field constriction, optic pallor or atrophy, and optic neuritis

*Not available in the United States.

bid, twice daily; D₅W, 5% dextrose in water; qid, four times daily; SIADH, syndrome of inappropriate secretion of antidiuretic hormone; tid, three times daily.

From Behrman RE: Nelson Textbook of Pediatrics, 17th ed. Philadelphia, Elsevier, 2004, p 2001.

Airway and Vital Signs

In what position is the patient?

If at all possible, the child should be positioned in the lateral decubitus position with suction readily available to prevent aspiration of gastric contents. Be prepared to restrain the child gently but firmly to prevent traumatic injury. Patency of the airway should be the first concern, followed by adequacy of ventilation. Apply oxygen by mask or nasal prongs.

What are the child's vital signs?

Tachycardia is expected with a seizure. It is virtually impossible to obtain an accurate cuff blood pressure reading during a tonic-clonic seizure. The child's perfusion tells as much as a blood pressure reading fraught with inaccuracy. A Dextrostix assessment is indicated because hypoglycemia commonly results in seizures (and is easily corrected).

Management I

How long has the child been seizing?

See earlier if the seizure has already stopped. If the seizure has lasted more than 3 minutes, first check the child's ABCs. Closely observe the seizure. Be sure that IV supplies are at hand if the child does not have a working IV line. Do not try to obtain IV access in a seizing patient unless it is absolutely necessary. Remember, the seizure is likely to be over in 2 to 3 minutes. Also remember that the antecubital fossa becomes a less attractive site for IV access in a patient who involuntarily flexes at the elbow. A hand, forearm, or saphenous site will be a better choice.

MEDICATIONS

Status epilepticus is defined as general or partial seizures lasting longer than 30 minutes without the patient regaining consciousness. Before administering any medication, remember that all anticonvulsants can depress the child's level of consciousness and respiratory drive. It is best to have airway support equipment at hand, including suctioning supplies, Ambu bag, appropriately sized masks, and a laryngoscopy tray. If the child has been seizing for 5 minutes, begin to prepare airway support equipment, administer an IV glucose bolus (5 mL/kg of 10% dextrose in water [$D_{10}W$]), change the IV solution to normal saline, and have anticonvulsant doses readied. Often, this process requires enough time for the seizure to stop spontaneously. In any case, most clinicians agree that treatment should probably be initiated after 10 to 15 minutes of continuous seizure activity. Do not let the presence of a frantic parent or nurse force you into treating the child pharmacologically before you are ready and comfortable doing so. The treatment is not without complications, and the risks of treatment should be considered along with the benefits.

The most important principle of anticonvulsant therapy is to choose a drug and use enough. Small doses of multiple drugs may be ineffective. Use full loading doses and do not administer additional drugs until you have reached the maximum recommended dose.

Diazepam and lorazepam are effective immediately in most children for tonic-clonic seizures. Diazepam has a short half-life, and seizures will tend to recur unless a longer-acting anticonvulsant is also administered. The starting dose of diazepam should be 0.1 to 0.3 mg/kg per dose intravenously (single-dose maximum of 5 mg for children younger than 5 years, 10 mg for children older than 5 years). This may be repeated every 10 to 15 minutes to a maximum of three doses. Lorazepam has the benefit of longer duration of action and is less likely than diazepam to result in hypotension and respiratory depression. An IV dose of 0.05 to 0.1 mg/kg of lorazepam should be used.

If an IV line cannot be established, both diazepam and lorazepam can be given rectally. The rectal dose of diazepam is 0.3 to 0.5 mg/kg diluted in 3 mL of normal saline. A rectal diazepam gel in standard doses of 2.5, 5, and 10 mg is now available. The rectal and IV doses of lorazepam are identical.

Phenytoin should be used next and is generally begun at a loading dose of 15 to 20 mg/kg at an infusion rate no faster than 1 mg/kg/min. All patients should be on a cardiorespiratory monitor when receiving phenytoin because of the risk for dysrhythmias. If bradycardia or hypotension results, the infusion must be slowed. The prodrug fosphenytoin has been used increasingly because it is more water soluble and less irritating when administered intravenously. If seizure activity persists, another dose of phenytoin may be given, up to a 25 mg/kg *total* loading dose. Remember that phenytoin forms a precipitate with glucose solutions and must therefore be administered in saline solution.

Phenobarbital is often the second-line drug for status epilepticus. The loading dose is 15 to 25 mg/kg infused no faster than 1 mg/kg/min. Monitor vital signs, especially respirations and pulse oximetry values. After phenobarbital loading, the child may remain sedated for a period of hours.

Persistent status seizure activity despite the administration of three anticonvulsants warrants transfer to the intensive care unit for the administration of a continuous diazepam infusion, general anesthetics (pentobarbital coma), or IV paraldehyde, 150 to 200 mg/kg slowly over a 15- to 20-minute period, followed by a continuous IV infusion of 20 mg/kg/hr. The use of paraldehyde rectally or intramuscularly is discouraged.

Once the child is no longer in status epilepticus, maintenance therapy depends on the type of seizure (see Table 29-3). Consultation with a pediatric neurologist is recommended, especially to help educate the family about seizure disorders, prognosis, and medication management. Further evaluation, including lumbar puncture, MRI or CT, or electroencephalography, may need to be pursued.

SUMMARY

Seizures are upsetting for all who witness them. The specific characteristics of the episode will help you determine whether the patient has in fact had a seizure and, if so, what type of seizure occurred. Because most seizures last less than 5 minutes, the most important emergency intervention is to prevent secondary injury, aspiration, and respiratory compromise. Remember to address the ABCs before proceeding to pharmacologic seizure management. In most cases the seizure will end before medications are administered. Status epilepticus is continuous seizure activity without regaining consciousness for 30 minutes. Treatment of status epilepticus should include the following, in order: address the ABCs; administer glucose intravenously; administer diazepam or lorazepam; administer phenytoin or fosphenytoin; administer phenobarbital; and transfer to the pediatric intensive care unit for respiratory support and further management, such as continuous diazepam infusion, pentobarbital, or paraldehyde.

Urine Output Abnormalities

Thomas H. Nichols, MD

Urine output abnormalities can be a challenging problem despite the fact that there are only two options: too little urine or too much. The challenge comes from the wide range of factors that influence urine output, including hydration status, cardiac output, intrinsic renal function, and urologic patency, to name a few. Because monitoring urine output is a useful way of assessing multiple factors and organ systems, it is usually closely measured by the nurses in all pediatric hospitalized patients. It is therefore common for the pediatric resident to be called regarding too little or too much urine output.

PHONE CALL

Questions

1. How old is the patient?
2. How much does the child weigh?
3. Why is the patient in the hospital?
4. How much urine has the patient produced in the last 24 hours?
5. How much fluid has the child taken in or been given over the last 24 hours?
6. What are the vital signs?
7. What is the child's admitting diagnosis?
8. When did the child last have an electrolyte panel checked?

Orders

1. Have the nurse total the amount of fluids in and out for the last 24-hour period and the day or night before that.
2. If the child has an indwelling Foley catheter and decreased urine output, ask the nurse to check the catheter for patency and flush the catheter with 10 to 20 mL of normal saline solution if necessary (see Chapter 26, Lines, Tubes, and Drains).
3. Order serum electrolyte, blood urea nitrogen (BUN), and creatinine determinations and urinalysis (pH and specific gravity).

4. If the child does not have an intravenous (IV) line, ask the RN to have an IV line started or to assemble the appropriate IV supplies for you.

5. If the child is receiving IV fluids and has decreased urine output, any potassium in the IV fluid should be removed or at least reduced. The rate of the IV fluids should be adjusted carefully in response to the urine output.

Inform RN

"Will arrive at the bedside in ... minutes."

Decreased urine output deserves fairly prompt evaluation because it can be a sign of decreased cardiac output, dehydration, or renal failure. Increased urine output also demands evaluation promptly, especially in neonates, infants, and small children. Keep in mind that decreased urine output in neonates may result from congenital anomalies of the genitourinary tract.

ELEVATOR THOUGHTS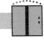

Decreased Urine Output

What are the causes?

Reduced cardiac output (prerenal)	Volume depletion
	Heart failure
	Cardiomyopathy
	Pericardial effusion
	Shock
Renal causes	Tubulointerstitial problems (acute tubulonecrosis, nephrotoxic drugs)
	Hemolytic-uremic syndrome
	Hemoglobinuria, myoglobinuria
	Acute crystalline nephropathy (oxalosis, hyperuricemia)
	Glomerulonephritis
	Renal artery thrombosis
	Renal artery embolization
Postrenal causes	Ureteropelvic junction (UPJ) obstruction
	Nephrolithiasis
	Bilateral ureteral obstruction
	Bladder outlet obstruction (blocked Foley catheter, urethral trauma, posterior urethral valves)
	Neurogenic bladder
	Syndrome of inappropriate antidiuretic hormone (SIADH) production (meningitis, trauma)

Increased Urine Output

What are the causes?
Urinary tract infection
Central diabetes insipidus (DI)
Diuretic use
Distal tubular dysfunction
Nephrogenic DI
High-output phase of acute tubular necrosis
Proximal tubular dysfunction
Aminoaciduria (cystinuria, Hartnup disease)
Familial hypophosphatemic rickets (vitamin D–refractory rickets)
Diabetes mellitus
Psychogenic polydipsia

MAJOR THREAT TO LIFE

- Renal failure
- Hyperkalemia
- Urosepsis

Decreased urine output for any cause can become a self-perpetuating situation, with progressive renal insufficiency leading to renal failure. Hyperkalemia is the most serious and life-threatening complication of renal insufficiency because of its high association with cardiac dysrhythmias.

BEDSIDE

Quick-Look Test

Does the patient appear well (comfortable), sick (uncomfortable or distressed), or critical (about to die)?
Sick or critical-appearing children usually have advanced renal failure. An uncomfortable child may have a distended bladder, flank pain, and/or cramps. Children with serious renal problems frequently appear deceptively well.

Airway and Vital Signs

Check for postural changes and signs of dehydration. A postural rise in heart rate greater than 15 beats per minute, a fall in systolic blood pressure greater than 15 mm Hg, or any decrease in diastolic pressure suggests significant hypovolemia. Baseline tachycardia is frequently a nonspecific indicator of volume depletion and/or stress. Fever suggests an infectious cause. Hypertension is suggestive of a renal artery problem or glomerulonephritis.

Selective Physical Examination

Approach the physical examination with prerenal, renal, and postrenal causes of decreased renal output in mind. Tachycardia, delayed capillary refill, and dry mucous membranes suggest intravascular depletion and thus a prerenal cause. Edema and hypertension suggest a renal cause, and a tender, distended bladder suggests a postrenal cause of decreased urine output.

HEENT	Icterus (hepatorenal syndrome), facial purpura and macroglossia (amyloidosis), periorbital edema (nephrotic syndrome), mucous membranes (dry or moist?)
Respiratory	Crackles, rales, dullness to percussion
Cardiovascular	Pulse rate and quality, capillary refill
Abdomen	Enlarged kidneys (horseshoe kidney, UPJ obstruction, polycystic kidney), bladder fullness (bladder outlet obstruction), bladder tenderness, flank or costovertebral angle tenderness
Rectal	Enlarged prostate (rare in children)
Genitourinary	Hypospadias
Pelvic (if indicated)	Cervical and/or adnexal masses (UPJ obstruction)
Skin	Morbilliform rash, purpura, bruising, turgor, jaundice
Extremities	Peripheral edema (nephrotic syndrome, renal failure)

Selective Chart Review

Does the child have a past history of urinary tract infection, vesicoureteral reflux, instrumentation, or trauma to the genitourinary tract?

Are there other congenital anomalies?

Has the child any history of renal failure?

What is the admitting diagnosis?

What medications is the child receiving?

Does the child have a condition that could lead to SIADH?

Has the child had laboratory studies recently that could indicate a prerenal, renal, or postrenal cause of decreased urine output?

What has been the child's fluid intake for the past 48 hours?

What was the urine output trend for the past 48 hours—was the decrease in urine output sudden or gradual?

A BUN-creatinine ratio greater than 20 suggests a prerenal cause, as does a urine specific gravity greater than 1.020 or a urine sodium level less than 20 mmol/L. Table 30-1 illustrates laboratory differences in children with prerenal, renal, and postrenal insufficiency.

If urine output is excessive, a form of DI may be the reason. Central DI may result from traumatic head injury, be a consequence of hypoxic-ischemic brain injury, or be a complication of meningitis or encephalitis. Nephrogenic DI may be primary (a rare X-linked recessive condition) or secondary to acute or chronic renal failure

TABLE 30–1 Laboratory Differential Diagnosis of Renal Insufficiency

	Prerenal		Renal		Postrenal
	Child	Neonate	Child	Neonate	
Urine Na+ (mEq/L)	<20	<20-30	>40	>40	Variable, may be >40
FE_Na * (%)	<1	<2-5	>2	>2-5	Variable, may be >2
Urine osmolality (mOsm/L)	>500	>300-50C	≈300	≈300	Variable, may be <300
RFI† (%)	<1	<2-5	>2	>2-5	Variable
Serum BUN-creatinine ratio	>20	≥10	≈10	>10	Variable, may be >20
Response to volume	Diuresis		No change	No change	No change
Response to furosemide	Diuresis		No change	No change	No change or diuresis
Urinalysis	Normal		RBC, WBC, casts, proteinuria		Variable or normal
Comments	Hx: diarrhea, vomiting, hemorrhage, diuretics		Hx: hypotension, anoxia, exposure to nephrotoxins		Hx: poor urine stream or output
	Px: volume depletion		Px: hypertension, edema		Px: flank mass, distended bladder

*FE_Na = fractional excretion of sodium (%) = (urine sodium/plasma sodium ÷ urine creatinine/plasma creatinine) × 100.
†RFI = renal failure index = (urine sodium ÷ urine creatinine/plasma creatinine) × 100.
BUN, blood urea nitrogen; Hx, history; Px, physical signs; RBC, red blood cell; WBC, white blood cell.
From Behrman RE, Kliegman R (eds): Nelson Essentials of Pediatrics, 2nd ed. Philadelphia, WB Saunders, 1994, p 602.

with loss of tubular concentrating ability or insensitivity to antidiuretic hormone at the tubules.

Management I: Decreased Urine Output

Prerenal

In hospitalized children, prerenal causes of decreased urine output are relatively common, and you should be able to conclude whether the cause is prerenal based on the history, the chart review, your examination, and the urinalysis. Euvolemia is the goal. Fluid-resuscitate a dehydrated child and diurese a child in congestive heart failure. In some cases it may be difficult to decide whether the child is "dry" or "wet." A modest fluid challenge may be helpful diagnostically if there is reduced urine output.

Fluid boluses should always consist of isotonic solutions such as 0.9% saline. Children in acute renal failure are unable to excrete potassium and thus are at risk for life-threatening hyperkalemia. As such, potassium-containing fluids should be withheld in favor of normal saline until the child's urine output has been restored.

Postrenal

Lower urinary tract obstruction is usually easily managed by placement of a Foley catheter in the bladder.

1. Bladder outlet obstruction in a newborn boy can be secondary to posterior urethral valves and requires urologic surgical intervention. A postobstructive diuresis can be observed once the bladder is decompressed.
2. Obstruction of an already indwelling Foley catheter can be relieved by flushing the catheter with 10 to 20 mL of normal saline solution to displace the catheter from the bladder wall or to dislodge bladder sediment (see Chapter 26, Lines, Tubes, and Drains).
3. Catheterization of the bladder rules out only bladder outlet obstruction and lower urinary tract obstruction. Upper urinary tract obstruction secondary to congenital anomalies or nephrolithiasis is best diagnosed by ultrasonography.

Renal

If prerenal and postrenal factors are not causing the patient's poor urine output, the cause is most likely within the lengthy list of renal or glomerular conditions.

Are any of the five potentially life-threatening complications or consequences of renal failure present?
   Hyperkalemia
   Congestive heart failure
   Severe metabolic acidosis (pH <7.2)
   Uremic encephalopathy
   Uremic pericarditis

Hyperkalemia is the most immediately threatening consequence of low urine output. A serum K^+ level should be checked and an electrocardiogram obtained to check for peaked T waves. Further indications that the serum potassium level is dangerously high are conduction abnormalities, such as PR and QRS prolongation and ST-T wave depression. Potassium-containing intravenous fluids, including parenteral nutrition, should be stopped (see treatment of hyperkalemia in Chapter 34, Electrolyte Abnormalities).

Congestive heart failure is suggested by the presence of jugular venous distention, tachypnea and rales, dependent edema, and an S_3 gallop. Treatment of congestive heart failure usually includes fluid restriction, inotropic support as needed, diuretics, and respiratory support as needed.

Metabolic acidosis is suggested by tachypnea as the child attempts to compensate by reducing P_{CO_2} (requires analysis of arterial blood gases, as noted in Chapter 32, Acidosis and Alkalosis).

Uremic encephalopathy is generally manifested as a gradual onset of confusion, stupor, or seizures and is almost always an indication for emergency dialysis. Seizures should be managed as discussed in Chapter 29 until dialysis can be initiated.

Uremic pericarditis also requires dialysis and is usually manifested as pleuritic chest pain radiating to the shoulder, pericardial friction rub, distant or muffled heart sounds, and diffuse ST-segment elevation on the electrocardiogram.

Is the patient taking any drug that may complicate renal insufficiency?
Potassium supplements

Potassium-sparing diuretics (aldactone, triamterene, amiloride)

Nephrotoxic drugs (nonsteroidal anti-inflammatory drugs [NSAIDs], aminoglycosides)

Review the indications for each carefully and consider alternative medications if possible. If aminoglycosides are necessary, serum peak and trough levels should be monitored closely.

Is the child in oliguric renal failure?
If a child produces less than 1 to 2 mL/kg/hr of urine, the child has oliguric renal failure. The first goal of therapy is to convert the patient to nonoliguric renal failure, which has a far better prognosis:

1. Correct prerenal and postrenal factors.
2. Give diuretics to increase urine output. Furosemide, 1 mg/kg per dose, may be given intravenously. If there is no response within 1 to 2 hours, a double dose should be administered. (Larger doses should be administered slowly to avoid ototoxicity.)
3. If there is no response to furosemide, the next diuretic recommended is bumetanide, 0.1 mg/kg intravenously. Frequently, the effectiveness of loop diuretics can be enhanced by administering hydrochlorothiazide, 1 to 2 mg/kg per dose, or metolazone, 0.25 mg/kg per dose.

Does the child need dialysis?

If the child does not respond to diuretics, the indications for urgent dialysis are any of the five complications of renal failure: hyperkalemia, congestive heart failure with pulmonary edema, metabolic acidosis, uremia, and complications of uremia, including pericarditis and encephalopathy. A nephrology consultation is necessary, and until dialysis can be arranged, it may be necessary to treat the child for the aforementioned conditions with measures that do not involve dialysis.

Hyperkalemia. Glucose with insulin infusion, $NaHCO_3$, and sodium polystyrene sulfonate temporarily reduce the serum potassium level by driving K^+ into intracellular fluid and binding K^+ within the gastrointestinal tract for excretion (see Chapter 34, Electrolyte Abnormalities). Calcium gluconate is used to treat dysrhythmias secondary to hyperkalemia.

Congestive heart failure. Inotropy, afterload reduction, and respiratory support should be provided as needed.

Metabolic acidosis. $NaHCO_3$ provides correction of pH, but it is only temporary.

Uremia. Uremic pericarditis rarely causes a sizable effusion that requires pericardiocentesis. Conservative measures are recommended, such as the use of NSAIDs, but they need to be used carefully with adequate hydration and close monitoring of renal function. Aspirin and indomethacin are contraindicated because they may worsen acidosis.

Specific therapy for a renal disease that has caused renal failure, such as glomerulonephritis, frequently depends on the results of renal biopsy. Routine urinalysis, renal ultrasound studies, and 24-hour urine sampling for protein and creatinine should be ordered. The urinalysis should be studied for the following:

Urine dipstick. Hematuria and proteinuria suggest glomerulonephritis. Remember, a positive dipstick result for blood can mean red blood cells, free hemoglobin, or myoglobin. Suspect rhabdomyolysis if the result is positive with few red blood cells by microscopic examination. (In this case, check the creatinine phosphokinase, calcium, phosphate, and urine myoglobin levels.) A positive urine protein test result should prompt investigation of serum albumin, and a 24-hour urine collection for protein and creatinine clearance should be started. When the urine sample is concentrated (specific gravity >1.015), the dipstick may be positive for protein in an otherwise normal child. In this case, a spot urine protein-creatinine ratio may be helpful (a ratio of 0.2 or less suggests normal renal function).

Urine microscopy. Red blood cell casts are diagnostic of glomerulonephritis. Oval fat bodies are suggestive of nephrotic syndrome. White blood cells are characteristic of pyelonephritis and can be seen with nephrolithiasis. Eosinophils are suggestive of acute interstitial nephritis.

Management II: Increased Urine Output

The major threat of any form of DI is dehydration. It is important to match urine output with adequate replacement fluid while searching for the cause. Administration of DDAVP (desmopressin acetate) intravenously or intranasally is both diagnostic (decreased urine output in central DI; no change in urine output in nephrogenic, antidiuretic hormone–insensitive DI) and therapeutic for central DI. If central DI is suspected, an endocrinology consultation is advisable to investigate hypothalamic or pituitary function.

Urinalysis and urine culture should be ordered if there is any suspicion of urinary tract infection or diabetes mellitus resulting in polyuria. Urine and serum electrolytes, creatinine, and osmolarity should also be determined. These tests can help differentiate causes of increased urine output.

Glucose in urine increases suspicion for diabetes mellitus. If glucosuria is present, you should check the serum glucose level, venous pH, and urine for ketones while remembering that diabetes mellitus in childhood is often manifested as diabetic ketoacidosis.

REMEMBER

Many medications are excreted by the kidneys and have effects on kidney function. All medications in an oliguric or anuric child must be scrutinized and discontinued if they are nephrotoxic. Similarly, drugs that require renal metabolism (digoxin, aminoglycosides) must have their doses and dosing schedules modified and levels closely monitored. **If this is overlooked, drug levels could reach toxic levels and result in significant problems for the patient.**

Vomiting

Rebecca S. Severe, MD

In hospitalized children, vomiting is often a nonspecific symptom accompanying any illness. A single episode of vomiting or a few instances of intermittent vomiting without additional significant gastrointestinal or neurologic symptoms or signs is unlikely to be indicative of a life-threatening problem. However, as with other problems that arise while on call, it is critical that pediatric house officers consider the potential for life-threatening causes of vomiting and at least assure themselves that such potential causes have been either excluded or evaluated and managed appropriately. It is also important to have an understanding of the complications of vomiting that may arise when vomiting has been excessive.

PHONE CALL

Questions

1. What is the child's age?
2. Has the child been vomiting previously, or is this a new symptom?
3. What is the child's admitting diagnosis?
4. Is fever or diarrhea associated with the vomiting?
5. Is there blood or bile in the vomitus?
6. Does the child have an intravenous (IV) line in place?
7. Does the child appear to be in pain or complaining of pain?
8. Does the child have a headache or other neurologic symptoms?

Orders

1. Have the nurse obtain a full set of vital signs.
2. If the child has not been weighed recently, have the nurse weigh the child and begin recording fluid intake and output.
3. If there is blood or bile in the vomitus, the child should be given NPO status immediately and IV fluids begun at maintenance doses.

Inform RN

"Will be at the bedside in … minutes."

Vomiting in a neonate or very young infant can frequently be a sign of a surgical problem and deserves evaluation promptly. In older children, one may adjust the urgency of evaluation according to the presence or absence of other complaints (pain) or symptoms (blood or bile).

ELEVATOR THOUGHTS

A brief review of the common causes of vomiting is best organized by age.

Neonatal vomiting *Anatomic*
   Gastroesophageal reflux
   Esophageal duplication cyst
   Duodenal atresia or stenosis
   Ileal atresia
   Ladd's bands
   Hirschsprung's disease
   Tracheoesophageal fistula (esophageal atresia)
   Pyloric stenosis
   Annular pancreas
   Malrotation
   Meconium ileus
   Anal atresia or imperforate anus
  Metabolic
   Inborn errors of metabolism
   Adrenogenital syndrome
  Intracranial
   Increased intracranial pressure (ICP) (hydrocephalus, subdural or subarachnoid hemorrhage)
  Infectious
   Urinary tract infection
   Necrotizing enterocolitis
   TORCH (toxoplasmosis, other agents, rubella, cytomegalovirus, herpes simplex) infection
  Toxic
   Perinatal drug exposure
   Therapeutic drug overdose

Infant and childhood vomiting *Anatomic*
   Congenital anomalies of the gastrointestinal tract
   Hirschsprung's disease
   Intussusception
   Swallowed foreign body (bezoar)

Infant and childhood vomiting—Cont'd

Intracranial
Brain tumor
Subdural hematoma
Hydrocephalus
Brain abscess

Metabolic
Inborn errors of metabolism
Uremia
Lactose intolerance
Adrenogenital syndrome
Toxic ingestion
Gluten intolerance

Infectious
Viral gastroenteritis
Parasitic gastroenteritis
Hepatitis
Appendicitis
Bacterial colitis
Mesenteric adenitis
Urinary tract infection
Pancreatitis
Pneumonia

Traumatic
Closed head injury
(concussion, subdural
hematoma)

Preadolescent and adolescent vomiting

Anatomic
Bowel obstruction

Intracranial
Brain tumor
Cerebrovascular accident

Metabolic
Uremia
Toxic ingestion
Diabetic ketoacidosis

Infectious
Viral gastroenteritis
Giardiasis
Bacterial colitis
Hepatitis
Pancreatitis

Traumatic
Postconcussive
Subdural hemorrhage

Psychogenic
Bulimia
School avoidance
Anxiety
Cyclic vomiting

MAJOR THREAT TO LIFE

- Increased ICP
- Surgical abdominal emergencies (intussusception, bowel obstruction, necrotizing enterocolitis)
- Dehydration with or without electrolyte abnormalities (pyloric stenosis)

The differential diagnosis of vomiting is best approached initially by the age of the child. In newborns and neonates, congenital malformations of the gastrointestinal tract must be considered, including duodenal or ileal atresia (associated with Down syndrome), pyloric stenosis, malrotation and midgut volvulus, tracheoesophageal fistula, annular pancreas, meconium ileus, and Hirschsprung's disease. In a preterm infant, especially one younger than 32 weeks' gestation and/or under 1500 g, vomiting may be a sign of necrotizing enterocolitis, which can progress rapidly to a perforated viscus, peritonitis, septic shock, and death. Nongastrointestinal diseases of the very young, including urinary tract infection, inborn errors of metabolism, adrenogenital syndrome, and increased ICP (hydrocephalus or subdural hematoma), can produce significant vomiting.

In older infants, infectious gastroenteritis becomes more common, including gastroenteritis secondary to rotavirus and influenza A. In toddlers and older children, toxic ingestion, bacterial food poisoning, hepatitis, and inflammatory bowel diseases are added to viral gastroenteritis. Nongastrointestinal disorders include urinary tract infection, as well as brain tumors, other causes of increased ICP, and postconcussive vomiting.

BEDSIDE

Quick-Look Test

Does the child appear well (comfortable), sick (uncomfortable or distressed), or critical (about to die)?

All children appear acutely uncomfortable when they are actively vomiting. They are anxious, tachycardic, and frequently diaphoretic. In infectious processes, nausea and vomiting tend to come in waves, with periods of relative calm and comfort in between, and almost invariably occur with fever. Acute surgical vomiting is usually accompanied by abdominal pain, which may or may not be well localized (see Chapter 6, Abdominal Pain). Vomiting associated with intracranial processes often appears early in the day and lessens as the day progresses.

Airway and Vital Signs

What are the temperature, pulse, and blood pressure?

Hypotension associated with vomiting is a late and ominous sign of hypovolemia and shock. Fever implies infectious or inflammatory processes and can worsen dehydration. Hypertension and bradycardia imply severe increased ICP.

Selective History and Chart Review

Is abdominal pain associated with the vomiting?

This is difficult to ascertain in infants but is quite helpful in older children. Although pain can occur with infectious gastroenteritis, it is unusual.

When did the vomiting start?

Vomiting can result from some medications, such as chemotherapeutic agents, as well as overdoses of digoxin and a variety of other medications. Vomiting after closed head injury can indicate a concussion or more serious complication, such as subarachnoid or subdural hemorrhage. Persistent or recurrent vomiting can represent cyclic vomiting, bulimia, or metabolic-endocrine disorders.

Is the vomiting forceful or effortless?

All babies spit up. All babies have some gastroesophageal reflux. Reflux is normal and is a medical problem only if (1) the volume of reflux is such that the child does not gain weight or (2) the child aspirates. Otherwise, all reflux does is create dirty laundry (the child's as well as the parents'). Reflux should be distinguished from vomiting. Reflux is effortless regurgitation in small infants and can occur immediately after feeding or 2 to 3 hours later. The child is not distressed; in fact, the child may be quite happy and content. Vomiting is forceful and uncomfortable. An infant with pyloric stenosis is often described as having "explosive or projectile" vomiting.

What is the nature of the emesis?

Bilious, brown, or feculent emesis is pathognomonic of bowel obstruction, either paralytic or mechanical. Frank blood implies upper gastrointestinal bleeding, especially a Mallory-Weiss tear, variceal bleeding, or gastric ulcer disease, except in a newborn, in whom it may reflect swallowed maternal blood. Vomiting food after fasting is consistent with gastric outlet obstruction and/or delayed gastric emptying.

Is there associated diarrhea?

Viral and/or bacterial enterocolitis is very common in children. Viral gastroenteritis tends to be seasonal, with specific causes common to summer (enteroviruses) and winter (rotavirus, influenza). Food poisoning with *Staphylococcus* or *Salmonella* can cause a particularly sudden onset of acute vomiting that tends to be followed by diarrhea. The absence of diarrhea and fever should always lead you to consider intracranial causes for the vomiting.

What medications is the child taking?

Emesis is a well-described side effect of certain cancer chemotherapeutic medications, including cyclophosphamide, doxorubicin, and vincristine. Vomiting is also well known with toxic levels of digoxin, aminophylline, β-blocking agents, and salicylates.

Selective Physical Examination

HEENT	Mucous membranes, dilated pupils, ketotic breath, nystagmus, and cranial nerve deficits may imply a nongastrointestinal cause of vomiting. In infants, the fontanelles should be checked
Neck	Nuchal rigidity
Respiratory	Left lower lobe pneumonia and/or empyema may cause vomiting
Abdomen	Quality and activity of bowel sounds, distention, localized or diffuse tenderness, masses, hepatosplenomegaly, costovertebral angle tenderness, rebound tenderness, rigidity
Rectal	Small rectum (Hirschsprung's disease), bleeding (Hemoccult positive)
Genitourinary	Hernia, scrotal masses, scrotal pain
Neurologic	Mental status, focal findings, visual fields, funduscopic examination, Romberg's sign

Management

Management of vomiting depends on the underlying cause. In many cases, the vomiting is mild, self limited, and not a sign of serious life-threatening problems, such as increased ICP or a surgical abdomen. Once you have excluded these possibilities, you may not need to do any more initially than ensure that the child remains hydrated and frequently re-evaluate the child via serial abdominal examinations. Remember that intra-abdominal processes may begin with isolated vomiting and lead to additional signs and symptoms over time. If there are signs of bowel obstruction, rapid gastrointestinal bleeding, or peritonitis, surgical consultation will be necessary. If there are signs of increased ICP, neuroimaging will be necessary, and transfer to the pediatric intensive care unit with institution of measures to decrease ICP may be required (see Chapter 7, Altered Mental Status). Vomiting in a newborn should be distinguished from reflux. Forceful or persistent vomiting deserves diagnostic evaluation and may require intervention. Flat and upright abdominal films may confirm the presence of intestinal obstruction with a double bubble (duodenal atresia), air-fluid levels (small bowel obstruction), or megacolon (meconium ileus or Hirschsprung's disease). Plain films may also confirm the presence of a radiopaque foreign body.

(Remember, many of the things that children swallow are not radiopaque.) Ultrasound studies are useful in neonates with hypochloremic, hypokalemic metabolic acidosis caused by hypertrophic pyloric stenosis and in older children with suspected appendicitis. Prompt surgical consultation should be obtained if there is a suggestion of bowel obstruction. Bowel obstruction in older children can result from an incarcerated hernia, volvulus, intussusception, or adhesions from previous abdominal surgery.

Dehydration should be addressed as discussed in Chapter 15, Diarrhea and Dehydration. Obviously, the usefulness of oral rehydration may be limited by severe vomiting. For this reason, IV access is very important and should be made a priority.

If the child has been vomiting excessively, keep in mind that electrolyte abnormalities may be developing, particularly hypokalemia. Checking the electrolytes and correcting abnormalities may be necessary (see Chapter 34, Electrolyte Abnormalities).

The use of antiemetic medications is controversial. When the cause of vomiting is clear, such as after chemotherapy, antiemetic medications may and should be used for symptomatic relief. However, in patients with vomiting of unknown cause, antiemetics must be used cautiously. Vomiting may become persistent in children with hepatitis, pancreatitis, and gastroenteritis, especially when there is an element of dehydration. The use of promethazine (Phenergan), chlorpromazine (Thorazine), prochlorperazine (Compazine), or trimethobenzamide (Tigan) may be accompanied by significant extrapyramidal side effects. Ondansetron and granisetron, serotonin antagonists, are effective treatment of a variety of causes of refractory vomiting, including the vomiting associated with chemotherapy.

REMEMBER

The most critical elements when evaluating a hospitalized child with vomiting are to rule out the surgical causes unique to each age group, consider the possibility of intracranial causes of the vomiting, and support the child's hydration status and electrolyte balance while keeping the child comfortable. Oral rehydration can be accomplished in most cases by giving small amounts frequently, such as Popsicles or ice chips. Consider the need for antiemetics very cautiously, especially in children with infectious causes of vomiting. **Don't forget that all forms of infectious vomiting are highly contagious. Do yourself and your next patient a big favor and wash your hands very well before and after evaluating *every* patient.**

Laboratory-Related Problems

32

Acidosis and Alkalosis

Elizabeth M. Galloway, MD

Multiple clinical conditions can affect a child's acid-base status. For example, a child with excessive vomiting may be expected to have a metabolic alkalosis secondary to loss of hydrogen ions from highly acidic gastric fluid. Likewise, diarrhea often results in a metabolic acidosis because of the loss of bicarbonate-rich intestinal fluid. In some instances, however, acidosis and alkalosis are discovered unexpectedly when the laboratory detects an abnormality in pH or serum bicarbonate. It is then necessary to determine the cause of the acidosis or alkalosis so that appropriate management to correct the disorder can be instituted.

In most cases, acidosis or alkalosis is mild, and correction of the underlying problem eventually improves the abnormality. When an abnormality is severe, direct treatment of the acidosis or alkalosis may be required.

Acid-base disorders can be separated into four primary categories: respiratory acidosis, metabolic acidosis, respiratory alkalosis, and metabolic alkalosis (Table 32-1). At the onset of any primary acid-base disorder, the body begins to predictably compensate (see Table 32-2). Respiratory compensation is rapid and accomplished by increasing or decreasing PCO_2 with changes in ventilation. Metabolic compensation is slower, beginning 12 to 24 hours after the onset of acidosis or alkalosis, and is accomplished by changing the renal loss or retention of bicarbonate.

ACIDOSIS

Acidosis is defined as an arterial pH less than 7.35. You should first determine whether the acidosis is respiratory or metabolic. A low serum bicarbonate value is consistent with metabolic acidosis, and a high PCO_2 is consistent with respiratory acidosis. Remember, too, that the acidosis may be a **combination** of metabolic and respiratory acidosis.

In a healthy person, normal metabolism generates acids, and these acids are excreted by buffering with extracellular bicarbonate

TABLE 32–1 **Primary Categories of Acidosis and Alkalosis**

	pH	[HCO$_3$] (mEq/L)	Pco$_2$ (mm Hg)	Common Conditions
Normal	7.35-7.45	24	40	
Respiratory acidosis	<7.35	≥24	>40	Hypoventilation
Metabolic acidosis	<7.35	<24	≤40	Ketoacidosis
Respiratory alkalosis	>7.45	≤24	<40	Hyperventilation
Metabolic alkalosis	>7.45	>24	≥40	Vomiting

and conversion to CO_2, which can then be eliminated through the lungs (recall the formula $[HCO_3^-] + [H^+] = CO_2 + H_2O$). These mechanisms maintain the concentration of hydrogen ion $[H^+]$ within a narrow range, thereby maintaining arterial pH within the "normal" range.

From the Henderson-Hasselbalch equation,

$$pH = pK_a + \log\ ([HCO_3^-]/[H_2CO_3])$$

The following relationship among hydrogen ion concentration, Pco$_2$, and HCO$_3^-$ can be derived:

$$[H^+] = 24 \times Pco_2/[HCO_3^-]$$

When abnormal conditions (illnesses, toxins) result in excessive concentrations of hydrogen ion (i.e., acidosis), the normal buffering system of the body is insufficient to prevent a change in pH; therefore, additional respiratory or metabolic compensation occurs. The normal response to respiratory acidosis is an increase in serum HCO$_3^-$ as a result of renal preservation. The normal response to metabolic acidosis is hyperventilation and a decrease in Pco$_2$. The degree of compensation is predictable, and specific rules allow you to determine whether the child has appropriately compensated for the primary disorder (Table 32-2). When compensation appears to be greater or less than expected, a mixed disorder should be suspected.

Respiratory Acidosis

Causes

1. Acute and chronic lung disease
   Airway obstruction
   Aspiration
   Bronchospasm
   Chronic obstructive lung disease (e.g., cystic fibrosis, bronchopulmonary dysplasia)
   Pneumonia
   Pulmonary edema
2. Abnormal chest or lung expansion
   Thoracic cage restriction (e.g., trauma, severe scoliosis)

TABLE 32–2 Expected Compensation for Primary Acid-Base Disorders

Disorder	Primary Event	Compensation	Rate of Compensation
Metabolic acidosis	$\downarrow [HCO_3^-]$	$\downarrow Pco_2$	For 1-mEq/L $\downarrow [HCO_3^-]$, $Pco_2 \downarrow$ 1-1.5 mm Hg
Metabolic alkalosis	$\uparrow [HCO_3^-]$	$\uparrow Pco_2$	For 1-mEq/L $\uparrow [HCO_3^-]$, $Pco_2 \uparrow$ 0.5-1 mm Hg
Respiratory acidosis			
Acute (<12-24 hr)	$\uparrow Pco_2$	$\uparrow HCO_3^-$	For 10–mm Hg $\uparrow Pco_2$, $[HCO_3^-] \uparrow$ 1 mEq/L
Chronic (3-5 days)	$\uparrow Pco_2$	$\uparrow\uparrow HCO_3^-$	For 10–mm Hg $\uparrow Pco_2$, $[HCO_3^-] \uparrow$ 4 mEq/L
Respiratory alkalosis			
Acute (<12 hr)	$\downarrow Pco_2$	$\downarrow [HCO_3^-]$	For 10–mm Hg $\downarrow Pco_2$, $[HCO_3^-] \downarrow$ 1-3 mEq/L
Chronic (1-2 days)	$\downarrow Pco_2$	$\downarrow\downarrow [HCO_3^-]$	For 10–mm Hg $\downarrow Pco_2$, $[HCO_3^-] \downarrow$ 2-5 mEq/L

Normal serum $[HCO_3^-]$ is 24 mEq/L and blood gas Pco_2 is 40 mm Hg.
From Brewer ED: Disorders of acid-base balance. Pediatr Clin North Am 37:432, 1990 with permission.

Pleural effusion

Pneumothorax

3. Central nervous system (CNS) or neuromuscular disorders and hypoventilation

Brainstem or spinal cord lesion

CNS depressant drugs (e.g., narcotics)

Muscular dystrophy

Myasthenia gravis

Guillain-Barré syndrome

Botulism

Werdnig-Hoffmann disease

Manifestations

Hypoxia often coincides with respiratory acidosis because of decreased alveolar ventilation. By 12 to 24 hours after the onset of respiratory acidosis, renal compensation begins, but serum HCO_3^- rarely rises above 32 mEq/L during the first few days of acidosis. After 3 or more days, serum HCO_3^- levels may increase further as a result of continued renal compensation and generally remain in the 35- to 45-mEq/L range until the respiratory acidosis is corrected.

Symptoms directly related to an increase in Pco_2 are not usually apparent until the Pco_2 rises to a value greater than 70 mm Hg and include

1. Decreased respiratory rate
2. Altered mental status
3. Papilledema
4. Asterixis

Management

Determine the severity:

Mild: pH = 7.30 to 7.35

Moderate: pH = 7.20 to 7.29

Severe: pH < 7.20

Management is directed at the underlying cause, and your evaluation should proceed to identify the possibilities just listed. Intubation, mechanical ventilation, and transfer to the intensive care unit may all be necessary for a child with moderate to severe respiratory acidosis. Any child with respiratory acidosis requires frequent monitoring with serial arterial blood gas determinations while you are identifying and treating the underlying cause. Monitoring oxygen saturation alone with a pulse oximeter is inadequate and may be falsely reassuring because preservation of oxygen saturation may continue despite a decline in ventilation. Tachypnea, labored breathing, and the use of accessory muscles may also initially prevent the development of acidosis, but eventual fatigue may lead to rapid decompensation.

Metabolic Acidosis

Causes

Metabolic acidosis results in a low serum HCO_3^- concentration and a PCO_2 that is normal or decreased. Once metabolic acidosis has been identified, you should determine the **anion gap**.

$$\text{Anion gap} = \text{Serum sodium} - (\text{Chloride} + HCO_3^-)$$

$$\text{Normal range} = 8 \text{ to } 16 \text{ mEq/L}$$

The causes of metabolic acidosis can be divided into those that produce a normal anion gap (hyperchloremic) and those that produce an increased anion gap (normochloremic). If the anion gap is normal, either loss of HCO_3^- has occurred through the gut or the kidneys or there has been rapid dilution of extracellular volume. If the anion gap is increased, acids have been added, either endogenously (e.g., via lactic acidosis or diabetic ketoacidosis) or exogenously (e.g., by ingestion). If the osmolal gap is also increased, you should suspect ingestion as the cause of the increased anion gap metabolic acidosis.

Osmolal gap =
  Measured serum osmolality − Calculated serum osmolality

$$\text{Calculated serum osmolality} = 2[\text{Na}] + \frac{\text{Blood urea nitrogen}}{2.8} + \frac{\text{Glucose}}{18}$$

Normal anion gap metabolic acidosis	Diarrhea
	Bowel, biliary, or pancreatic tube or fistula drainage
	Exogenous chloride-containing compounds (NH_4Cl, HCl)
	Renal tubular acidosis
	Carbonic anhydrase inhibitor treatment
	Mineralocorticoid deficiency
Increased anion gap metabolic acidosis	Lactic acidosis (hypoxia, shock, inborn errors of carbohydrate or pyruvate metabolism)
	Ketoacidosis (diabetes, starvation, aminoacidemia, organic aciduria)
	Uremia
	Ingestion (salicylates, ethylene glycol, methanol, paraldehyde)

Manifestations

Hyperventilation may be present with metabolic acidosis as the child attempts to eliminate the CO_2 that accumulates as a result of excessive hydrogen ion concentration. Ketotic breath or other odors may be clues to a metabolic cause of the acidosis, such as diabetes or an inborn error of metabolism. If the acidosis is severe, altered mental status, decreased cardiac contractility, and shock may all occur.

Management

Determine the severity:
    Mild: pH = 7.30 to 7.35
    Moderate: pH = 7.20 to 7.29
    Severe: pH < 7.20

As with other acid-base disorders, treating the underlying cause is essential. For most children, maintaining adequate hydration, maximizing cardiac output and perfusion, correcting other electrolyte abnormalities, removing potential toxins, and providing supportive care prevent progression of the acidosis. If the acidosis is severe, it may be necessary to administer $NaHCO_3$ to rapidly improve arterial pH to a value greater than 7.20. It is not necessary to return the pH to normal in this circumstance, and the goal should be to attain a pH of approximately 7.25. The dose of bicarbonate to be given can be calculated by using the following formula:

$$NaHCO_3 \text{ dose (mEq)} = (\text{Desired } [HCO_3^-] - \text{Observed } [HCO_3^-]) \\ (\text{Weight in kg})(0.4)$$

The desired $[HCO_3^-]$ should be 18 mEq/L in cases of normal anion gap acidosis and 12 mEq/L with increased anion gap acidosis. Aiming for a higher concentration in children with normal anion gap acidosis is reasonable because losses of bicarbonate (as with diarrhea) can usually be expected to continue. When administering bicarbonate it is important to remember the following:

1. Careful attention must be paid to the serum potassium concentration. In an acidotic child with normal amounts of potassium, the serum potassium concentration should increase as intracellular potassium shifts out of cells. Administration of bicarbonate shifts this potassium intracellularly and thereby returns the serum concentration to normal. If an acidotic child is normokalemic or hypokalemic, life-threatening hypokalemia may be precipitated by the administration of bicarbonate.
2. In this situation, bicarbonate should be diluted and administered slowly. Rapid infusion may result in dysrhythmias.
3. $NaHCO_3$ may be contraindicated if the child is severely hypernatremic and/or hyperosmolar.

ALKALOSIS

Alkalosis is defined as an arterial pH greater than 7.45. You should first determine whether the alkalosis is respiratory or metabolic. A low P_{CO_2} is consistent with respiratory alkalosis, and a high serum bicarbonate level is consistent with metabolic alkalosis (Table 32-1).

The normal response to respiratory alkalosis is a decrease in serum HCO_3^- as a result of the law of mass action (recall the formula $[HCO_3^-] + [H^+] = CO_2 + H_2O$) and renal excretion of bicarbonate. The normal response to metabolic alkalosis is hypoventilation and an increase in arterial and venous PCO_2. The degree of compensation is predictable (see Table 32-2), and when compensation is greater or less than expected, a mixed acid-base disorder should be suspected.

Respiratory Alkalosis

Causes

Anxiety
Sepsis
Pneumonia
Congestive heart failure
Hepatic failure
Salicylates
Fever
High altitude
Pulmonary emboli
CNS disorders (trauma, tumor)
Hyperthyroidism

Manifestations

Hyperventilation may lead to circumoral paresthesias or even tetany secondary to increased calcium binding to albumin and a decrease in serum ionized calcium. In addition, altered mental status may ensue if the alkalosis is severe enough.

Management

Determine the severity:
Mild: pH = 7.45 to 7.55
Moderate: pH = 7.56 to 7.69
Severe: pH > 7.70
Most instances of respiratory alkalosis are mild and short lived. Management of respiratory alkalosis depends on relieving the underlying cause. In cases of hyperventilation secondary to anxiety, rebreathing into a paper bag may be beneficial.

Metabolic Alkalosis

Causes

1. Loss of H^+ ions
    Vomiting
    Nasogastric suction
    Congenital chloride-wasting diarrhea
    Renal loss (diuretics, hyperaldosteronism, Cushing's disease, adrenogenital syndrome, licorice ingestion, Bartter syndrome)

2. Exogenous alkali (citrate, lactate, acetate)
3. Contraction of extracellular volume (vomiting, cystic fibrosis in infants)

Vomiting is the most common cause of metabolic alkalosis in children ("contraction alkalosis"). With vomiting, hydrogen ion is lost directly in gastric fluid but is also lost as a result of renal sodium-hydrogen exchange in response to extracellular volume contraction. Renal failure, potassium depletion, and chloride depletion are other factors that contribute to a state of metabolic alkalosis.

When a metabolic alkalosis is accompanied by a low serum chloride concentration, measuring the urinary chloride level can be helpful in determining the cause. A value less than 10 mEq/L suggests that the kidney is reabsorbing chloride in response to losses that may occur with vomiting, nasogastric suction, chloride-wasting diarrhea, or cystic fibrosis in infants. A value greater than 20 mEq/L suggests diuretics, excessive mineralocorticoid, or Bartter syndrome.

Manifestations

Severe alkalosis may result in altered mental status. Otherwise, the signs and symptoms are those of the underlying disorder.

Management

Determine the severity:
 Mild: pH = 7.45 to 7.55
 Moderate: pH = 7.56 to 7.69
 Severe: pH > 7.70

Metabolic alkalosis associated with volume depletion (low urinary chloride) responds to the administration of normal saline solution. Once the fluid and chloride deficits are repleted, renal excretion of bicarbonate allows resolution of the alkalosis. Remember that an associated hypokalemia must also be corrected before normal saline solution is effective. As with other acid-base disorders, correcting the underlying cause is usually sufficient.

Anemia, Thrombocytopenia, and Coagulation Abnormalities

Teresa M. Uy, MD

Anemia is a common problem in the pediatric age group and is often discovered during hospitalization for an acute illness. Many systemic illnesses are accompanied by mild to moderate anemia and do not require extensive evaluation or specific treatment. Similarly, anemia may be expected to be present with many chronic illnesses, and appropriate management of the underlying illness generally prevents progressive worsening of the anemia. When anemia is severe or when cardiac or pulmonary disease mandates that hemoglobin (and oxygen-carrying capacity) be maintained, specific treatment of anemia may be necessary.

Thrombocytopenia and abnormalities in coagulation are much less common than anemia in the pediatric population. These abnormalities require further evaluation and often specific treatment. A low platelet count or abnormal clotting study result generally reflects significant illness; therefore, when notified of such abnormalities, your response should be prompt.

ANEMIA

Causes

The potential causes of anemia can be narrowed by considering the signs and symptoms of the patient and the initial laboratory evaluation, which should include hemoglobin, hematocrit, reticulocyte count, red blood cell (RBC) indices (mean corpuscular volume [MCV], mean corpuscular hemoglobin [MCH], mean corpuscular hemoglobin concentration [MCHC]), and RBC morphology. Further evaluation should then be more selective and the choice of additional tests based on the initial results. It is important to remember that normal values for some of these measurements vary with age (Table 33-1).

TABLE 33–1 Estimated Normal Mean Values and Lower Limits of Normal (95% Range) for Hemoglobin, Hematocrit, Mean Corpuscular Volume, and Mean Corpuscular Hemoglobin

Age (yr)	Hemoglobin (g/L)		Packed Cell Volume (%)		MCV (fL)		MCH (pg)	
	Mean	Lower Limit	Mean	Lower Limit	Mean	Lower Limit	Mean	Lower Limit
0.5-4	125	110	36	32	80	72	28	24
5-10	130	115	38	33	83	75	29	25
11-14, F	135	120	39	34	85	77	29	26
11-14, M	140	120	41	35	85	77	29	26
15-19, F	135	120	40	34	88	79	30	27
15-19, M	150	130	43	37	88	79	30	27
20-44, F	135	120	40	35	90	80	31	27
20-44, M	155	135	45	39	90	80	31	27

Anemias can be divided into two large categories by analyzing the reticulocyte count:

1. Inadequate production of hemoglobin (low reticulocyte count)
2. Increased loss of hemoglobin (high reticulocyte count)

Inadequate Production (Low Reticulocyte Count)

MICROCYTIC ANEMIAS (LOW MCV)

1. Iron deficiency
2. Thalassemias
3. Lead toxicity
4. Sideroblastic anemia
5. Chronic disease (infection, inflammation, renal disease)

NORMOCYTIC ANEMIAS (NORMAL MCV)

1. Transient erythroblastopenia of childhood
2. Aplastic anemia (congenital or acquired, e.g., drugs)
3. Pure RBC aplasia
4. Bone marrow suppression or replacement (leukemia, tumors, storage diseases, infections)
5. Chronic disease

MACROCYTIC ANEMIAS (HIGH MCV)

1. Vitamin B_{12} deficiency
2. Folate deficiency
3. Aplastic anemia
4. Pure RBC aplasia (Diamond-Blackfan)
5. Hypothyroidism

Increased Loss (High Reticulocyte Count)

BLEEDING

1. Trauma
2. Gastrointestinal (GI) bleeding

3. Splenic sequestration
4. Pulmonary hemorrhage
5. Ruptured aneurysm
6. Ruptured ectopic pregnancy
7. Intraventricular hemorrhage (in premature infants)

HEMOLYSIS

1. Hemoglobinopathies
   Sickle cell disease
   Hemoglobin SC
2. RBC membrane defects
   Spherocytosis
   Elliptocytosis
   Paroxysmal nocturnal hemoglobinuria
3. Enzymopathies
   Pyruvate kinase deficiency
   Glucose-6-phosphate dehydrogenase
4. Extracellular defects
   Isoimmune hemolysis (Coombs positive)
   Fragmentation (disseminated intravascular coagulopathy
      [DIC], hemolytic-uremic syndrome [HUS], thrombotic
      thrombocytopenic purpura [TTP])
   Splenomegaly

Keep in mind that in children with chronic anemia, exacerbations may develop as a result of another cause (e.g., splenic sequestration or aplastic crisis in those with sickle cell disease) and that a single cause may lead to other causes (e.g., chronic GI blood loss leading to iron deficiency).

Manifestations

The manifestations of anemia are those of the underlying cause. Pallor is often the initial clue that an anemia is present. The palpebral conjunctivae, mucous membranes, and nail beds are the most obvious sites to look for pallor. Specific manifestations of the anemia depend on whether the anemia is acute or chronic. Acute and rapid onset of anemia secondary to hemorrhage results in signs and symptoms of hypovolemia and/or shock:

1. Tachycardia, hypotension
2. Cool, clammy extremities
3. Delayed capillary refill
4. Diaphoresis, tachypnea

Acute hemolysis may result in tachycardia, tachypnea, and pallor but does not usually produce the same degree of hypovolemia that is seen with hemorrhage. Jaundice secondary to hyperbilirubinemia, dark urine (hemoglobinuria), and/or splenomegaly may be clues to hemolysis.

Chronic anemia results in less obvious signs and symptoms:

1. Pallor
2. Fatigue, lethargy

3. Dyspnea with exertion
4. Mild tachycardia, tachypnea

Management

Determine the severity. The clinical status of the patient, *not* the laboratory value, should be used to determine the severity. For example, acute hemorrhage may initially result in a mild decrease or even no decrease in the hemoglobin level. If the patient is dehydrated, hemoconcentration may falsely increase the hemoglobin and hematocrit despite a significant reduction in RBCs. Conversely, many patients are asymptomatic despite profound anemia, especially if the anemia has developed over time.

A patient who is hypovolemic or in shock has severe anemia and needs prompt intervention. A patient with normal vital signs and a physical examination that does not indicate hypovolemia may need intervention if (1) the hemoglobin level is very depressed and a further drop is anticipated or (2) the hemoglobin level is very depressed and other factors (heart or lung disease) mandate intervention to improve oxygen-carrying capacity. A child with no symptoms and mild to moderate anemia may need further evaluation but probably does not need intervention in the middle of the night.

Hypovolemia

The same principles that apply in other conditions of hypovolemia and shock apply in a patient with hypovolemia and anemia (see Chapter 15, Diarrhea and Dehydration, and Chapter 25, Hypotension and Shock). Rapid expansion of the intravascular space is the initial goal.

1. Notify your senior resident.
2. Make sure that the child has at least one (ideally two) large-bore intravenous (IV) lines placed. "Large bore" is defined as the largest that you can place, usually a 16-gauge line in an older child and an 18-gauge line in a younger child or infant.
3. Send blood to the blood bank for a stat cross-match for packed RBCs (PRBCs). Always err on the side of requesting more. The blood is not wasted if you decide later not to use it.
4. Expand the intravascular space. The ideal fluid in this situation, when acute anemia and hypovolemia coincide, presumably because of massive blood loss (hemorrhage or hemolysis), is whole cross-matched blood. If the situation is critical (ongoing rapid blood loss in a patient in shock), O-negative blood should be given. If blood is not yet available, normal saline or lactated Ringer's solution should be infused, starting at 20 mL/kg and additional boluses administered according to the blood pressure response, heart rate, and clinical signs (pulse, capillary refill). Once blood is available, it should be used in place of crystalloid. After volume has been restored and the child is normotensive, the hemoglobin level and hematocrit should be determined,

with additional infusion of blood or PRBCs dependent on the degree of anemia.

5. Determine the cause of the blood loss. Search for obvious sites of hemorrhage, as well as occult sources. Periumbilical (Cullen's sign) or flank (Grey Turner's sign) ecchymoses may indicate abdominal hemorrhage. A careful abdominal and rectal examination with Hemoccult determination is mandatory. A chest radiograph should be obtained if pulmonary hemorrhage is a consideration. Review the child's medication list for anticoagulants and the chart for potential coagulopathies or recent surgery.

6. Surgical consultation may be necessary if intra-abdominal bleeding is suspected.

Normovolemia

A normovolemic child does not require immediate intervention but may need a transfusion if symptomatic or the degree of anemia is profound.

1. Determine the cause of the anemia. As noted earlier, a complete blood count with RBC indices, reticulocyte count, and review of the peripheral smear (Fig. 33-1) should allow you to narrow the possibilities or make a definitive diagnosis. Remember that even though hypovolemia is not present, blood loss may have

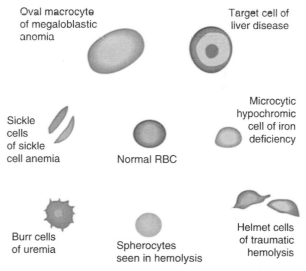

Figure 33–1 Examples of blood smears demonstrating helpful diagnostic features associated with specific anemias. (From Marshall SA, Ruedy J: On Call: Principles and Protocols, 4th ed. Philadelphia, Elsevier, 2004, p 325.)

occurred or may be ongoing and the potential exists for rapid decompensation if the patient is hemorrhaging. As in hypovolemic patients, your physical examination should be directed toward signs of obvious or occult bleeding.
2. If a transfusion is necessary, the amount of cross-matched PRBCs to be transfused can be calculated by using the formula

Volume of PRBCs (mL) = Estimated blood volume (mL) × (Desired Hct − Observed Hct)/Hct of PRBCs

where the hematocrit (Hct) of PRBCs can be estimated to be 65 and blood volume is estimated as follows:

Premature infants	100 mL/kg
Neonates	85 mL/kg
Infants (>1 mo)	75 mL/kg
Children	70 mL/kg
Adolescents	65 mL/kg

Alternatively, an arbitrary transfusion of 10 to 15 mL/kg of PRBCs can be administered. With either approach, rechecking the hemoglobin concentration and hematocrit in 4 to 6 hours allows you to determine the adequacy of the replacement.

THROMBOCYTOPENIA

Causes

The cause of a low platelet count can be divided into two categories:
1. Inadequate production (bone marrow infiltration or suppression)
2. Increased destruction or sequestration

Inadequate production	Malignancies (e.g., leukemia, neuroblastoma)
	Storage diseases (e.g., Gaucher's disease)
	Wiskott-Aldrich syndrome
	Thrombocytopenia: absent radius syndrome
	Infections (e.g., viral marrow suppression, fungemia, congenital infections)
	Drugs (resulting in marrow suppression)
Increased destruction	Idiopathic thrombocytopenic purpura (ITP)
	Systemic lupus erythematosus (SLE)
	HUS
	TTP
	DIC (e.g., with infection)
	Cavernous hemangiomas (Kasabach-Merritt syndrome)
	Drugs (immune mediated)
	Splenomegaly

Manifestations

Thrombocytopenia may be asymptomatic, result in petechiae only, or be associated with significant bleeding. The underlying disorder, rather than the specific platelet count, determines the severity of the clinical manifestations. Hemorrhage is generally rare unless the platelet count is less than 20,000/mm³.

Bleeding secondary to thrombocytopenia tends to involve the skin and mucous membranes rather than deeper internal organs. Petechiae, purpura, bruising, and bleeding from gums or IV sites are seen most often. This is in contrast to bleeding that results from an abnormality in clotting factors, in which deeper bleeding (e.g., hemarthroses) is more common. If thrombocytopenia is severe enough, however, children may be at increased risk for intracranial or other internal bleeding. Purpura secondary to thrombocytopenia is **nonpalpable** and should be distinguished from palpable purpura, which is more suggestive of vasculitis.

Additional clinical findings and laboratory studies should help you narrow the list of potential causes of a low platelet count. If anemia and/or leukopenia is also present, marrow suppression should be further considered. Isolated thrombocytopenia is more suggestive of a problem causing increased destruction of platelets (e.g., ITP). The presence of an associated hemolytic anemia increases the likelihood of an autoimmune (SLE, Evans syndrome) or microangiopathic (DIC, HUS, TTP) cause. Reviewing the peripheral smear may suggest a microangiopathy if schistocytes, helmet cells, and other fragmented cells are evident. In such a context, an elevated blood urea nitrogen and/or creatinine level with other signs of renal failure should increase your suspicion for HUS; the additional presence of neurologic symptoms should alert you to the possibility of the much less common diagnosis of TTP. An associated prolongation of the prothrombin time (PT) and partial thromboplastin time (PTT) should raise your suspicion for DIC.

Management

Treatment of thrombocytopenia varies, depending on the underlying cause. Generally, platelet transfusions are more beneficial in conditions in which thrombocytopenia is a result of inadequate production. In conditions involving increased destruction, platelet transfusions may temporarily increase the platelet count, but as long as the pathogenic mechanisms leading to increased destruction continue, the platelet count eventually falls again. Nonetheless, if life-threatening hemorrhage is present, platelets should be transfused in these situations, even if it is only a temporary measure. In children with TTP, some evidence suggests that platelet transfusions may actually exacerbate the illness; therefore, decisions regarding platelet transfusions for TTP should be made carefully and in consultation with a pediatric hematologist.

If a platelet transfusion is necessary, it is customary to transfuse 6 to 8 units of platelets at a time (or 4 U/m²). Each unit per square meter can be expected to increase the platelet count by approximately 10,000/mm³.

Platelet count increase (per mm^3) =
$$30,000 \times \text{Units transfused/Total blood volume (L)}$$

The platelet count should be checked 1 hour after transfusion to evaluate the response.

Idiopathic Thrombocytopenic Purpura

Treatment is not required when the patient is asymptomatic and the platelet count is greater than 35,000 mm^3. Common treatments include IV gamma globulin, anti-Rh D therapy (in patients who are Rh D positive), and steroids. Decisions regarding treatment of ITP should be made in consultation with a pediatric hematologist.

Thrombotic Thrombocytopenic Purpura

Children with TTP are usually quite ill and generally require management in the intensive care setting. Plasmapheresis, corticosteroids, and IV immune globulin may all be considered, but any treatment plan should be undertaken in consultation with a pediatric hematologist.

COAGULATION ABNORMALITIES: PROLONGED PT AND PTT

Causes

The PT tests the **extrinsic** pathway of the clotting cascade (Fig. 33-2). The PTT tests the **intrinsic** pathway. The extrinsic pathway is most affected by deficiencies in factors I (fibrinogen), II (prothrombin), V, VII, and X, whereas the intrinsic pathway is most affected by deficiencies in factors VIII, IX, XI, and XII.

Disorders prolonging the PT	Clotting factor deficiencies (factors I, II, V, VII, X)
	Oral anticoagulants (warfarin sodium [Coumadin])
	Vitamin K deficiency (e.g., hemorrhagic disease of the newborn)
	Liver disease
	DIC
	Heparin (sometimes)
Disorders prolonging the PTT	Clotting factor deficiencies (factors VIII, IX, XI, XII)
	Anticoagulants (heparin; sometimes oral)
	Circulating endogenous anticoagulant (e.g., lupus anticoagulant)
	DIC
	von Willebrand's disease (sometimes)

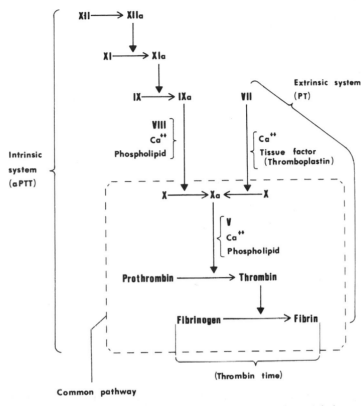

Figure 33–2 The coagulation cascade. aPTT, activated partial thromboplastin time. (From Marshall SA, Ruedy J: On Call: Principles and Protocols, 4th ed. Philadelphia, Elsevier, 2004, p 337.)

Factor deficiencies can be suspected or excluded by the results of mixing studies, in which normal plasma is mixed 1:1 with the child's plasma. The PT or PTT should "correct" if a deficient factor has been replaced by the addition of normal plasma. Failure to correct is consistent with an anticoagulant.

Manifestations

With the exception of lupus anticoagulant, bleeding is the obvious manifestation. Bleeding associated with a prolongation of the PT and/or PTT tends to involve deeper parts of the body, including visceral organs and joints.

Lupus anticoagulant is not associated with bleeding but rather predisposes one to **thrombosis**. The prolongation of the PTT that is usually (but not always) discovered is the result of in vitro phenomena in which the presence of lupus anticoagulant interferes with the test itself.

Management

Factor Deficiencies

Fresh frozen plasma (10 to 15 mL/kg) or specific factor concentrates can be infused to replace the deficient factor, once identified. Cryoprecipitate (0.5 bag/kg) contains high concentrations of fibrinogen and factor VIII and can also be used when these factors are deficient. If the bleeding is minor, IV or intranasal desmopressin (DDAVP) may be administered to increase plasma factor VIII levels. In children with severe bleeding, the use of products such as coagulation factor VIIa (recombinant) should be considered. However, DDAVP should not be administered without consulting specialists familiar with its use, such as hematologists.

von Willebrand's Disease

In most cases, bleeding is minor and may be treated with DDAVP, which releases von Willebrand's factor (vWF). Less commonly, von Willebrand's disease causes major bleeding that may be treated with Humate-P, a factor VIII concentrate that contains high levels of vWF. Cryoprecipitate or fresh frozen plasma is also effective. Use of these products should always be undertaken in consultation with a pediatric hematologist.

Vitamin K Deficiency

Hemorrhagic disease of the newborn occurs during the first week of life when an exaggeration of the normally mild decrease in vitamin K–dependent factors occurs. Prophylactic administration of intramuscular vitamin K at the time of birth usually prevents hemorrhagic disease but is less effective in premature infants. If bleeding ensues, IV vitamin K, 1 to 5 mg, is effective, and a response should be seen within a few hours.

Intestinal malabsorption and prolonged antibiotic treatment may result in vitamin K deficiency beyond the neonatal period. Vitamin K should be administered orally, subcutaneously, or intravenously (1 mg for infants, 2 to 3 mg for children, 10 mg for adolescents and adults). If vitamin K is ineffective, fresh frozen plasma should then be administered.

Liver Disease

Liver disease may result in decreased synthesis of clotting factors and subsequent factor deficiencies. For mild bleeding, administration of vitamin K, as just outlined, may be all that is necessary. If bleeding is severe, fresh frozen plasma (10 to 15 mL/kg) corrects all clotting factor deficiencies except fibrinogen deficiency. Cryoprecipitate (0.5 bag/kg) can be infused to correct the fibrinogen deficiency.

Disseminated Intravascular Coagulopathy

While the underlying cause is being treated, supportive care should include infusions of fresh frozen plasma, cryoprecipitate, and platelets when bleeding, thrombocytopenia, and PT and PTT abnormalities are severe.

34

Electrolyte Abnormalities

James J. Nocton, MD

HYPERNATREMIA (SERUM SODIUM >150 mEq/L)

Causes

Sodium excess
    Improperly mixed formula
    Excessive sodium bicarbonate administration for acidosis
    Ingestion of ocean water
    Hyperaldosteronism
Water deficit
    Inadequate intake
    Renal losses
        Diabetes insipidus (central or nephrogenic)
        Diabetes mellitus
        Osmotic diuresis
        Obstructive uropathy
        Renal dysplasia
    Extrarenal losses
        Diarrhea
        Excessive sweating
        Excessive insensible losses (burns, phototherapy)

Manifestations

Hypernatremia is usually the result of abnormal water loss in excess of sodium loss rather than an increase in total body sodium. In children, diarrhea is the most common cause and results in dehydration. With hypernatremic dehydration, the shift of water into the extracellular space tends to preserve intravascular volume; therefore, urine output may remain close to normal and such children may initially be less symptomatic than those with other forms of dehydration. Polyuria should suggest diabetes insipidus or diabetes mellitus. In an infant who does not appear dehydrated and has normal urine output, you should carefully determine how the infant is being fed and how the formula has been mixed. Errors in mixing are a common cause of hypernatremia in this age group.

The clinical manifestations of hypernatremia are those that result from the osmotic shift of water from the intracellular compartment to the extracellular compartment. Pulmonary edema may ensue, and its effects on brain cells may result in lethargy, irritability, coma, seizures, hypertonicity, and muscle spasms. Brain hemorrhage is the most serious potential consequence of hypernatremia.

Management

Determine the hydration status of the child and the severity of the hypernatremia. Most infants and children with hypernatremia are dehydrated. Management of a dehydrated patient with hypernatremia is discussed in Chapter 15, Diarrhea and Dehydration.

If the patient is normovolemic (or volume overloaded) and hypernatremic, as in instances in which sodium intake has been excessive, diuresis may be useful. Furosemide, 1 mg/kg intravenously (IV) initially with repeated doses at 2- to 4-hour intervals, promotes urinary sodium loss. If a large volume must be diuresed to return the sodium level to normal, urinary losses may be measured and replaced with 5% dextrose in water (D_5W). **Frequent** monitoring of the patient's hydration status and serum sodium level is mandatory. Remember that serum sodium levels must be corrected slowly (10 to 15 mEq/L/day) because cerebral edema may develop if free water shifts rapidly intracellularly as the extracellular sodium concentration falls.

Severe hypernatremia (>200 mEq/L) may require peritoneal dialysis or hemodialysis and consultation with a pediatric nephrologist.

HYPONATREMIA (SERUM SODIUM <130 mEq/L)

Causes

The potential causes of hyponatremia that you should consider depend on the volume status of the patient. An estimate of volume status and the urinary sodium concentration allows you to limit the list of possibilities (Fig. 34-1). A **hypovolemic** patient is losing sodium (and free water) either through urine or from extrarenal sites. The urinary sodium concentration should allow you to distinguish renal from extrarenal losses. A **euvolemic** patient may also have urinary sodium losses, but they are lower than in a hypovolemic patient, and water loss is minimal or absent. In some cases (e.g., syndrome of inappropriate antidiuretic hormone [SIADH]), there may be an increase in free water. The urine sodium level in those with euvolemic hyponatremia is concentrated at greater than 20 mEq/L. A **hypervolemic** patient has edema from heart, liver, or renal disease or overt

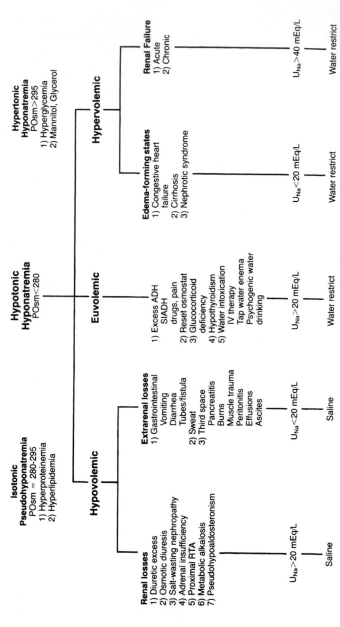

Figure 34-1 Classification, diagnosis, and treatment of hyponatremic states. ADH, antidiuretic hormone; RTA, renal tubular acidosis; SIADH, syndrome of inappropriate antidiuretic hormone. (From Berry PL, Belsha CW: Hyponatremia. Pediatr Clin North Am 37:354, 1990, with permission)

renal failure. The urinary sodium concentration is usually very high in those with renal failure.

Keep in mind that pseudohyponatremia or factitious hyponatremia may also occur. **Pseudohyponatremia** is a laboratory measurement error that occurs when excessive protein or lipid is present in plasma. Hyperproteinemia or hyperlipidemia increases plasma volume by decreasing the percentage of plasma that is free water. Some laboratory machines measure and report the sodium concentration in terms of the volume of *total plasma* rather than plasma water, and therefore the sodium concentration is artificially low. A clue to the presence of pseudohyponatremia is normal plasma osmolality despite a low serum sodium concentration. **Factitious hyponatremia** is redistribution of water from the intracellular to the extracellular compartment because of excessive extracellular osmolality. Hyperglycemia or the administration of mannitol increases plasma osmolality, thereby resulting in a shift of free water and a fall in the sodium concentration. Generally,

Decrease in sodium (mEq/L) =
$$1.6 \text{ mEq/L} \times \text{Increase in blood glucose}/100 \text{ mg/dL}$$

Manifestations

The clinical manifestations depend in part on the volume status of the child and the underlying cause of the hyponatremia. When hyponatremia develops rapidly (<24 hours) and when it is severe (<120 mEq/L), the following may occur as a result of the intracellular shift of water:
1. Altered mental status
2. Seizures
3. Nausea and vomiting
4. Muscle cramps and weakness
5. Coma

Management

Determine the hydration status of the child and the severity of the hyponatremia.

Hypovolemic Patients

Most children with hyponatremia are dehydrated and hypovolemic, without symptoms such as altered mental status or seizures. These children can be managed as outlined in Chapter 15, with gradual replacement of the sodium and water deficit over a 24-hour period.

If altered mental status or seizures are present, more rapid correction of the decreased concentration may be necessary. In this situation, hypertonic saline solution (either 3% or 5%, containing 513 and 855 mEq/L of sodium, respectively) should be administered, with the goal of raising the serum sodium concentration to 125 mEq/L.

The following formula can be used to calculate the number of milliequivalents of sodium necessary to achieve this concentration:

Sodium (mEq) required =
$$(125 - \text{Current serum Na}) \times 0.6 \times \text{Weight (kg)}$$

The total required should be infused over a period of approximately 4 hours or at a rate of 5 mEq/kg/hr. Once the serum sodium concentration reaches approximately 125 mEq/L, further correction of the sodium deficit can proceed as discussed in Chapter 15.

Euvolemic Patients

Euvolemic patients or those with slight increases in extracellular volume usually require water restriction. SIADH production (most often associated with meningitis) or water intoxication is the most likely cause. Restriction to two thirds of the maintenance fluid requirement is the usual initial treatment, but adjustments may be necessary, with frequent monitoring of the serum sodium level. If the child is symptomatic, with seizures or altered mental status, the serum sodium concentration may be increased by combining hypertonic saline solution and diuresis with IV furosemide. In this way, excessive free water is diuresed as you are infusing a more hypertonic solution, thereby preventing a further increase in extracellular volume. The same formula discussed for hypovolemic patients may be used to calculate the required amount of sodium to be administered. Serum electrolytes (including potassium) should be measured frequently during such treatment because hypokalemia may ensue during diuresis.

Hypervolemic Patients

Salt and water restriction is required for those with edema-forming states or renal failure. Diuresis with furosemide also helps decrease extracellular volume. As with hypovolemia and euvolemia, a child with severe, symptomatic hyponatremia may require hypertonic saline solution, which should be combined with diuretics. Dialysis may be necessary for those in renal failure.

HYPERKALEMIA (SERUM POTASSIUM >5.5 mEq/L)

Causes

Decreased excretion
  Renal failure (acute or chronic)
  Potassium-sparing diuretics (amiloride, triamterene, spironolactone)
  Adrenal insufficiency
  Distal tubular dysfunction (type IV renal tubular acidosis)
Impaired extrarenal regulation
  Diabetes mellitus

Drugs (β-blockers, succinylcholine, angiotensin-converting enzyme inhibitors)
Shift from intracellular to extracellular fluid
    Acidosis
    Tissue destruction (trauma, hemolysis, burns, tumor lysis, rhabdomyolysis)
    Hyperkalemic periodic paralysis
Increased intake
    Potassium supplements (IV or orally)
    Blood transfusions
    Salt substitutes
Factitious
    Difficulty drawing blood (hemolysis, as with a heel puncture)
    Thrombocytosis

Manifestations

The effects of hyperkalemia on the cardiac conduction system are the most significant and may be fatal. The progressive changes that can be seen on an electrocardiogram (ECG) as the serum potassium concentration rises are, in order,
1. Peaked T waves (serum potassium, 6 to 7 mEq/L)
2. Depressed ST segments
3. Decreased R wave amplitude
4. Prolonged PR interval (serum potassium, 7 to 8 mEq/L)
5. Small or absent P waves
6. Wide QRS complexes (serum potassium, 8 to 9 mEq/L)
7. Sine wave pattern
8. Asystole or dysrhythmias

In addition, hyperkalemia may cause paresthesias, muscle weakness, and decreased tendon reflexes as a result of depolarization of muscle cells.

Management

Determine the severity of the hyperkalemia. All patients with hyperkalemia should have an ECG performed immediately to search for the signs just listed. Continuous ECG monitoring is also necessary until the problem is corrected.

Severe Hyperkalemia

If the serum potassium level is greater than 8 mEq/L or ECG changes other than peaked T waves are seen, you should proceed as follows:
1. Notify your senior resident.
2. Remove any potassium from the IV fluids
3. Administer 10% calcium gluconate, 0.5 mL/kg IV over a 2- to 5-minute period. This does not change the serum potassium level but protects the heart from the effects of hyperkalemia. The onset of action is immediate, and effects last approximately 1 hour.

4. Administer sodium bicarbonate, 2 to 3 mEq/kg IV over a 3- to 5-minute period. Make sure to flush the calcium gluconate from the line before giving bicarbonate because the two may be incompatible. The sodium bicarbonate shifts potassium intracellularly; its effect is immediate and lasts for 1 to 2 hours.
5. Administer glucose, 0.5 g/kg, with 0.3 unit of insulin per gram of glucose over a period of 2 hours.
6. Nebulized albuterol will move potassium intracellularly by stimulating β_1-adrenergic receptors.
7. Sodium polystyrene sulfonate (Kayexalate), 1 to 2 g/kg, with 3 mL of sorbitol per gram of resin divided every 6 hours orally **or** 5 mL of sorbitol per gram of resin as an enema over a period of 4 to 6 hours. **This is the only drug treatment that removes potassium from the body.** It is estimated that 1 g/kg decreases the serum potassium concentration by 1 mEq/L.
8. If these measures are unsuccessful, hemodialysis is necessary.
9. The serum potassium concentration should be determined every hour until it is less than 6.5 mEq/L.

Moderate Hyperkalemia

If the serum potassium level is between 6.5 and 8 mEq/L and the ECG reveals only peaked T waves, you should proceed as follows:
1. Notify your senior resident.
2. Remove any potassium from the IV fluids.
3. Administer sodium bicarbonate, glucose and insulin, and Kayexalate in the doses outlined earlier.
4. Monitor the serum potassium level every hour until it is less than 6.5 mEq/L.

Mild Hyperkalemia

If the serum potassium level is less than 6.5 mEq/L and the ECG is normal or has peaked T waves only, you should consider correcting other contributing factors (e.g., acidosis), as well as administering Kayexalate as previously outlined. Potassium should again be removed from any IV fluids. If the cause is identified and is not progressive, the serum potassium measurement can be repeated in 4 hours.

HYPOKALEMIA (SERUM POTASSIUM <3.5 mEq/L)

Causes

Excessive renal losses
 Diuretics
 Antibiotics (penicillins, amphotericin, aminoglycosides)
 Glucocorticoid excess
 Renal tubular acidosis type I

Hyperaldosteronism
Vomiting, nasogastric suctioning leading to alkalosis
Extrarenal losses
  Vomiting
  Diarrhea
  Laxative abuse
Shift from extracellular to intracellular space
  Alkalosis
  Insulin
  β-Catecholamines
  Lithium
Inadequate intake

Manifestations

As with hyperkalemia, the cardiac effects are the most significant and include the following:

1. Premature atrial contractions
2. Premature ventricular contractions (PVCs)
3. Flattened T waves
4. Appearance of U waves
5. ST-segment depression

In addition, neuromuscular symptoms and signs may appear, such as weakness, paresthesias, ileus, and depressed tendon reflexes.

Management

Determine the severity of the hypokalemia. All patients should have an ECG performed and undergo continuous ECG monitoring until the problem is corrected.

Severe Hypokalemia

If the serum potassium level is less than 2.5 mEq/L **and** there are PVCs, U waves, or ST-segment changes, IV supplementation of potassium should be considered. Potassium chloride, 0.5 mEq/kg, up to 10 mEq maximum, can be given IV over a 1-hour period while the patient is continually monitored. The serum potassium level should be measured again in 1 hour. Further supplementation can proceed more slowly by adding up to 40 mEq/L of potassium to an IV solution and infusing at the standard maintenance rate.

Moderate or Mild Hypokalemia

In those with a serum potassium level greater than 2.5 mEq/L and no ECG changes, hypokalemia may often respond to correction of the underlying cause, with no need for supplementation. If supplementation is necessary, oral supplements should be sufficient. The serum potassium level should be measured again in 4 to 6 hours to ensure that it does not continue to fall.

HYPERCALCEMIA

Causes

Increased intake
  Vitamin D or A intoxication
  Excessive calcium supplementation
  Milk-alkali syndrome (antacid ingestion)
Increased production or mobilization from bone
  Hyperparathyroidism (primary or tertiary)
  Hyperthyroidism
  Immobilization
  Malignancies (bone metastases, tumor lysis syndrome)
  Sarcoidosis
Decreased excretion
  Thiazide diuretics
  Familial hypocalciuric hypercalcemia
Miscellaneous
  Williams syndrome
  Pheochromocytoma
  Adrenal insufficiency

Manifestations

"Stones, bones, groans, and psychic moans" refer to some of the manifestations of hypercalcemia. Renal stones may develop, and polyuria and polydipsia are also common because hypercalcemia reduces the ability to concentrate urine. Bone pain ("bones") and abdominal symptoms ("groans"), such as pain, nausea, constipation, vomiting, and pancreatitis, may also occur. "Psychic moans" may be manifested as delirium, dementia, psychosis, lethargy, and even coma.

The ECG may reveal a short QT interval and a prolonged PR interval. Dysrhythmias may develop if the hypercalcemia is severe enough.

Management

Determine the severity of the hypercalcemia. Approximately half the total serum calcium is bound to albumin, and the other half is present in a free or ionized form. The clinical effect of hypercalcemia depends on the amount that is unbound, or the **ionized calcium**. Most laboratories routinely report total calcium, which reflects both ionized calcium and calcium that is bound to albumin. Thus, in hypoalbuminemic states, there may be an **increase** in ionized calcium despite normal serum total calcium. A useful assumption that can allow you to estimate the ionized calcium is that each 1-g/dL decrease in serum albumin decreases bound calcium (and total calcium) by approximately 0.8 mg/dL.

Severe Hypercalcemia

A serum calcium level greater than 14 mg/dL or the presence of symptoms requires immediate treatment. The serum calcium concentration can be reduced by rapid expansion of intravascular volume. Infusing a bolus of 20 mL/kg of normal saline solution results in a reduction in serum calcium concentration as a result of hemodilution and the increase in urinary calcium excretion that accompanies the excess sodium excreted in urine. Urinary calcium excretion can also be promoted with IV furosemide, 1 mg/kg every 2 to 4 hours. While you are monitoring the child's volume status closely, the normal saline boluses and furosemide may be repeated and should result in a fall in the serum calcium concentration. If it does not begin to decrease soon after volume expansion and diuresis, hemodialysis should be considered. Hemodialysis should be considered initially if the serum calcium concentration is greater than 15 mg/dL or the child has severe symptoms (e.g., coma).

Mild or Moderate Hypercalcemia

If the serum calcium concentration is less than 14 mg/dL, you may proceed at a less urgent pace. As with severe hypercalcemia, volume expansion and diuresis help increase urinary excretion of calcium. Increasing the IV rate to slightly expand intravascular volume after an initial 20-mL/kg bolus of normal saline solution may be sufficient. Likewise, IV furosemide, 1 mg/kg every 3 to 4 hours, should result in a gradual fall in the serum calcium concentration. Prednisone, 1 mg/kg/day, may be helpful because it decreases intestinal absorption of calcium by blocking the effect of 1,25-dihydroxyvitamin D. The effect of prednisone should be apparent within 2 to 3 days. Bisphosphonates and calcitonin are additional potential therapies because they inhibit bone resorption, but they should be used only after consultation with a pediatric endocrinologist.

HYPOCALCEMIA

Causes

Decreased intake
  Vitamin D deficiency (malabsorption, nutritional deficiency, abnormal vitamin D metabolism, lack of sunlight)
  Short-bowel syndrome
Decreased production or mobilization
  Hypoparathyroidism
  Pseudohypoparathyroidism
  Vitamin D deficiency
  Hyperphosphatemia
  Magnesium deficiency

       Pancreatitis
       Rhabdomyolysis
       Alkalosis
    Increased excretion
       Chronic renal failure
       Drugs (loop diuretics, aminoglycosides)
    Exchange transfusion in neonates

Manifestations

Papilledema, abdominal pain, mental status changes, laryngospasm (stridor), carpopedal spasm, seizures, and paresthesias may all occur. The ECG may reveal a prolonged QT interval. Chvostek's sign and Trousseau's sign may be present (Figs. 34-2 and 34-3).

Management

Determine the severity of the hypocalcemia by the presence and type of symptoms. An asymptomatic patient does not require urgent correction of the calcium concentration. IV calcium administration entails some special risks (see later); therefore, it should be reserved for those who cannot take oral calcium or whose symptoms demand immediate correction.

As with hypercalcemia, first correct for the serum albumin concentration. Hypoalbuminemia is common in hospitalized children, and

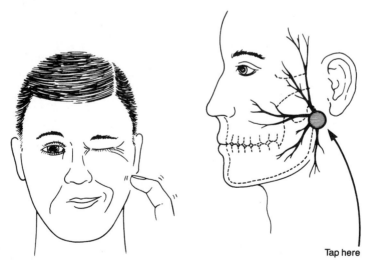

Tap here

Figure 34–2 Chvostek's sign: facial muscle spasm elicited by tapping the facial nerve anterior to the earlobe and below the zygomatic arch. (From Marshall SA, Ruedy J: On Call: Principles and Protocols, 4th ed. Philadelphia, Elsevier, 2004, p 331.)

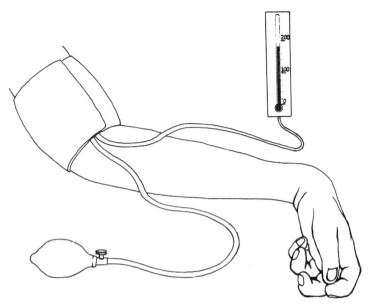

Figure 34–3 Trousseau's sign: carpal spasm elicited by occluding arterial blood flow to the forearm for 3 to 5 minutes. (From Marshall SA, Ruedy J: On Call: Principles and Protocols, 4th ed. Philadelphia, Elsevier, 2004, p 332.)

the ionized calcium concentration may be normal despite a significant reduction in the total serum calcium concentration.

Remember also to check the serum phosphate concentration. If it is markedly elevated, you need to consider correcting the phosphate concentration before administering calcium. Metastatic calcification may occur if the serum phosphate concentration remains high as calcium is administered.

A symptomatic child should be treated with 10% IV calcium gluconate, 100 to 200 mg/kg over a period of 5 to 10 minutes. Additional doses can be given if necessary. If possible, peripheral infusion of calcium should be avoided. Extravasation of calcium may result in significant tissue necrosis. Scalp veins and other small peripheral veins should never be used to infuse calcium solutions. Hypotension and bradycardia are also potential effects of calcium infusion; therefore, all patients should be monitored while receiving an infusion. Once the symptoms of hypocalcemia have resolved, oral calcium supplementation can be started. Elemental calcium can be given in a dosage of 50 mg/kg/day divided into three to four doses.

An asymptomatic child with hypocalcemia may be treated with oral elemental calcium in the same doses as just listed.

There are several circumstances in which caution is necessary in the treatment of hypocalcemia. In children with abnormal calcium mobilization, such as those with pancreatitis or rhabdomyolysis, care should be taken when correcting the serum calcium concentration because hypercalcemia may eventually result from the release of complexed calcium when the pancreatitis or rhabdomyolysis resolves. In a child with acidosis, the ionized calcium concentration will be increased because of displacement of calcium from albumin. Correction of the acidosis may cause the ionized calcium level to fall even further. Finally, in those with hypomagnesemia, parathyroid hormone release is impaired and the tissue response to parathyroid hormone is also diminished. The magnesium concentration will need to be corrected to treat the hypocalcemia effectively.

REMEMBER

The most important element of the management of any electrolyte problem is close monitoring with repeated measurement of electrolytes to gauge the effect of your treatment plan. The approaches outlined in this chapter allow you to begin thinking about the problem and to initiate a treatment plan, but repeated re-evaluation of the patient's clinical status and laboratory studies is essential. Keep in mind that you will eventually need to see the morning "lytes."

Glucose Disorders

Caroline C. Shieh, MD

There are many potentially serious consequences of a serum glucose imbalance. Certain pediatric patient populations are particularly susceptible, including patients with newly diagnosed diabetes, noncompliant diabetic patients, premature neonates, and infants of diabetic mothers. Each of these populations can experience life-threatening hypoglycemia or hyperglycemia. It is important for the house officer to keep glucose disorders in the differential diagnosis of many diverse conditions, including seizures, altered mental status, dehydration, and metabolic acidosis.

HYPERGLYCEMIA

Causes

Patients with known diabetes mellitus (DM)
  Poorly controlled type 1 or type 2 DM
  Stress (septic shock, surgery, trauma)
  Medications (thiazide diuretics, steroids, salicylates)
  Total parenteral nutrition (TPN) administration
Patients without previously documented DM
  New-onset type 1 or type 2 DM
  Stress (septic shock, surgery, trauma)
  Medications (thiazide diuretics, steroids, salicylates)
  TPN administration

Note: Serum glucose measurement has traditionally been reported as milligrams per deciliter. The current *Système International* (SI) reports serum glucose as millimoles per liter. When discussing serum levels throughout this chapter, SI units are used. However, for the following classification of hyperglycemia and the similar classification of hypoglycemia, both sets of units are included for reference.

Acute Manifestations

Mild hyperglycemia (fasting blood glucose level of 6.1 to 11.0 mmol/L [120 to 200 mg/dL])
  Polyuria, polydipsia, thirst

Moderate hyperglycemia (fasting blood glucose level of 11.1 to 22.5 mmol/L [200 to 410 mg/dL])

    Volume depletion (tachycardia, decreased perfusion, decreased blood pressure)

    Polyuria, polydipsia, thirst

Severe hyperglycemia (fasting blood glucose level >22.5 mmol/L [410 mg/dL])

    Type 1 DM

        Polyuria, polydipsia, thirst

        Ketotic breath

        Kussmaul breathing (deep, regular, pauseless respirations seen with pH <7.2)

        Volume depletion

        Anorexia, nausea, vomiting, abdominal pain, ileus

        Delirium, confusion, hyporeflexia, hypotonia, coma

    Type 2 DM

        Polyuria, polydipsia

        Volume depletion

        Confusion, hyperosmolar nonketotic coma (glucose levels of 50 to 110 mmol/L [900 to 2000 mg/dL])

Management

Many hyperglycemic patients require the administration of insulin either subcutaneously or intravenously. Bovine, porcine, and human insulin is available, each with different antigenicity. Bovine insulin is the most antigenic, whereas human is the least. Human insulin is associated with fewer adverse reactions (e.g., insulin allergy, antibody-mediated insulin resistance, lipoatrophy) and should be the preparation of choice, especially when treatment is intermittent. If the child is already receiving bovine or porcine insulin without problems, the same preparation should be continued and dosage adjustments made accordingly.

Assess the Severity

Although a Chemstrip or glucometer reading is fairly accurate, a serum glucose determination should also always be obtained (Table 35-1). The blood glucose level must then be closely monitored as it drops to avoid overshooting into the hypoglycemic range.

Mild, Asymptomatic Hyperglycemia

Mild asymptomatic hyperglycemia does *not* require urgent treatment. Make sure that the child is not receiving any glucose-containing intravenous (IV) fluids. In addition, a diagnosis of DM requires that no concurrent stress be present that can precipitate hyperglycemia. Any of the following is diagnostic of DM:

    Fasting blood glucose level greater than 126 mg/dL on two measurements

    Random blood glucose level greater than 200 mg/dL for two measurements (venous plasma) or symptoms of polyuria, polydipsia with a single measurement greater than 200 mg/dL

TABLE 35-1 **Blood Glucose Levels**

	Fasting or Preprandial Blood Glucose, mmol/L	2-Hour Postprandial Blood Glucose, mmol/L
Hypoglycemia	<3.5 (60 mg/dL)	
Normal range	3.5-6.0 (60-110 mg/dL)	<11.0 (200 mg/dL)
Mild hyperglycemia	6.1-11.0 (110-200 mg/dL)	11.1-16.5 (200-300 mg/dL)
Moderate hyperglycemia	11.1-22.5 (200-405 mg/dL)	16.6-27.5 (300-500 mg/dL)
Severe hyperglycemia	>22.5 (>405 mg/dL)	>27.5 (>500 mg/dL)

A glucose tolerance test with a fasting glucose level less than 126 mg/dL and a 2-hour postprandial glucose level of 200 mg/dL or more (venous plasma)

Moderate Hyperglycemia

Moderate hyperglycemia may require treatment, either by starting insulin or by adjusting the insulin dose already being given. Indications for treatment include osmotic diuresis, as evidenced by increased urine output and the presence of glucose in the urine. In the neonatal intensive care unit this is frequently seen in premature infants receiving TPN. Starting insulin is preferable to decreasing the total glucose load in the TPN in order to maximize caloric intake. Likewise, in a patient with known diabetes, the insulin dose is adjusted rather than altering the diet further.

For example, if you are called at night because of a Chemstrip or glucometer reading of 25 mmol/L (450 mg/dL) in a 12-year-old patient known to have diabetes, you should proceed as follows:

1. Order a stat blood glucose determination to confirm the Chemstrip or glucometer reading.
2. Be certain that a good IV line is in place.
3. Check to see whether recent stress (infection, trauma, surgery) may be contributing to the hyperglycemia or whether the child received medications that may cause hyperglycemia.
4. Give 0.1 U/kg of regular insulin subcutaneously or intravenously. The main consideration is not to devise a schedule that achieves perfect blood glucose control for the rest of the child's hospital stay. Short-term control of blood glucose levels has not been shown to decrease complications in diabetic patients. When the blood glucose concentration is elevated at night, it is important to prevent ketoacidosis in a type 1 DM patient or a hyperosmolar state in a type 2 DM patient without precipitating hypoglycemia overnight. (The worst time for anyone to become hypoglycemic is overnight, when mental status changes might develop and not be noticed for some time.)

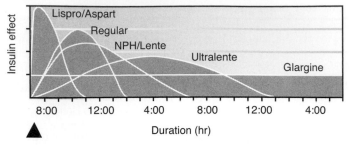

Figure 35–1 Insulin effect profiles. The following relative peak effect and duration units are used: lispro/aspart, peak 20 for 4 hours; regular, peak 15 for 7 hours; NPH/lente, peak 12 for 12 hours; ultralente, peak 9 for 19 hours; and glargine, peak 5 for 24 hours. (From Behrman RE: Nelson Textbook of Pediatrics, 17th ed. Philadelphia, Elsevier, 2004, p 1957.)

5. Determination of the reason for poor control of blood glucose before breakfast may aid in an ongoing adjustment of the patient's insulin regimen. A Chemstrip or glucometer finding of hypoglycemia at 3:00 AM suggests that the hyperglycemia seen before breakfast is due to the Somogyi effect: hyperglycemic rebound caused by a surge of counter-regulatory hormones that increase glucose production in response to nocturnal hypoglycemia. This rebound is a result of giving too much long-lasting or NPH insulin at dinnertime. Likewise, hyperglycemia at 3:00 AM suggests that too much short-acting insulin was given at dinnertime as compared with NPH (Fig. 35-1 and Table 35-2).

TABLE 35–2 **Insulin Preparations**

Type	Onset (hr)	Peak Action (hr)	Duration (hr)
Short-acting insulin Regular Semilente	0.5-20	2-4	6-12
Intermediate insulin NPH Lente	1-4	4-12	16-28
Long-acting insulin Protamine zinc Ultralente	4-6	8-20	24-36

From Behrman RE, Kliegman R (eds): Nelson Essentials of Pediatrics, 2nd ed. Philadelphia, WB Saunders, 1994, p 648.

Severe Hyperglycemia

Severe hyperglycemia should be considered a medical emergency requiring immediate intervention. The two states that result from severe hyperglycemia are diabetic ketoacidosis (DKA) and hyperosmolar non-ketotic hyperglycemic coma (HONKC).

Type 1 Diabetes Mellitus: Diabetic Ketoacidosis. Commonly seen in newly diagnosed patients or those with poorly controlled type 1 DM, DKA results from an absolute deficiency of insulin, which causes poor utilization of glucose and increased release of free fatty acids; the fatty acids are then converted to acidic ketone bodies (hence, acidosis and ketosis).

1. Correct the volume depletion.

   Aggressive correction of dehydration is vital to reversing the hypovolemic shock and poor tissue perfusion in patients with DKA. Normal saline solution, 20 mg/kg as a rapid IV bolus, should be followed by a continuous infusion of at least 1.5 times maintenance fluids (initially without dextrose).

2. Administer insulin

   Give regular insulin in a continuous insulin infusion (in normal saline solution) at a rate of 0.1 U/kg/hr. Monitor blood glucose, sodium, and potassium levels and pH closely (hourly) until the serum glucose level is below 14 mmol/L (250 mg/dL). At that point slow the insulin infusion to 0.025 to 0.05 U/kg/hr, and change the maintenance fluids to 5% dextrose in 0.5 normal saline with potassium acetate and potassium chloride (provided that the patient is making urine). Ideally, blood sugar should fall no faster than 80 to 100 mg/dL/hr. When the serum glucose level has been stabilized at 8 to 10 mmol/L (140 to 180 mg/dL) and the ketoacidosis has resolved, subcutaneous insulin should be resumed and the insulin infusion subsequently stopped after 1 to 2 hours. Continue to monitor glucose levels every 4 hours and add supplemental subcutaneous regular insulin as needed to keep the blood glucose level at 8 to 10 mmol/L.

3. Monitor serum glucose and electrolytes, urine ketones and glucose, and arterial blood gases (ABGs) frequently.

   Hyperglycemic patients tend to have metabolic acidosis and hypokalemia. As normal saline solution and insulin are administered, the acidosis is corrected and potassium shifts into cells from the extracellular space. This can result in significant hypokalemia, with cardiac dysrhythmias as a consequence. Determination of ABGs, electrolytes, blood urea nitrogen, creatinine, and glucose should be repeated frequently. If the patient has normal renal function, potassium should be added to the IV fluids as a combination of potassium acetate and potassium chloride. Caution must be used in a child with renal failure to avoid hyperkalemia.

4. Search for the precipitating cause.

Infection, dehydration, acute stress, and noncompliance with diet may be the cause.

Type 2 Diabetes Mellitus: Hyperosmolar Nonketotic Hyperglycemic Coma. HONKC is a rare condition in children and adolescents, but it does occur. There can be any variety of exacerbating factors, including infections, pancreatitis, sepsis, or medications. The blood glucose level is usually *very* high (e.g., >55 mmol/L [1000 mg/dL]).

1. Correct the volume depletion and water deficit.

The goal of fluid management in a patient with HONKC is to correct both the hyperosmolar state and the dehydration. Once the volume deficit has been corrected with normal saline solution, the remaining water deficits, as indicated by persistent hyperglycemia and hypernatremia, are best corrected with hypotonic IV solutions, such as 0.5 normal saline.

2. Begin an insulin infusion.

See the approach to DKA outlined earlier. Merely rehydrating the child frequently causes a substantial fall in the blood glucose concentration through osmotic diuresis. As a result, patients with HONKC often require less insulin than do patients with type 1 DM and DKA.

3. Monitor glucose, ABGs, and electrolytes.

Manage as noted earlier for DKA.

4. Search for the precipitating cause.

Manage as noted earlier for DKA.

HYPOGLYCEMIA

Causes

Patients with documented DM
Excess ingestion of insulin or oral hypoglycemic agents
Decreased caloric intake
Increased exercise
Patients without documented DM
Surreptitious intake of insulin or oral hypoglycemic agents
Insulin overproduction (insulinoma, Zollinger-Ellison syndrome)
Medications: ethanol, pentamidine, disopyramide, monoamine oxidase inhibitors, salicylates
Hepatic failure
Adrenal insufficiency

Manifestations

Adrenergic Response

The adrenergic response consists of catecholamine release as a result of a rapid decrease in the glucose level. Diaphoresis, tremulousness, palpitations, hunger, tachycardia, perioral numbness, anxiety, delirium, confusion, seizures, and coma may result.

Central Nervous System Response

The central nervous system response is slower than the adrenergic response and develops over a period of 1 to 3 days. Headache, diplopia, bizarre behavior, nonfocal neurologic signs, confusion, delirium, seizures, and coma may all be seen. Patients taking oral hypoglycemic agents may not experience an adrenergic response. Mental status change may arise solely because of hypoglycemia.

Management

Assess the severity. Any symptomatic patient with suspected hypoglycemia requires immediate treatment. Symptoms may be precipitated by either a rapid fall in the blood glucose level or an absolute low level of glucose.

1. Obtain a serum glucose determination. Confirm the diagnosis of hypoglycemia, and if the cause is not obvious, draw about 10 mL of blood for future analysis, including serum insulin level and C peptide measurement. Insulin produced endogenously includes the C peptide fragment, in contrast to commercial insulin, which does not. A high insulin level with a high C peptide level suggests endogenous overproduction, whereas a high insulin level associated with a low C peptide level is diagnostic of exogenous insulin administration.

2. If the child is awake and cooperative, oral glucose in the form of orange juice or sugar-containing soda may be given. However, if the child has an altered mental status, IV glucose in the form of 50% dextrose in water ($D_{50}W$) (1 to 2 mL/kg) or $D_{25}W$ (2 mL/kg) should be administered. In infants, 2 to 4 mL/kg $D_{10}W$ is usually given. If there is no IV access and the patient is unable to take oral glucose (e.g., unconscious), glucagon, 0.5 to 1.0 mg by subcutaneous or intramuscular injection, should be given. Use caution with glucagon because vomiting may follow its administration and could result in airway compromise in a patient with depressed mental status.

3. If there is ongoing hypoglycemia or if the patient's symptoms were severe (e.g., seizures, coma), a continuous glucose infusion should be started with D_5W or $D_{10}W$ at a maintenance dose initially. Reassess the blood glucose level hourly until a steady state is attained. Hypoglycemia caused by the ingestion of oral hypoglycemic agents may require additional boluses as a result of the prolonged metabolism of these medications.

The differential diagnosis of hypoglycemia in infants and children includes the entities shown in Table 35-3. The work-up is complex, but for the house officer at night, the best plan of action is to obtain an extra red-top tube of at least 5 mL for later testing of insulin levels, thyroid screen, and serum toxicology studies. Urine should also be obtained, especially to screen for toxic ingestion.

TABLE 35–3 **Causes of Childhood Hypoglycemia**

I. Decreased availability of glucose
    A. Decreased intake: fasting, malnutrition, illness
    B. Decreased absorption: acute diarrhea
    C. Inadequate glycogen reserves: defects in enzymes of glycogen synthetic pathways
    D. Ineffective glycogenolysis: defects in enzymes of glycogenolytic pathways
    E. Inability to mobilize glycogen: glucagon deficiency
    F. Ineffective gluconeogenesis: defects in enzymes of gluconeogenic pathway
II. Increased utilization of glucose
    A. Hyperinsulinism: islet cell adenoma or hyperplasia, nesidioblastosis, ingestion of oral hypoglycemic agents, insulin therapy
    B. Large tumors: Wilms' tumor
III. Diminished availability of alternative fuels
    A. Decreased or absent fat stores
    B. Inability to oxidize fats: enzymatic defects in fatty acid oxidation
IV. Unknown or complex mechanisms
    A. Sepsis or shock
    B. Reye's syndrome
    C. Salicylate ingestion
    D. Ethanol ingestion
    E. Adrenal insufficiency
    F. Hypothyroidism
    G. Hypopituitarism

From Fleisher GR, Ludwig S (eds): Textbook of Pediatric Emergency Medicine. Baltimore, Williams & Wilkins, 1988, p 742.

SUMMARY

Hyperglycemia is common in infants and children and may be seen as a complication of many other conditions. It is rarely life threatening but can cause significant morbidity and thus should be treated promptly. Hypoglycemia is much rarer and more dangerous and frequently arises as a complication of therapy for hyperglycemia. The house officer on call needs to act quickly to normalize the blood glucose level to ensure adequate glucose delivery to meet the metabolic demands of the child.

Hyperbilirubinemia

Katrina R. Ubell, MD

Jaundice in adults is a condition that brings to mind any number of ominous hepatic disorders and a host of unpleasant complications. In children, although almost all of these conditions may be seen, the vast majority of cases are transient and without significant consequences. Jaundice is frequently noted by some observer other than the child's parents, who do not appreciate the subtle and often gradual accumulation of pigment. Jaundice or hyperbilirubinemia is a symptom and not a disease unto itself. The house officer must define the underlying cause in order to plan an appropriate intervention. Although jaundice in a hospitalized child rarely has an acute onset, the on-call house officer may sometimes be the first to address the issue of hyperbilirubinemia. This is most common in the newborn nursery.

PHONE CALL

Questions

1. What is the child's age?
2. What are the child's vital signs?
3. What is the child's admitting diagnosis?
4. Has the child ever been jaundiced before?
5. Is the child receiving any medications?

Orders

Obtain the following laboratory tests as soon as possible:
1. Total and direct serum bilirubin level
2. Alkaline phosphatase, alanine transaminase (ALT), aspartate transaminase (AST), γ-glutamyltransferase (GGT), and lactate dehydrogenase (LDH)
3. Complete blood count, reticulocyte count, and peripheral blood smear
4. In a newborn, the mother's and infant's blood types and a Coombs test

Inform RN

"Will arrive at the bedside in … minutes."

Hyperbilirubinemia is rarely life threatening, but in younger children it deserves evaluation within several hours. In neonates, the evaluation should be immediate because in some instances the rise in bilirubin may be rapid and severe and accompanied by life-threatening anemia or placing the newborn at risk for kernicterus.

ELEVATOR THOUGHTS

The differential diagnosis of jaundice is extensive. Jaundice in a neonate is usually the result of different factors than jaundice in an older child. Direct (conjugated) hyperbilirubinemia and indirect (unconjugated) hyperbilirubinemia are also associated with different causes (see Fig. 36-1 and Tables 36-1 and 36-2).

MAJOR THREAT TO LIFE

- Hemolytic anemia–mediated heart failure or nephropathy
- Kernicterus

Hyperbilirubinemia is generally most threatening when its onset is rapid and the bilirubin is unconjugated. In the relatively immature central nervous system of a neonate, especially if premature, unconjugated bilirubin may be deposited in the basal ganglia, hippocampus, and subthalamic nuclei of the brain and can result in severe brain damage.

BEDSIDE

Quick-Look Test

Does the patient appear well (comfortable), sick (uncomfortable or distressed), or critical (about to die)?

A general rule to follow in estimating the serum bilirubin level in a neonate is that the sclerae become icteric at a bilirubin level of 2 to 4 mg/dL, the face and mucous membrane at a level of 4 to 7, the chest and abdomen at a level of 8 to 10, the legs at levels above 12, and the soles of the feet at levels above 15. Remember, this is a very rough estimate, and a serum level must be obtained to accurately assess the magnitude of the jaundice. Does the patient exhibit any signs of hemodynamic instability or neurologic deficits?

Airway and Vital Signs

Tachycardia, pallor, respiratory distress, and poor perfusion can be seen with severe hemolytic processes that can cause heart failure. Children with severe hepatic dysfunction usually appear quite ill.

Selective Physical Examination

HEENT　　　　The sclerae and mucous membranes are very
　　　　　　　　good places to assess jaundice, particularly in

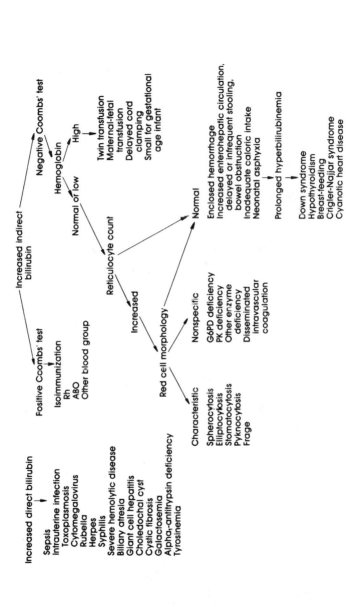

Figure 36–1 Schematic approach to the diagnosis of neonatal jaundice. G6PD, glucose-6-phosphate dehydrogenase; PK, pyruvate kinase. (From Oski FA: Differential diagnosis of jaundice. In Taeusch HW, Ballard RA, Avery MA (eds): Schaffer and Avery's Diseases of the Newborn, 6th ed. Philadelphia, WB Saunders, 1991, p 774.)

TABLE 36–1 Diagnostic Features of the Various Types of Neonatal Jaundice

Diagnosis	Nature of van den Bergh Reaction	Jaundice Appears	Jaundice Disappears	Peak Bilirubin Concentration mg/dL	Peak Bilirubin Concentration Age (Days)	Bilirubin Rate of Accumulation (mg/dL/day)	Remarks
"Physiologic jaundice"							Usually related to degree of maturity
Full-term	Indirect	2-3 days	4-5 days	10-12	2-3	<5	
Preterm	Indirect	3-4 days	7-9 days	15	6-8	<5	Metabolic factors: hypoxia, respiratory distress, lack of carbohydrate
Hyperbilirubinemia as a result of metabolic factors							Hormonal influences: cretinism, hormones
Full-term	Indirect	2-3 days	Variable	<2	1st wk	<5	Genetic factors: Crigler-Najjar syndrome, transient familial hyperbilirubinemia
Premature	Indirect	3-4 days	Variable	<15	1st wk	<5	Drugs: vitamin K, novobiocin

Hemolytic states and hematoma	Indirect	May appear in 1st 24 hr	Variable	Unlimited	Variable	Usually >5	Erythroblastosis: Rh, ABO Congenital hemolytic states: spherocytic, nonspherocytic Infantile pyknocytosis Drugs: vitamin K Enclosed hemorrhage: hematoma
Mixed hemolytic and hepatotoxic factors	Indirect and direct	May appear in 1st 24 hr	Variable	Unlimited	Variable	Usually >5	Infection: bacterial sepsis, pyelonephritis, hepatitis, toxoplasmosis, cytomegalic inclusion disease, rubella Drugs: vitamin K
Hepatocellular damage	Indirect and direct	Usually 2-3 days	Variable	Unlimited	Variable	Variable, can be >5	Biliary atresia, galactosemia, hepatitis and infection

From Brown AK: Neonatal jaundice. Pediatr Clin North Am 9:589, 1962.

TABLE 36–2 Differential Diagnosis of Jaundice in Childhood

Unconjugated Hyperbilirubinemia				Conjugated Hyperbilirubinemia			
Hemolysis and Reticulocytosis							
Positive Coombs Test	Negative Coombs Test	No Hemolysis	Obstructive	Infectious	Metabolic	Toxic	Idiopathic	Autoimmune
ABO and Rh incompatibility Autoimmune, systemic lupus erythematosus Drug-induced and idiopathic acquired hemolytic anemia	RBC enzyme defect (G6PD deficiency) Hemoglobinopathy (sickle cell anemia) RBC membrane defect (hereditary spherocytosis) Hemolytic-uremic syndrome Wilson's disease	Gilbert syndrome Physiologic jaundice of the newborn Breast milk jaundice Crigler-Najjar syndrome Hypothyroidism Pyloric stenosis Internal hemorrhage	Biliary atresia Choledochal cyst Cholelithiasis Tumor/neoplasia Bile duct stenosis Spontaneous bile duct perforation Bile-mucus plug	Hepatitis A, B, C, D, E Cytomegalovirus Herpes simplex 1, 2, 6 Epstein-Barr virus Coxsackievirus Echovirus Measles Varicella Syncytial giant cell (paramyxovirus) Toxoplasmosis Syphilis Leptospirosis Bacterial sepsis/urinary tract infection (especially gram negative) Cholecystitis Fitz-Hugh-Curtis syndrome	Wilson's disease α₁-Antitrypsin deficiency Galactosemia Tyrosinemia Fructosemia Niemann-Pick disease Gaucher's disease Zellweger syndrome Wolman's disease Cystic fibrosis Neonatal iron storage disease Indian childhood cirrhosis Trihydroxyprostanic acidemia	Total parenteral nutrition Acetaminophen Ethanol Salicylates Iron Halothane Isoniazid Valproic acid Veno-occlusive disease	Idiopathic neonatal hepatitis Alagille syndrome Nonsyndrom·c paucity of intrahepatic bile ducts Progressive familial intrahepatic cholestasis Familial benign recurrent cholestasis Cholestasis with lymphedema (Aagenaes syndrome) Cholestasis with hypopituitarism Familial erythrophagocytic lymphohistiocytosis	Autoimmune chronic hepatitis Sclerosing cholangitis Graftversus-host disease

G6PD, glucose-6-phosphate dehydrogenase; RBC, red blood cell.
From Behrman RE, Kliegman RM: Nelson Essentials of Pediatrics, 2nd ed. Philadelphia, WB Saunders, 1994.

HEENT—Cont'd	darkly pigmented children; cephalohematoma or excessive bruising in the newborn
Cardio-vascular	Heart rate, pulse volume, blood pressure, perfusion, jugular venous distention
Abdomen	Distention, hepatomegaly, masses, tenderness, ascites (fluid wave), caput medusa, incision scars
Neurologic	Cranial nerves, tone (axial as well as segmental in infants), quality of cry, primitive reflexes (Moro, grasp, tonic-neck, stepping, placing), motor function, mental status

Acute cardiac failure can occur with severe hemolytic processes. A change in color of the urine would also be expected with severe hemolysis.

Management

Diagnostic investigation depends largely on the age of the child and the presence of associated findings besides jaundice. The two most common scenarios are discussed in this chapter: (1) a neonate in the nursery or on the infant floor whose daytime laboratory results indicating a high bilirubin level are brought to the attention of the on-call house officer and (2) a child in whom jaundice develops acutely during a hospitalization.

Neonatal Hyperbilirubinemia

It is not uncommon for an infant to be admitted to rule out sepsis immediately after birth because of prolonged rupture of membranes, fetal distress, meconium aspiration, or respiratory distress. Likewise, a newborn may be admitted to the observation nursery or the neonatal unit for evaluation of some form of congenital anomaly or syndrome. In any case, laboratory studies are often ordered and not reported until after hours to the on-call house staff. Adequate sign-out should anticipate the results and a plan of action, but this is not always the case. Therefore, the on-call house officer may have to evaluate the laboratory results and the patient and determine the next action.

Hyperbilirubinemia within the first 24 hours of birth is worrisome. A rapid rise in unconjugated bilirubin in the first 24 hours is common in hemolytic processes involving ABO incompatibility between the infant and the mother, concealed hematoma or hemorrhage, cytomegalovirus infection, sepsis, congenital rubella, or congenital toxoplasmosis. Laboratory evaluation should be initiated immediately and include a complete blood count and peripheral smear, reticulocyte count, typing and screening with direct and indirect Coombs tests, total and direct bilirubin, and serum albumin. Acute hemolytic anemia in a newborn may require not only simple transfusion but also partial or complete exchange transfusion. A cord hemoglobin level of 10 g/dL, a bilirubin level of 5 mg/dL or greater on the first day of life, and a reticulocyte count of 15% or more suggest severe hemolytic anemia and may require at least partial exchange transfusion.

Exchange transfusion is a technique that requires experience. It is entirely appropriate to summon at least a senior resident, if not a neonatal fellow or attending physician, to supervise this procedure.

Blood for exchange transfusion should be as fresh as possible and be completely cross-matched if possible. In acute settings, type O-negative blood may be used. The blood should be warmed to 37°C and should be continuously mixed or gently agitated during the transfusion. The exchange requires large intravenous lines, which in a newborn generally means umbilical venous catheterization (see Chapter 26, Lines, Tubes, and Drains, for the details of umbilical catheterization). When proper positioning of the umbilical line or lines has been confirmed by radiograph, 10- to 20-mL aliquots of blood are withdrawn, alternating with equal volumes of donor blood. Calculation of the total volume of the exchange is based on an estimated total circulating blood volume of 85 mL/kg body weight.

The therapy of choice for mild indirect hyperbilirubinemia is phototherapy. The infant is placed in a diaper only, or a surgical mask may be used to create a "bikini diaper" so that the maximal amount of skin surface area can be bathed in blue (420- to 470-nm wavelength) light. Bilirubin in the skin absorbs this wavelength, and photoisomerization converts toxic 4Z, 15Z-bilirubin into the unconjugated, configurational isomer 4Z, 15E-bilirubin, which can be excreted without the need for conjugation. Besides the familiar banks of lights frequently seen in neonatal units, fiberoptic "bili-blankets" allow "home phototherapy." One must be conscientious about shielding the eyes of newborn infants from this intense light exposure, regardless of their gestational age. Remember that phototherapy increases the infant's insensible water loss by as much as 20%, and therefore the maintenance fluid requirements of the baby must be adjusted.

The risk to the infant of specific serum bilirubin levels relative to age can be determined by using a nomogram (Fig. 36-2). Risk factors for the development of severe hyperbilirubinemia are shown in Table 36-3.

In an infant who is 2 to 3 days of age, hyperbilirubinemia may be physiologic and require no intervention if the level remains reasonable. Table 36-1 details several types of jaundice and their onset, along with ranges of bilirubin levels and some of their causes. Levels of 15 mg/dL or less total bilirubin in a full-term infant rarely require intervention. So-called physiologic jaundice, or icterus neonatorum, may be influenced by maternal diabetes, polycythemia, race, male sex, trisomy 21, bruising or cephalohematoma, delayed stooling, oxytocin induction, breast-feeding, and a host of other nonspecific factors.

The diagnosis of physiologic jaundice in term or preterm infants can be established by excluding known causes of jaundice by history and clinical and laboratory findings, as in Table 36-2. The cause of jaundice should be pursued if (1) hyperbilirubinemia occurs within 24 hours of birth, (2) the level exceeds 12 mg/dL in the absence of risk factors, (3) the level rises at a rate greater than 5 mg/dL/24 hr, or (4) the jaundice persists for longer than 2 weeks.

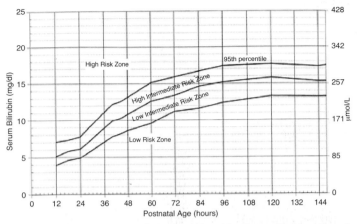

Figure 36–2 Nomogram to determine the risk of specific elevations in serum bilirubin. (From American Academy of Pediatrics Subcommittee on Hyperbilirubinemia: Management of hyperbilirubinemia in the newborn infant 35 or more weeks of gestation. Pediatrics 114:297-316, 2004.)

If the percentage of direct to total bilirubin rises, one must suspect a cholestatic process, hepatocellular damage, or a metabolic disorder (galactosemia, tyrosinemia, α_1-antitrypsin deficiency). Further laboratory testing is necessary, including a prothrombin time (PT) and partial thromboplastin time (PTT) to assess hepatic synthetic function, as well as measurement of the transaminases AST (also known as serum glutamic-oxaloacetic transaminase [SGOT]), ALT (also known as serum glutamate pyruvate transaminase [SGPT]), LDH, alkaline phosphatase, and GGT to assess hepatocellular damage. Testing for cystic fibrosis is indicated, as are abdominal ultrasound studies to determine the integrity of the biliary tree (biliary atresia, choledochal cyst). Disorders such as the latter are also suggested by persistent jaundice in the face of acholic stools and poor weight gain.

Table 36-4 presents an algorithm for the treatment of indirect hyperbilirubinemia in healthy term infants. In addition, some recommend starting phenobarbital to activate the conjugation pathway nonspecifically and the cytochrome P-450 pathways in hepatocytes. This therapy has the unwanted side effect of sedating the infant, which may decrease feeding and thereby slow stool excretion and increase enterohepatic reabsorption of bilirubin. It also does nothing to enhance the phototherapy and is not recommended for routine "physiologic jaundice."

Acute Jaundice in Children

Fortunately a fairly rare event, acute jaundice in children, especially conjugated hyperbilirubinemia, is almost always a manifestation of

TABLE 36–3 **Risk Factors for the Development of Severe Hyperbilirubinemia in Infants of 35 or More Weeks' Gestation (in Approximate Order of Importance)**

Major Risk Factors

Predischarge TSB or TcB level in the high-risk zone (Fig. 36-2)
Jaundice observed in the first 24 hours
Blood group incompatibility with a positive direct antiglobulin test, other
  known hemolytic disease (e.g., G6PD deficiency)
Gestational age of 35-36 weeks
Previous sibling received phototherapy
Cephalohematoma or significant bruising
Exclusive breast-feeding, particularly if nursing is not going well
  and weight loss is excessive
East Asian race

Minor Risk Factors

Predischarge TSB or TcB level in the high intermediate-risk zone (Fig. 36-2)
Gestational age of 37-38 weeks
Jaundice observed before discharge
Previous sibling with jaundice
Macrosomic infant of a diabetic mother
Maternal age ≥25 years
Male gender

Decreased Risk*

TSB or TcB level in the low-risk zone (Fig 36-2)
Gestational age ≥41 weeks
Exclusive bottle feeding
Black race[†]
Discharge from hospital after 72 hours

*Factors associated with a decreased risk for significant jaundice, listed in order of decreasing importance.
[†]Race as defined by mother's description.
G6PD, glucose-6-phosphate dehydrogenase; TcB, transcutaneous bilirubin; TSB, total serum bilirubin.
From American Academy of Pediatrics Subcommittee on Hyperbilirubinemia: Management of hyperbilirubinemia in the newborn infant 35 or more weeks of gestation. Pediatrics 114:297-316, 2004, with permission.

severe hepatocellular damage from a hypoxic-ischemic insult, accumulation of a hepatotoxin (acetaminophen ingestion), or acute hepatitis. As in neonates, accumulation of unconjugated bilirubin is usually due to hemolysis of red blood cells. Hemoglobinopathies, erythrocyte enzyme defects, and erythrocyte membrane defects account for a large percentage of the hemolytic processes.

Diagnostic evaluation is much the same as for a neonate. Synthetic hepatic function, as well as hepatocellular injury, must be investigated, as should cholestasis. Acute hepatocellular injury is manifested by an elevation in aminotransferases (AST, ALT, LDH, GGT), regardless of the cause. The most marked transaminase elevations are seen with

TABLE 36–4 **Approach to Indirect Hyperbilirubinemia in Healthy Term Infants without Hemolysis***

Age (hr)	Phototherapy	Phototherapy and Preparation for Exchange Transfusion†	Exchange Transfusion If Phototherapy Fails‡
<24	§	§	§
24-48‖	≥15-18	≥25	≥20
49-72	≥18-20	≥30	≥25
>72	≥20	≥30	≥25
>2 wk	¶	¶	¶

*With hemolysis, exchange transfusion is initiated with an indirect bilirubin level of 20 or greater at any age. The precise level of unconjugated bilirubin in healthy breast-fed term infants that requires therapy is unknown. Treatment options include observation, continued breast-feeding, and initiation of phototherapy or interrupted breast-feeding (use formula as substitute) with or without phototherapy. If there are any signs of kernicterus during the evaluation or treatment as suggested anywhere in the table or at any level of bilirubin, emergency exchange transfusion must be performed.

†If the bilirubin level at initial evaluation is high, intense phototherapy should be initiated and preparation made for exchange transfusion. If phototherapy fails to reduce bilirubin to the levels noted on the column to the right, initiate exchange transfusion.

‡Intensive phototherapy usually reduces serum bilirubin levels 1 to 2 mg/dL in 4 to 6 hours; this is often associated with the administration of intravenous fluids at 1 to 1.5 times maintenance. Oral alimentation should also continue.

§Jaundice in the first 24 hours of life is not seen in "healthy" infants.

‖Hyperbilirubinemia of this degree within 48 hours of birth is unusual and should suggest hemolysis, concealed hemorrhage, or causes of conjugated (direct) hyperbilirubinemia.

¶Jaundice suddenly appearing in the second week of life or continuing beyond the second week of life with significant hyperbilirubinemia levels to warrant therapy should be investigated in detail because it is most probably due to a serious underlying cause, such as biliary atresia, galactosemia, hypothyroidism, or neonatal hepatitis.

From Behrman RE, Kliegman RM, Arvin AM (eds). Nelson Textbook of Pediatrics, 15th ed. Philadelphia, WB Saunders, 1996.

acute viral hepatitis, hypoxic-ischemic injury, hepatotoxin exposure, and Reye's syndrome. A differential rise in ALT or AST can suggest a variety of processes, but usually the two are elevated similarly. Elevation of alkaline phosphatase, 5'-nucleotidases, cholesterol, and conjugated bilirubin suggests obstruction and/or inflammation of the hepatobiliary tract.

Assessment of the synthetic function of the liver is important. The PT and PTT are important functional assays for the various serum globulins manufactured in the liver, particularly vitamin K–dependent clotting factors (II, VII, IX, X).

For the on-call physician, little in the way of intervention can be done in an older child with acute jaundice other than supportive care and initiation of the diagnostic work-up. In particular, children who have suffered hepatocellular damage are subject to shock and disseminated intravascular coagulation and can die if not aggressively supported early in their disease.

SUMMARY

Hyperbilirubinemia in a newborn may be physiologic, but a wide variety of pathologic conditions must be considered and ruled out by history, physical examination, and laboratory evaluation. Although rarely life threatening, hyperbilirubinemia may have serious consequences. In older children, hepatocellular injury from infection, toxins, or a hypoxic-ischemic event must be ruled out and aggressive supportive treatment instituted at once to allow time to make the diagnosis and initiate more definitive therapy.

Pediatric Procedures

James J. Nocton, MD
Rainer G. Gedeit, MD

Procedures are a great source of anxiety for the house officer or medical student. As a pediatric house officer, you may have limited opportunities to perform some procedures; consequently, it may be difficult to feel a sense of competence when you find yourself in the position of needing to obtain intravenous (IV) access or intubate a child. However, if you take advantage of every opportunity to try procedures, you will increase your chances of becoming proficient at such techniques as peripheral IV line placement, venipuncture, arterial blood gas sampling, lumbar puncture, intubation, umbilical line placement, joint aspiration, interosseous line placement, femoral line placement, and peripheral arterial line placement.

The key to success with any procedure involving a sharp object (e.g., a needle) is comfort of the person **holding** the sharp object. Set up for every procedure in the same way so that the routine is comfortable and automatic. Know the supplies that you will need and prepare them in advance, whether they are blood tubes, culture bottles, slides, or swabs.

For almost every procedure involving needles there is a choice regarding the use of local anesthesia. Obviously, this is not a consideration in a dire emergency, but that is the exception, not the rule. Small children are fearful and move and resist, thereby reducing the likelihood of success. If properly anesthetized, the child resists and moves less, and you will be a hero when the IV goes in on the first try!

Topical EMLA, an anesthetic, can be used for any procedure in which numbing of the skin will be helpful. EMLA is a white cream that must be applied 20 to 30 minutes before the procedure and covered with an occlusive dressing. It works quite well, but you must know what sites to apply it to ahead of time. It is ideal for lumbar puncture or joint aspiration, especially in older children. Remember to consider the child's comfort during every procedure; the child's comfort may increase your own.

Intravenous Access

IV access is an important ingredient in intervention and stabilization of any patient in the hospital. The following is a brief overview of the options available, some helpful technical tips, and a general approach to this procedure in pediatrics.

The legendary house officers who can get an IV line into anyone always have a routine that they follow with every patient, regardless of age. First, try to perform all procedures in a treatment or procedure room. All the supplies are there, and it maintains the patient's room as a sanctuary where the child is free from harm. Second, make sure that all your favorite supplies are set up before bringing the patient into the room. Third, get help from the patient's nurse or your medical student. **Don't ever ask a parent to hold a child for a procedure.** First, they might faint, whereupon you will have two patients. Second, the parents should "rescue" their child from you afterward, not assist you. Regarding whether parents should observe procedures, if you are not comfortable having the parents in the room, tell them that honestly and explain that you are more likely to be successful if they are not present. Most parents respond favorably if you express your desire to make the procedure easier for their child.

The person holding the patient is as important to this process as the person holding the needle! Give the nurse or student clear instructions about how to restrain the child and assist you best. This is true in both a dire emergency and routine replacement of a peripheral IV line. Apply a rubber tourniquet above the potential site tight enough to occlude the veins but not so tight that you cannot palpate a pulse distally. Look and feel for the veins in the same places that you have veins, starting at the most distal point. Veins feel hollow, like a straw. Tendons are tense and cord-like. Arteries are firm and deep and should be pulsatile. Look at several different sites before making an attempt. It pays to shop around a little. Remove the tourniquet until you are ready to make your attempt.

The sites that should be explored in any patient include the dorsal hand veins, the radial vein of the wrist, the anterior ulnar vein of the forearm, the median cephalic vein in the lateral antecubital fossa, the median basilic vein in the medial antecubital fossa (Fig. A-1), the superficial veins of the dorsum of the foot, and the saphenous vein anterior and superior to the medial malleolus of the ankle and along its proximal length on the medial aspect of the foreleg (Fig. A-2). Next, the external jugular should be considered (Fig. A-3). Remember, neck lines in any child and scalp IV lines in infants are very distressing to parents and should be choices of last resort. IV line placement is

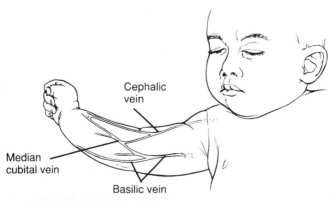

Figure A–1 Veins of the upper extremity. (Reproduced with permission. Textbook of Pediatric Advanced Life Support, 1994. Copyright American Heart Association.)

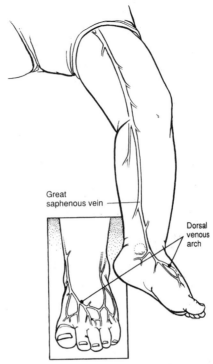

Great
saphenous vein

Dorsal
venous
arch

Figure A–2 Veins of the lower extremity. (Reproduced with permission. Textbook of Pediatric Advanced Life Support, 1994. Copyright American Heart Association.)

not a benign intervention. Children suffer more complications from IV lines than from any other medical intervention in the hospital.

Selecting the catheter for a peripheral IV line is very important, not only to the success of your attempt but also to the longevity of the line that you place. Whatever size you originally think of, choose one size larger. Larger IV catheters will go in easier and last longer. In most full-term infants, regardless of hydration status, a 22-gauge catheter can be placed in any vein. Frequently in infants, a 20-gauge catheter or even an 18-gauge catheter can be placed in the antecubital, distal saphenous, or external jugular veins. Save the 24-gauge catheters for preterm infants. Smaller IV catheters do not advance into veins easily, cannot handle high flow rates, and cause a jet-like stream within the vessel that damages endothelium and causes infiltration into the surrounding tissues. The bigger needle may appear to hurt more, but it also goes in better and lasts longer, which means fewer IV attempts and less discomfort for your patient.

Once you have selected the site, put on your gloves and prepare the site with povidone-iodine scrub and alcohol. Apply the tourniquet again and

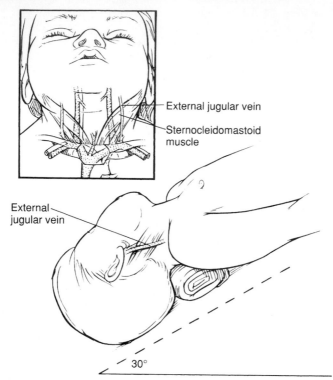

External jugular vein

Sternocleidomastoid muscle

External jugular vein

30°

Figure A–3 External jugular vein cannulation. (Reproduced with permission. Textbook of Pediatric Advanced Life Support, 1994. Copyright American Heart Association.)

confirm that this is a good site. Then ask your assistant to gently but firmly hold the child. The IV starter should hold the extremity to ensure its position. Make the attempt boldly to get through the skin in one quick stab. Anticipate the withdrawal reaction and then advance into the vessel.

An IV catheter is a needle within a plastic tube. When you see blood return in the needle, you know that the *lumen of the needle* is within the lumen of the vessel; it does not necessarily mean that *the catheter* is within the lumen of the vessel. Because the needle tip extends 2 to 3 mm beyond the catheter, you must advance the needle and catheter a bit more before the catheter can be advanced into the vessel as you withdraw the needle. The blood return in the catheter should remind you to release the tourniquet and place the needle in a safe place away from the field and the child. Instruct your assistant to maintain control over the child until the IV line is safely and securely taped into place. Be meticulous about how you tape the IV line, and do it the same way every time. This ensures that the nurse will not be calling you again in 30 minutes to replace the same IV line.

In conclusion, do not approach placement of an IV line timidly. Confidence begets success. Be systematic, consistent, methodical, and caring, and pick a larger catheter. Also, know your limitations. If you are not successful, call someone else to attempt the line placement. Rather than leave once help arrives, stay and observe "the master" at work. You may learn more than you expect. Remember that you want to help the patient to be healed and be comfortable. "Getting" a difficult IV line is a big confidence boost, but it should not come at the expense of causing more discomfort to the patient than is acceptable.

If a peripheral IV line cannot be established, a deep or central line may be required. Again, *know your limitations*. Central lines require experience, time, sterile technique, and sedation and are not to be pursued casually or without supervision. In an extreme emergency, an intraosseous line can be life saving and should be considered within 90 seconds, even in a hospitalized patient. The best tool for this is the Baxter bone marrow aspiration/interosseous line needle. In children younger than 3 years, the anterior tibial plateau is prepared with povidone-iodine and alcohol. The needle is directed 1 to 3 cm below the tibial tuberosity at a 30-degree angle caudally to avoid the epiphyseal growth plate (Fig. A-4). Insertion requires firm, steady pressure with a twisting motion through the bone. Less resistance is felt as the marrow cavity is entered. Frequently, no marrow is aspirated. Infusion with a syringe should be free of resistance or soft tissue swelling. In older children, the distal end of the femur can be used, with the needle angled 30 degrees cephalad. Once in place, the needle must be secured and the extremity restrained. Again, medical students or house officers must know their own limitations, be willing to learn, and be concerned for the welfare and comfort of the patient.

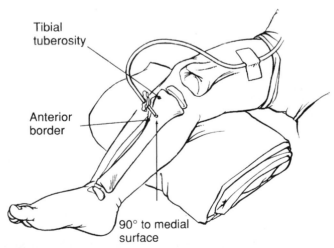

Figure A–4 Intraosseous cannulation technique. (Reproduced with permission. Textbook of Pediatric Advanced Life Support, 1994. Copyright American Heart Association.)

Femoral Line Placement

There are any number of reasons why a central venous line may be the best choice for a pediatric inpatient. Lack of peripheral access, need for a high dextrose concentration, parenteral nutrition, use of cardiotonic infusions, and need for large-volume fluid resuscitation or exchange are among the most common. The femoral vein is an excellent site for obtaining central venous access.

Position the patient supine with the arms and legs adequately restrained. It is preferable that the patient be sedated for this procedure; thus, airway support supplies must be at the bedside. Place a double-folded towel under the buttocks to extend the hips and bring the vein and artery into a straight position. Mark the following landmarks with a waterproof pen: the pubic tubercle, the anterior superior iliac spine, and the femoral artery (Fig. A-5A). Scrub both sides of the groin with povidone-iodine (Betadine) solution. Infuse 1 to 2 mL of 1% lidocaine (without epinephrine) subcutaneously and deeper to the periosteum; be careful to aspirate frequently to ensure that you have not entered a vessel.

Direct the needle medial to the femoral pulse, 1 cm caudal to the inguinal ligament at a 45-degree angle toward the umbilicus (Fig. A-5B). Advance slowly, aspirating as you advance, until free flow of dark, venous blood is obtained. Remove the syringe to allow free backflow of blood. If using the Seldinger technique, advance the soft tip or "J" tip of the wire into the needle and into the vessel. Note: if the guidewire is in the vessel, it should advance with little or no resistance. **Never push or force the wire. If it does not "fall into the vessel" with minimal resistance, you must start again.** Perforating the vessel wall in the retroperitoneum can cause significant intra-abdominal bleeding and must be avoided. Once the wire has advanced without resistance, withdraw the needle while leaving the wire in place. Never advance more than half the wire length into the patient because you must thread the catheter over the wire and have enough wire left to grasp after passing the catheter to the insertion site. First use a No. 11 scalpel blade and then the appropriate dilator or dilators from your central line kit to enlarge the wire entry site. Next place the preflushed catheter over the wire to the desired length. Remove the wire, aspirate and flush the catheter, and obtain an abdominal radiograph to confirm its position. Unless you are in an emergency resuscitation situation, always confirm the position of the line before using it.

Sometimes an "over-the-needle catheter," or angiocatheter, will be used for femoral line placement, especially in small infants and children. The same procedure is used until free flow of blood is obtained from the needle. The needle should be advanced another millimeter and the catheter threaded off the needle and into the femoral vein. This catheter should give free backflow of venous blood and also must be both aspirated and flushed.

Regardless of how it was placed, a femoral venous catheter should be securely sutured, dressed with a clear occlusive dressing, and dated. Always write a succinct procedure note explaining the justification for the procedure, your technique, the results, and any complications.

Lumbar Puncture

A lumbar puncture, or spinal tap, is likely to be the most common procedure performed by a pediatric house officer. Obtaining cerebrospinal fluid (CSF) for culture, microscopy, and biochemical analysis is an essential part of every work-up for sepsis.

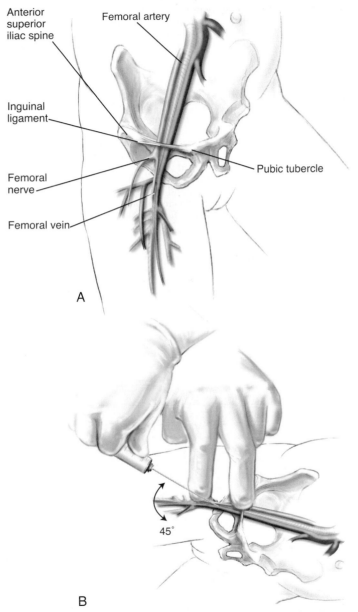

Anterior
superior
iliac spine

Femoral artery

Inguinal
ligament

Pubic tubercle

Femoral
nerve

Femoral vein

A

45°

B

Figure A–5 A, Anatomy of the femoral vein. **B**, Technique for placing a femoral line.

For a right-handed person performing a lumbar puncture, the patient's head should be positioned to the left, with the supply kit to the right. This allows you to position your left hand so that your fingers are on the iliac crest and your thumb is on the desired interspace. The right hand is then free to insert the needle and fill the tubes.

The person holding the child is equally important. This person must also monitor the child's condition, especially the respiratory pattern in infants. Infants can be held quite effectively in the left lateral decubitus position or in the upright sitting position (Fig. A-6). Older children, if uncooperative, may require a second holder. **Remember, never attempt a lumbar puncture without adequate help.**

Once you have set up the supply tray and have given your holder or holders their instructions, put on gloves in sterile fashion. With the child in the desired position, prepare the lower part of the back vigorously with povidone-iodine. Place the cover drape, and find the anatomic landmarks by position-ing your left fingers on the iliac crest and feeling for the posterior iliac spines with your left thumb. The level of the crest should be L2-3, and the level of the posterior spine should be L5. Feel for the L3-4 interspace and keep your

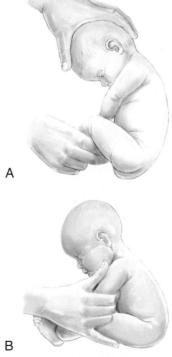

A

B

Figure A–6 A, Lateral recumbent position for restraining an infant for lumbar puncture. View from above the infant. **B,** Sitting position for restraining an infant for lumbar puncture. Lateral view.

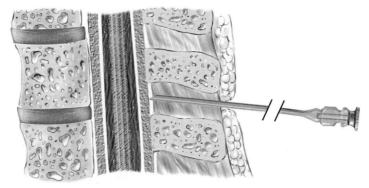

Figure A–7 The needle should be inserted in a slightly cephalad direction to avoid the vertebral bodies.

left thumb at that level. Using a prefilled 3-mL syringe, inject a small amount of 1% lidocaine subcutaneously. Be prepared for the child to move, and make sure that your holder is also prepared. Once the child settles, advance the needle, aspirate, and inject about 0.5 mL of lidocaine. **There is no good reason to not use local anesthesia for a lumbar puncture. It will help immensely in avoiding a traumatic or bloody tap because of movement of the child.** Return the lidocaine syringe to your sterile tray and insert the spinal needle at a 15- to 20-degree angle cephalad to avoid the posterior vertebral spines (Fig. A-7). If resistance is met, withdraw and angle more cephalad. In a term infant, the needle will advance 1 to 1.5 cm, and then resistance will be felt before the "pop" as the needle penetrates the dura (Fig. A-8). Withdraw the

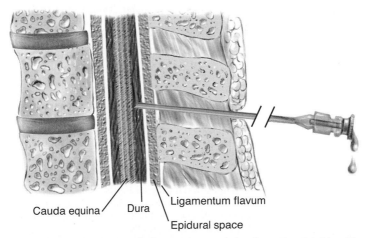

Cauda equina / Dura \ Ligamentum flavum

Epidural space

Figure A–8 Once the needle has penetrated the dura, the stylet is withdrawn to allow spinal fluid to flow freely.

stylet and watch for CSF backflow. If an opening pressure is desired, attach the manometer via the three-way stopcock and determine the CSF level in centimeters. Then proceed to collect about 5 mL of CSF in sterile test tubes. Replace the stylet, withdraw the needle, and apply pressure on the site with the left thumb. The holder should allow the child to straighten and relax. A small bandage should be placed and the date written on it.

As with every procedure, a succinct procedural note should be written immediately to document the indications for the lumbar puncture, the technique, the results, and any complications.

Peripheral Arterial Line Placement

Not infrequently, a patient requires invasive blood pressure monitoring to maintain close control of fluid resuscitation, inotropic medication monitoring, or vasodilator use. Other children require frequent arterial blood gas monitoring, such as for severe asthma exacerbation or diabetic ketoacidosis. An arterial line usually requires the patient to be in a pediatric intensive care unit (PICU), but it may be placed in the emergency room or on the floor before transfer to the PICU.

The first step in placement of a peripheral arterial line is to palpate the various sites available for the best pulse. The radial artery is a common choice, as are the posterior tibial and the dorsalis pedis arteries. Before placement of any arterial line, it is vital for you to establish that the artery you are planning to use is not the only arterial blood supply to the distal end of that extremity. With the hand, one should perform the Allen test by holding pressure over both the ulnar and radial arteries for 5 to 10 seconds. Release the ulnar artery. If the hand becomes pink rapidly, there is adequate collateral circulation to allow the radial artery to be used.

As with every procedure, have all of your supplies ready, including precut pieces of tape, IV connector tubing with a three-way stopcock, a syringe of heparinized saline flush, and an armboard. Again, review with your holders what they need to do. Some people prefer to attach the limb to the armboard first. Do it whichever way you are more comfortable. If you are right handed, set up your supplies to your right. Hold the limb firmly with your gloved left hand. Make sure that you can easily palpate the pulse in this position. Prepare the area vigorously with povidone-iodine. Anesthetize the skin and shallow subcutaneous tissue with 1% lidocaine via a 26- or 25-gauge needle. For infants under 2.5 kg, a 24-gauge catheter should be used. For almost all other children, a 22-gauge catheter should suffice. Insert the catheter about 3 to 4 mm distal to the pulse just through the skin. Advance the catheter and needle until a flash of blood appears in the needle. **Remember, the tip of the needle extends 1 to 2 mm beyond the tip of the catheter, which means that you must advance the needle and catheter an additional 1 to 2 mm to ensure that the catheter tip is within the artery.** Pull the needle back from the catheter; if there is backflow of blood into the catheter, advance the catheter into the artery. If there is no backflow, pull back on the catheter until blood flows back and then advance. Remove the needle and attach the flush syringe and stopcock. Secure the arterial catheter in place with tape, with or without sutures, and dress it with a clear plastic occlusive dressing. Date the dressing so that nursing personnel can monitor its condition. As always, immediately write an appropriate procedural note.

Resuscitation Calculations

James J. Nocton, MD
Rainer G. Gedeit, MD

Intubation Equipment

Age/Weight	Endotracheal Tube Size	Laryngoscope Blade
Newborn/3-5 kg	2.5-3.5 mm	0-1 straight
Infant/6-9 kg	3.5 mm uncuffed	1 straight
Toddler/10-11 kg	4.0 mm uncuffed	1 straight
Small child/12-14 kg	4.5 mm uncuffed	2 straight
Child/15-18 kg	5.0 mm uncuffed	2 straight or curved
Child/19-22 kg	5.5 mm uncuffed	2 straight or curved
Large child/24-28 kg	6.0 mm cuffed	2-3 straight or curved
Adult/>30 kg	6.5 mm cuffed	3 straight or curved

Resuscitation Medications

Drug	Dosage
Epinephrine	First dose IV/IO: 0.01 mg/kg (1:10,000, 0.1 mL/kg) ETT: 0.1 mg/kg (1:1000, 0.1 mL/kg) Subsequent doses Repeat every 3-5 minutes during CPR Consider higher dose: 0.1-0.2 mg/kg (1:1000, 0.1-0.2 mL/kg)
Amiodarone	IV/IO: 5 mg/kg
Lidocaine	IV/IO/ETT: 1 mg/kg
Glucose	IV/IO: 0.5-1 g/kg (1-2 mL/kg of 50% solution)

CPR, cardiopulmonary resuscitation; ETT, endotracheal tube; IO, intraosseous; IV, intravenous.

C

Posteroanterior and Lateral Chest X-Ray Projections

James J. Nocton, MD
Rainer G. Gedeit, MD

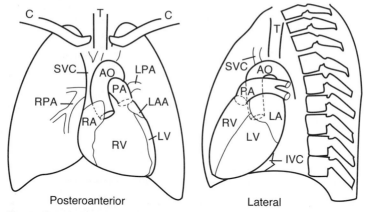

Posteroanterior   Lateral

Figure C–1 Posteroanterior and lateral chest x-ray projections. AO, aorta; C, clavicle; IVC, inferior vena cava; LA, left atrium; LAA, left atrial appendage; LPA, left pulmonary artery; LV, left ventricle; PA, pulmonary artery; RA, right atrium; RPA, right pulmonary artery; RV, right ventricle; SVC, superior vena cava; T, trachea.

Oxyhemoglobin Dissociation Curve of Normal Blood

James J. Nocton, MD
Rainer G. Gedeit, MD

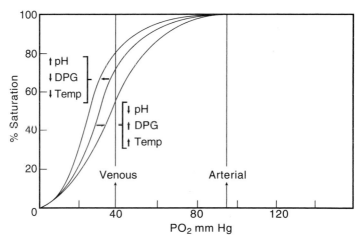

Figure D–1 Oxyhemoglobin dissociation curve of normal blood. The major factors influencing the position of the curve are temperature, pH, and the intracellular concentration of 2,3-diphosphoglycerate (DPG). The curve shifts if there are changes in these factors, as indicated in the figure.

E

Calculation of Creatinine Clearance

James J. Nocton, MD
Rainer G. Gedeit, MD

Calculation of Creatinine Clearance

$$\mathrm{CrCl\,(mL/min)} = \frac{\mathrm{U_{Cr}\,(mg/mL) \times V\,(mL/min)}}{\mathrm{P_{Cr}\,(mg/mL)}}$$

CrCl = creatinine clearance
U_{Cr} = urinary concentration of creatinine
V = urinary flow rate
P_{Cr} = Plasma concentration of creatinine
To correct clearance for body surface area (BSA):

Corrected CrCl = CrCl (mL/min) $\times$ 1.73/BSA (m^2)

Calculation of Alveolar-Arterial Oxygen Gradient

James J. Nocton, MD
Rainer G. Gedeit, MD

The alveolar-arterial oxygen gradient, or P $(A-a)o_2$, can be calculated easily from the arterial blood gas (ABG) results. It is useful for confirming the presence of a shunt.

$$P(A-a)o_2 = Pao_2 - Pao_2$$

- Pao_2 = alveolar oxygen tension calculated as shown subsequently
- Pao_2 = arterial oxygen tension measured by ABG determination

Pao_2 can be calculated by the following formula:

$$Pao_2 = (PB - PH_2O)(Fio_2) - Paco_2/R$$

- PB = barometric pressure (760 mm Hg at sea level)
- PH_2O = 47 mm Hg
- Fio_2 = fraction of O_2 in inspired gas
- $Paco_2$ = arterial CO_2 tension measured by ABG determination
- R = respiratory quotient (0.8)

Normal P(A-a)o_2 ranges from 12 mm Hg or less for infants, children, and adolescents.

In pure ventilatory failure, P(A-a)o_2 will remain 12 to 20 mm Hg. In oxygenation *failure, it will increase.*

Adapted from Marshall SA, Ruedy J: On Call: Principles and Protocols, 4th ed. Philadelphia, WB Saunders, 2004, p 425.

Blood Tubes

James J. Nocton, MD
Rainer G. Gedeit, MD

Blood Tubes

Lavender Top (Ethylenediaminetetraacetic Acid [EDTA])

Complete blood count (CBC) and differential
Reticulocyte count
Direct Coombs test
Glucose-6-phosphate dehydrogenase (G6PD)
Sickle cell
Malaria stain
Adrenocorticotropic hormone (ACTH)

Red/Gray ("Tiger Top")

Sequential Multiple Analyzer plus Computer (SMAC) (glucose)*
Cardiac enzymes
Liver enzymes
Drug concentrations (alcohol, digoxin, gentamicin)
C peptide/insulin
Protein electrophoresis
C3, C4, cryoglobulins
Osmolality
Pregnancy test

Red Top

Cross-match
Haptoglobin
Tricyclic antidepressant (TCA) concentrations
Rheumatoid arthritis (RA)
Antinuclear antibody (ANA)

Green Top

Lactate*
Ammonia*

Blue Top (Citrate)

Prothrombin time (PT), activated partial thromboplastin time (aPTT)
Circulating anticoagulants
Coagulation factor assays
Fibrinogen

Blue Top (for FDPs only)

Fibrin degradation products (FDPs)

*These specimens must be delivered to the laboratory immediately or put on ice for transportation.

From Marshall SA, Ruedy J: On Call: Principles and Protocols, 4th ed. Philadelphia, Elsevier, 2004, pp 419-420.

H

Assessment of Neonatal Maturity (Ballard Score)

James J. Nocton, MD
Rainer G. Gedeit, MD

NEUROMUSCULAR MATURITY

	−1	0	1	2	3	4	5
Posture							
Square Window (wrist)	>90°	90°	60°	45°	30°	0°	
Arm Recoil		180°	140°–180°	110°–140°	90–110°	<90°	
Popliteal Angle	180°	160°	140°	120°	100°	90°	<90°
Scarf Sign							
Heel to Ear							

Figure H–1 Assessment of neonatal maturity (Ballard score).

Continued

PHYSICAL MATURITY

Skin	sticky friable transparent	gelatinous red, translucent	smooth pink, visible veins	superficial peeling &/or rash. few veins	cracking pale areas rare veins	parchment deep cracking no vessels	leathery cracked wrinkled
Lanugo	none	sparse	abundant	thinning	bald areas	mostly bald	
Plantar Surface	heel-toe 40-50mm: -1 <40mm: -2	>50mm no crease	faint red marks	anterior transverse crease only	creases ant. 2/3	creases over entire sole	
Breast	imperceptible	barely perceptible	flat areola no bud	stippled areola 1-2mm bud	raised areola 3-4mm bud	full areola 5-10mm bud	
Eye/Ear	lids fused loosely:-1 tightly:-2	lids open pinna flat stays folded	sl. curved pinna; soft; slow recoil	well-curved pinna; soft but ready recoil	formed &firm instant recoil	thick cartilage ear stiff	
Genitals male	scrotum flat, smooth	scrotum empty faint rugae	testes in upper canal rare rugae	testes descending few rugae	testes down good rugae	testes pendulous deep rugae	
Genitals female	clitoris prominent labia flat	prominent clitoris small labia minora	prominent clitoris enlarging minora	majora & minora equally prominent	majora large minora small	majora cover clitoris & minora	

Scoring system: Ballard JL, Khoury JC, Wedig K, Wang L, Eilers-Walsman BL, Lipp R. New Ballard Score, expanded to include extremely premature infants. *J Pediatr.* 1991;119:417-423.

Figure H-1 Cont'd

Body Surface Nomogram

James J. Nocton, MD
Rainer G. Gedeit, MD

See next page for nomogram for estimation of surface area (SA).

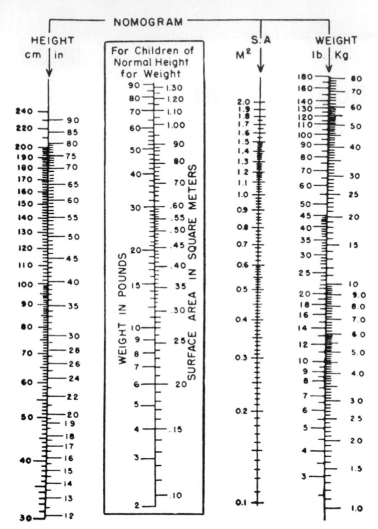

Figure I–1 Nomogram for estimation of surface area (SA). SA is indicated at the point where a straight line that connects the height and weight levels intersects the SA column. If the patient is roughly of average size, SA can be estimated from the weight alone (*enclosed area*). (Nomogram modified from data of E. Boyd by C.D. West. From Behrman RE, Kliegman RM [eds]: Nelson Essentials of Pediatrics, 2nd ed. Philadelphia, WB Saunders, 1994.)

Vital Signs at Various Ages

James J. Nocton, MD
Rainer G. Gedeit, MD

Age	Heart Rate (Beats/min)	Blood Pressure (mm Hg)	Respiratory Rate (Breaths/min)
Premature	120-170*	55-75/35-45[†]	40-70[‡]
0-3 mo	100-150*	65-85/45-55	35-55
3-6 mo	90-120	70-90/50-65	30-45
6-12 mo	80-120	80-100/55-65	25-40
1-3 yr	70-110	90-105/55-70	20-30
3-6 yr	65-110	95-110/60-75	20-25
6-12 yr	60-95	100-120/60-75	14-22
> 12 yr	55-85	110-135/65-85	12-18

*In sleep, infant heart rates may drop significantly lower, but if perfusion is maintained, no intervention is required.

[†] A blood pressure cuff should cover approximately two thirds of the arm; too small a cuff yields spuriously high pressure readings, and too large a cuff yields spuriously low pressure readings.

[‡] Many premature infants require mechanical ventilatory support, thus making their spontaneous respiratory rate less relevant.

From Behrman RE, et al (eds): Nelson Textbook of Pediatrics, 17th ed. Philadelphia, Elsevier, 2004, p 280.

Blood Pressure in Children

James J. Nocton, MD
Rainer G. Gedeit, MD

Blood pressure levels for boys and girls by age and height percentiles are listed in the following tables.

TABLE K–1 Blood Pressure Levels for Boys by Age and Height Percentiles

Age (Yr)	Blood Pressure Percentile	Systolic Blood Pressure by Percentile of Height (mm Hg)							Diastolic Blood Pressure by Percentile of Height (mm Hg)						
		5%	10%	25%	50%	75%	90%	95%	5%	10%	25%	50%	75%	90%	95%
1	50th	80	81	83	85	87	88	89	34	35	36	37	38	39	39
	90th	94	95	97	99	100	102	103	49	50	51	52	53	53	54
	95th	98	99	101	103	104	106	106	54	54	55	56	57	58	58
	99th	105	106	108	110	112	113	114	61	62	63	64	65	66	66
2	50th	84	85	87	88	90	92	92	39	40	41	42	43	44	44
	90th	97	99	100	102	104	105	106	54	55	56	57	58	58	59
	95th	101	102	104	106	108	109	110	59	59	60	61	62	63	63
	99th	109	110	111	113	115	117	117	66	67	68	69	70	71	71
3	50th	86	87	89	91	93	94	95	44	44	45	46	47	48	48
	90th	100	101	103	105	107	108	109	59	59	60	61	62	63	63
	95th	104	105	107	109	110	112	113	63	63	64	65	66	67	67
	99th	111	112	114	116	118	119	120	71	71	72	73	74	75	75
4	50th	88	89	91	93	95	96	97	47	48	49	50	51	51	52
	90th	102	103	105	107	109	110	111	62	63	64	65	66	66	67
	95th	106	107	109	111	112	114	115	66	67	68	69	70	71	71
	99th	113	114	116	118	120	121	122	74	75	76	77	78	78	79
5	50th	90	91	93	95	96	98	98	50	51	52	53	54	55	55
	90th	104	105	106	108	110	112	112	65	65	66	67	68	69	69

Continued

TABLE K–1 Blood Pressure Levels for Boys by Age and Height Percentiles—Cont'd

Age (Yr)	Blood Pressure Percentile	Systolic Blood Pressure by Percentile of Height (mm Hg)							Diastolic Blood Pressure by Percentile of Height (mm Hg)						
		5%	10%	25%	50%	75%	90%	95%	5%	10%	25%	50%	75%	90%	95%
	95th	108	109	110	112	114	115	116	69	70	71	72	73	74	74
	99th	115	116	118	120	121	123	123	77	78	79	80	81	81	82
6	50th	92	94	96	98	99	100	100	53	53	54	55	56	57	57
	90th	105	106	108	110	111	113	113	68	68	69	70	71	72	72
	95th	109	110	112	114	115	117	117	72	72	73	74	75	76	76
	99th	116	117	119	121	123	124	125	80	80	81	82	83	84	84
7	50th	94	95	97	99	100	101	102	55	55	56	57	58	59	59
	90th	106	107	109	111	113	114	115	70	70	71	72	73	74	74
	95th	110	111	113	115	117	118	119	74	74	75	76	77	78	78
	99th	117	118	120	122	124	125	126	82	82	83	84	85	86	86
8	50th	94	95	97	99	100	102	102	56	57	58	59	60	60	61
	90th	107	109	110	112	114	115	116	71	72	72	73	74	75	76
	95th	111	112	114	116	118	119	120	75	76	76	78	79	79	80
	99th	119	120	122	123	125	127	127	83	84	85	86	87	87	88
9	50th	95	96	98	100	102	103	104	57	58	59	60	61	61	62
	90th	109	110	112	114	115	117	118	72	73	74	75	76	76	77
	95th	113	114	116	118	119	121	121	76	77	78	79	80	81	81
	99th	120	121	123	125	127	128	129	84	85	86	87	88	88	89

Age (Year)	BP Percentile	SBP							DBP						
10	50th	97	98	100	102	103	105	106	58	59	60	61	61	62	63
	90th	111	112	114	115	117	119	119	73	73	74	75	76	77	78
	95th	115	116	117	119	121	122	123	77	78	79	80	81	81	82
	99th	122	123	125	127	128	130	130	85	86	86	88	88	89	90
11	50th	99	100	102	104	105	107	107	59	59	60	61	62	63	63
	90th	113	114	115	117	119	120	121	74	74	75	76	77	78	78
	95th	117	118	119	121	123	124	125	78	78	79	80	81	82	82
	99th	124	125	127	129	130	132	132	86	86	87	88	89	90	90
12	50th	101	102	104	106	108	109	110	59	60	61	62	63	63	64
	90th	115	116	118	120	121	123	123	74	75	75	76	77	78	79
	95th	119	120	122	123	125	127	127	78	79	80	81	82	82	83
	99th	126	127	129	131	133	134	135	86	87	88	89	90	90	91
13	50th	104	105	106	108	110	111	112	60	60	61	62	63	64	64
	90th	117	118	120	122	124	125	126	75	75	76	77	78	79	79
	95th	121	122	124	126	128	129	130	79	79	80	81	82	83	83
	99th	128	130	131	133	135	136	137	87	87	88	89	90	91	91
14	50th	106	107	109	111	113	114	115	60	61	62	63	64	65	65
	90th	120	121	123	125	126	128	128	75	76	77	78	79	79	80
	95th	124	125	127	128	130	132	132	80	80	81	82	83	84	84
	99th	131	132	134	136	138	139	140	87	88	89	90	91	92	92
15	50th	109	110	112	113	115	117	117	61	62	63	64	65	66	66
	90th	122	124	125	127	129	130	131	76	77	78	79	80	80	81
	95th	126	127	129	131	133	134	135	81	81	82	83	84	85	85
	99th	134	135	136	138	140	142	142	88	89	90	91	92	93	93
16	50th	111	112	114	116	118	119	120	63	63	64	65	66	67	67
	90th	125	126	128	130	131	133	134	78	78	79	80	81	82	82

Continued

TABLE K–1 Blood Pressure Levels for Boys by Age and Height Percentiles—Cont'd

Age (Yr)	Blood Pressure Percentile	Systolic Blood Pressure by Percentile of Height (mm Hg)							Diastolic Blood Pressure by Percentile of Height (mm Hg)						
		5%	10%	25%	50%	75%	90%	95%	5%	10%	25%	50%	75%	90%	95%
17	95th	129	130	132	134	135	137	137	82	83	83	84	85	86	87
	99th	136	137	139	141	143	144	145	90	90	91	92	93	94	94
	50th	114	115	116	118	120	121	122	65	66	66	67	68	69	70
	90th	127	128	130	132	134	135	136	80	80	81	82	83	84	84
	95th	131	132	134	136	138	139	140	84	85	86	87	87	88	89
	99th	139	140	141	143	145	146	147	92	93	93	94	95	96	97

From National High Blood Pressure Education Program; National Heart, Lung, and Blood Institute; National Institutes of Health; U.S. Department of Health and Human Services: NIH Publication No. 05-5267; originally printed September 1996 (96-3790); revised May 2005.

TABLE K–2 Blood Pressure Levels for Girls by Age and Height Percentiles

Age (Yr)	Blood Pressure Percentile	Systolic Blood Pressure by Percentile of Height (mm Hg)							Diastolic Blood Pressure by Percentile of Height (mm Hg)						
		5%	10%	25%	50%	75%	90%	95%	5%	10%	25%	50%	75%	90%	95%
1	50th	83	84	85	86	88	89	90	38	39	39	40	41	41	42
	90th	97	97	98	100	101	102	103	52	53	53	54	55	55	56
	95th	101	101	102	104	105	106	107	56	57	57	58	59	59	60
	99th	108	108	109	111	112	113	114	64	64	65	65	66	67	67
2	50th	85	85	87	88	89	91	91	43	44	44	45	46	46	47
	90th	98	99	100	101	103	104	105	57	58	58	59	60	61	61
	95th	102	103	104	105	107	108	109	61	62	62	63	64	65	65
	99th	109	110	111	112	114	115	116	69	69	70	70	71	72	72
3	50th	86	87	88	89	91	92	93	47	48	48	49	50	50	51
	90th	100	100	102	103	104	106	106	61	62	62	63	64	64	65
	95th	104	104	105	107	108	109	110	65	66	66	67	68	68	69
	99th	111	111	113	114	115	116	117	73	73	74	74	75	76	76
4	50th	88	88	90	91	92	94	94	50	50	51	52	52	53	54
	90th	101	102	103	104	106	107	108	64	64	65	66	67	67	68
	95th	105	106	107	108	110	111	112	68	68	69	70	71	71	72
	99th	112	113	114	115	117	118	119	76	76	76	77	78	79	79
5	50th	89	90	94	93	94	95	96	52	53	53	54	55	55	56
	90th	103	103	105	106	107	109	109	66	67	67	68	69	69	70

TABLE K-2 Blood Pressure Levels for Girls by Age and Height Percentiles—Cont'd

Age (Yr)	Blood Pressure Percentile	Systolic Blood Pressure by Percentile of Height (mm Hg)							Diastolic Blood Pressure by Percentile of Height (mm Hg)						
		5%	10%	25%	50%	75%	90%	95%	5%	10%	25%	50%	75%	90%	95%
	95th	107	107	108	110	111	112	113	70	71	71	72	73	73	74
	99th	114	114	116	117	118	120	120	78	78	79	79	80	81	81
6	50th	91	92	93	94	96	97	98	54	54	55	56	56	57	58
	90th	104	105	106	108	109	110	111	68	68	69	70	70	71	72
	95th	108	109	110	111	113	114	115	72	72	73	74	74	75	76
	99th	115	116	117	119	120	121	122	80	80	80	81	82	83	83
7	50th	93	93	95	96	97	99	99	55	56	56	57	58	58	59
	90th	106	107	108	109	111	112	113	69	70	70	71	72	72	73
	95th	110	111	112	113	115	116	116	73	74	74	75	76	76	77
	99th	117	118	119	120	122	123	124	81	81	82	82	83	84	84
8	50th	95	95	96	98	99	100	101	57	57	57	58	59	60	60
	90th	108	109	110	111	113	114	114	71	71	71	72	73	74	74
	95th	112	112	114	115	116	118	118	75	75	75	76	77	78	78
	99th	119	120	121	122	123	125	125	82	82	83	83	84	85	86
9	50th	96	97	98	100	101	102	103	58	58	58	59	60	61	61
	90th	110	110	112	113	114	116	116	72	72	72	73	74	75	75
	95th	114	114	115	117	118	119	120	76	76	76	77	78	79	79
	99th	121	121	123	124	125	127	127	83	83	84	84	85	86	87

Age	BP Percentile		Systolic BP							Diastolic BP					
10	50th	98	99	100	102	103	104	105	59	59	59	60	61	62	62
	90th	112	112	114	115	116	118	118	73	73	73	74	75	76	76
	95th	116	116	117	119	120	121	122	77	77	77	78	79	80	80
	99th	123	123	125	126	127	129	129	84	84	85	86	86	87	88
11	50th	100	101	102	103	105	106	107	60	60	60	61	62	63	63
	90th	114	114	116	117	118	119	120	74	74	74	75	76	77	77
	95th	118	118	119	121	122	123	124	78	78	78	79	80	81	81
	99th	125	125	126	128	129	130	131	85	85	86	87	87	88	89
12	50th	102	103	104	105	107	108	109	61	61	61	62	63	64	64
	90th	116	116	117	119	120	121	122	75	75	75	76	77	78	78
	95th	119	120	121	123	124	125	126	79	79	79	80	81	82	82
	99th	127	127	128	130	131	132	133	86	86	87	88	88	89	90
13	50th	104	105	106	107	109	110	110	62	62	62	63	64	65	65
	90th	117	118	119	121	122	123	124	76	76	76	77	78	79	79
	95th	121	122	123	124	126	127	128	80	80	80	81	82	83	83
	99th	128	129	130	132	133	134	135	87	87	88	89	90	90	91
14	50th	106	106	107	109	110	111	112	63	63	63	64	65	66	66
	90th	119	120	121	122	124	125	125	77	77	77	78	79	80	80
	95th	123	123	125	126	127	129	129	81	81	81	82	83	84	84
	99th	130	131	132	133	135	136	136	88	88	89	90	90	91	92
15	50th	107	108	109	110	111	113	113	64	64	64	65	66	67	67
	90th	120	121	122	123	125	126	127	78	78	78	79	80	81	81
	95th	124	125	126	127	129	130	131	82	82	82	83	84	85	85
	99th	131	132	133	134	136	137	138	89	89	90	91	91	92	93
16	50th	108	108	110	111	112	114	114	64	64	65	66	66	67	68
	90th	121	122	123	124	126	127	128	78	78	79	80	81	81	82

Continued

TABLE K-2 Blood Pressure Levels for Girls by Age and Height Percentiles—Cont'd

Age (Yr)	Blood Pressure Percentile	Systolic Blood Pressure by Percentile of Height (mm Hg)							Diastolic Blood Pressure by Percentile of Height (mm Hg)						
		5%	10%	25%	50%	75%	90%	95%	5%	10%	25%	50%	75%	90%	95%
17	95th	125	126	127	128	130	131	132	82	82	83	84	85	85	86
	99th	132	133	134	135	137	138	139	90	90	90	91	92	93	93
	50th	108	109	110	111	113	114	115	64	65	65	66	67	67	68
	90th	122	122	123	125	126	127	128	78	79	79	80	81	81	82
	95th	125	126	127	129	130	131	132	82	82	83	84	85	85	86
	99th	133	133	134	136	137	138	139	90	90	91	91	92	93	93

From National High Blood Pressure Education Program; National Heart, Lung, and Blood Institute; National Institutes of Health; U.S. Department of Health and Human Services: NIH Publication No. 05-5267; originally printed September 1996 (96-3790); revised May 2005.

Normal Values and SI Units

James J. Nocton, MD
Rainer G. Gedeit, MD

SI units is the abbreviation for *Système International d'Unités*. The system is an outgrowth of the metric system and provides a uniform system of reporting laboratory data between nations. Most laboratory values in *On Call Pediatrics* are presented in SI units. Because some laboratories have not yet converted to this system of reporting, a conversion table for commonly measured laboratory parameters is provided.

Table L-1

Laboratory Test	Previous Reference Intervals	Previous Units	Conversion Factor	SI Reference Intervals	SI Unit Symbol
Alanine aminotransferase (ALT)	6-50	U/L	×1	6-50	U/L
Albumin (serum)		g/dL	×10		g/L
Premature	1.8-3.0			18-30	
Term newborn <6 days	2.5-3.4			25-34	
<5 years	3.9-5.0			39-50	
5-19 years	4.0-5.3			40-53	
Alkaline phosphatase		U/L	×1		U/L
1-9 years	145-420			145-420	
10-11 years	130-560			130-560	
12-13 years					
Male	200-495			200-495	
Female	105-420			105-420	
14-15 years					
Male	130-525			130-525	
Female	70-230			70-230	
16-19 years					
Male	65-260			65-260	
Female	50-130			50-130	
Amylase (serum)	35-127	U/L	×1	35-127	U/L
Aspartate aminotransferase (AST)		U/L	×1		U/L
Neonate	35-140			35-140	
1-9 years	15-55			15-55	
10-19 years	5-45			5-45	

Bicarbonate					
Arterial	21-28	mmol/L	×1	21-28	mmol/L
Venous	22-29			22-29	
Bilirubin		mg/dL	×17.1		μmol/L
Total					
Preterm					
Cord blood	<2.0			<34	
0-1 day	<8.0			<137	
1-2 days	<12.0			<205	
2-5 days	<16.0			<274	
>5 days	<20.0			<340	
Full-term					
Cord blood	<2.0			<34	
0-1 day	<6.0			<103	
1-2 days	<8.0			<137	
2-5 days	<12.0			<205	
>5 days	<10.0			<171	
Conjugated	0-0.2			0-3.4	
Calcium, total (serum)		mg/dL	×0.25		mmol/L
Newborn	9.0-10.6			2.3-2.7	
1-2 days	7.0-12.0			1.8-3.0	
4-7 days	9.0-11.0			2.3-2.7	
Child to adult	8.4-10.8			2.1-2.7	
Calcium, ionized (serum)		mg/dL	×0.25		mmol/L
Newborn	4.3-5.1			1.1-1.3	
1-2 days	4.0-4.7			1.0-1.2	
Child to adult	4.8-5.0			1.2-1.25	

Continued

Table L-1—Cont'd

Laboratory Test	Previous Reference Intervals	Previous Units	Conversion Factor	SI Reference Intervals	SI Unit Symbol
Carbon dioxide					
Partial pressure (Pco_2)		mm Hg	×0.1333		kPa
Infant	27-41			3.6-5.5	
Child: male	35-48			4.7-6.4	
Child: female	32-45			4.3-6.0	
Total τCO_2		mmol/L	×1		mmol/L
Premature	14-27			14-27	
Newborn	13-22			13-22	
Child	20-28			20-28	
Thereafter	23-30			23-30	
Carbon monoxide (carboxyhemoglobin HbCO)	<5	%	×0.01	HbCO fraction	<0.05
CSF leukocyte count		cells/mm³	×10⁶		×10⁶ cells/L
Premature infant	0-25 mononuclear			0-25 mononuclear	
	0-10 polymorphs			0-10 polymorphs	
	0-1000 RBCs			0-1000 RBCs	
Term newborn	0-20 mononuclear			0-20 mononuclear	
	0-10 polymorphs			0-10 polymorphs	
	0-800 RBCs			0-800 RBCs	
<3-month infant	0-5 mononuclear			0-5 mononuclear	
	0-10 polymorphs			0-10 polymorphs	
	0-50 RBCs			0-50 RBCs	
Child	0-5 mononuclear			0-5 mononuclear	
Chloride (serum)	97-110	mmol/L	×1	97-110	mmol/L
Cholesterol, total (serum)		mg/dL	×0.0259		mmol/L

	Conventional		Conversion	SI	SI Unit
1-3 years	45-182			1.15-4.70	
4-6 years	109-189			2.80-4.80	
6-9 years					
Male	126-191			3.25-4.94	
Female	122-210			3.20-5.40	
10-14 years					
Male	130-205			3.40-5.30	
Female	124-220			3.20-5.60	
15-19 years					
Male	115-200			2.90-5.10	
Female	125-210			3.20-5.50	
Complement (serum)		mg/dL	×10		mg/L
C3					
Neonate	53-130			530-1300	
Infant (<1 year)	62-180			620-1800	
Child	77-195			770-1950	
Adult	83-177			830-1770	
C4					
Neonate	7-27			70-270	
Child	7-40			70-400	
Adult	15-45			150-450	
Creatinine (serum)		mg/dL	×88.4		µmol/L
Newborn	0.3-1.0			27-88	
Infant	0.2-0.4			18-35	
Child	0.3-0.7			27-62	
Adolescent	0.5-1.0			44-88	
Adult	0.5-1.2			44-106	

Continued

Table L-1—Cont'd

Laboratory Test	Previous Reference Intervals	Previous Units	Conversion Factor	SI Reference Intervals	SI Unit Symbol
Creatinine clearance		$mL/min/1.73\ m^2$	×1		$mL/min/1.73\ m^2$
Newborn	40-65			40-65	
Child to adult	88-137			88-137	
Creatinine kinase (CPK)		U/L	×1		U/L
<12 hours	70-1175			70-1175	
24-36 hours	130-1200			130-1200	
3-4 days	85-725			85-725	
Child to adult	5-130			5-130	
Digoxin		ng/mL	×1.281		nmol/L
Therapeutic (12 hours after dose)	0.8-2.0			1.0-2.6	
Toxic					
Child	>2.5			>3.2	
Adult	>3.0			>3.8	
Erythrocyte count		$10^6\ cells/mm^3$	×1		$10^{12}\ cells/L$
Cord blood	3.9-5.5			3.9-5.5	
1-3 days (capillary)	4.0-6.6			4.0-6.6	
1-2 weeks	3.6-6.2			3.6-6.2	
1-2 months	2.7-5.4			2.7-5.4	
3-6 months	3.1-4.5			3.1-4.5	
1-2 years	3.7-5.3			3.7-5.3	
2-6 years	3.9-5.3			3.9-5.3	
6-12 years	4.0-5.2			4.0-5.2	
12-18 years					

Test	Conventional Value	Conventional Units	Conversion	SI Value	SI Units
Female	4.1-5.1			4.1-5.1	
Male	4.5-5.3			4.5-5.3	
Erythrocyte sedimentation rate (ESR)		mm/hr	×1		mm/hr
Westergren or Wintrobe					
Child	0-10			0-10	
Adult	0-20			0-20	
Ferritin (serum)		ng/mL	×1		µg/L
Newborn	25-200			25-200	
1 month	200-600			200-600	
2-5 months	50-200			50-200	
6 months-15 years	7-140			7-140	
Adult					
Male	15-200			15-200	
Female	12-150			12-150	
Fibrinogen		mg/dL	×0.01		g/L
Newborn	125-300			1.25-3.00	
Adult	200-400			2.00-4.00	
Folate		ng/mL	×2.265		nmol/L
Newborn	7.0-32			15.9-72.4	
Adult	1.8-9.0			4.1-20.4	
Gamma-glutamyltransferase (GGT)		U/L	×1		U/L
Newborn	37-193			37-193	
1-2 months	12-147			12-147	
2-4 months	8-90			8-90	
4 months-15 years	5-30			5-30	

Continued

Table L-1—Cont'd

Laboratory Test	Previous Reference Intervals	Previous Units	Conversion Factor	SI Reference Intervals	SI Unit Symbol
Glucose		mg/dL	×0.0555		mmol/L
Newborn	40-60			2.2-3.3	
Infant	50-90			2.8-5.0	
Child	60-100			3.3-5.5	
Adult	70-105			3.9-5.8	
Hematocrit (Hct)		Percent packed red cells	×0.01		Volume fraction (vol RBCs/vol whole blood)
0-3 days	44-72			0.44-0.72	
2 months	28-42			0.28-0.42	
6-12 years	35-45			0.35-0.45	
12-18 years					
Male	37-49			0.37-0.49	
Female	36-46			0.36-0.46	
Hemoglobin (Hgb)		g/dL	×0.155		mmol/L
Newborn	14.5-22.5			2.25-3.5	
2 months	9.0-14.0			1.4-2.2	
6-12 years	11.5-15.5			1.8-2.4	
12-18 years					
Male	13.0-16.0			2.0-2.5	
Female	12.0-16.0			1.9-2.5	
Iron		µg/dL	×0.179		µmol/L
Newborn	100-250			17.9-44.8	
Infant	40-100			7.2-17.9	

Child	50-120	μg/dL	×0.179	9.0-21.5	μmol/L
Adult	40-160			7.2-28.6	
Iron-binding capacity (TIBC)					
Infant	100-400			17.9-71.6	μmol/L
Child to adult	250-400			44.8-71.6	
Lactate		mmol/L	×1		mmol/L
Venous	0.5-2.2			0.5-2.2	
Arterial	0.5-1.6			0.5-1.6	
Lead	<10	μg/dL	×0.0483	<0.48	μmol/L
Leukocyte count (WBC)		×1000 cells/mm³	×10⁶		×10⁹ cells/L
Newborn	9.0-30.0			9.0-30.0	
1 month	5.0-19.5			5.0-19.5	
1-3 years	6.0-17.5			6.0-17.5	
4-7 years	5.5-15.5			5.5-15.5	
8-13 years	4.5-13.5			4.5-13.5	
Adult	4.5-11.5			4.5-11.5	
Lipase (serum)		U/L	×1		U/L
1-4 years	18-95			18-95	
5-14 years	21-128			21-128	
15-19 years	28-149			28-149	
Magnesium (serum)		mg/dL	×0.4114		mmol/L
0-6 days	1.2-1.6			0.49-0.66	
7 days-2 years	1.6-2.6			0.66-1.05	
2-14 years	1.5-2.3			0.60-0.95	
14 years-adult	1.8-3.0			0.74-1.23	
Osmolality		mOsm/kg H₂O			
Serum	275-295				
Urine	50-1400				

Continued

Table L-1—Cont'd

Laboratory Test	Previous Reference Intervals	Previous Units	Conversion Factor	SI Reference Intervals	SI Unit Symbol
Oxygen, partial pressure (PO_2), arterial		mm Hg	×0.133		kPa
Birth	8-24			1.1-3.2	
<1 hour	33-85			4.4-11.3	
1 day	55-95			7.3-12.6	
Thereafter (decreases with age)	80-108			11.0-14.4	
Partial thromboplastin time (PTT)		Seconds (differs by method)			
Nonactivated	60-85				
Activated	25-35				
pH (arterial)					
Cord blood	7.22-7.34				
Premature	7.35-7.50				
Full-term newborn	7.11-7.36				
1 day	7.29-7.45				
Thereafter	7.35-7.45				
Phosphate (PO_4)	2.5-5.0	mg/dL	×0.3229	0.80-1.60	mmol/L
Platelet count		×10^3/mm^3	×10^6		×10^9/L
Newborn	84-478			84-478	
Child to adult	130-400			130-400	
Potassium (K^+)		mmol/L	×1		mmol/L
<2 months	3.0-7.0			3.0-7.0	
2-12 months	3.5-6.0			3.5-6.0	
>12 months	3.5-5.0			3.5-5.0	

Prealbumin		mg/L	×1		mg/L
2-6 months	142-330			142-330	
6-12 months	120-274			120-274	
1-3 years	108-259			108-259	
Protein, total		g/dL	×10		g/L
Premature	4.3-7.6			43-76	
Newborn	4.6-7.4			46-74	
1-7 years	6.1-7.9			61-79	
8-12 years	6.4-8.1			64-81	
13-19 years	6.6-8.2			66-82	
Prothrombin time (PT)		Seconds			
One stage (quick)	11-15				
Two stage modified	18-22				
Sodium (Na⁺)		mmol/L	×1		mmol/L
Newborn	134-146			134-146	
Infant	139-146			139-146	
Child	138-145			138-145	
Adult	136-146			136-146	
Thyroid-stimulating hormone (TSH)		mIU/L	×1		mIU/L
Newborn	0.7-39			0.7-39	
Thereafter	0.7-6.4			0.7-6.4	
Thyroxine (T₄)		µg/dL	×12.870		nmol/L
Full-term newborn	8.2-19.9			106-256	
1 week	6.0-15.9			77-205	
1-12 months	6.1-14.9			79-192	
1-3 years	6.8-13.5			88-174	
4-10 years	5.5-12.8			71-165	
Adolescents to adults	4.2-13.0			54-167	

Continued

Table L-1—Cont'd

Laboratory Test	Previous Reference Intervals	Previous Units	Conversion Factor	SI Reference Intervals	SI Unit Symbol
Transferrin		mg/dL	×0.01		g/L
1-3 years	218-347			2.18-3.47	
4-9 years	208-378			2.08-3.78	
10-19 years	224-444			2.24-4.44	
Triglycerides (serum after fasting)	Male (female)	mg/dL	×0.01	Male (female)	g/L
Cord blood	10-98 (10-98)			0.10-0.98 (0.10-0.98)	
0-5 years	30-86 (32-99)			0.30-0.86 (0.32-0.99)	
6-11 years	31-108 (35-114)			0.31-1.08 (0.35-1.14)	
12-15 years	36-138 (41-138)			0.36-1.38 (0.41-1.38)	
16-19 years	40-163 (40-128)			0.40-1.63 (0.40-1.28)	
Urea nitrogen (BUN)		mg/dL	×0.357		mmol/L
Cord blood	21-40			7.5-14.3	
Premature (1 week)	3-25			1.1-9.0	
Newborn	3-12			1.1-4.3	
Infant/child	5-18			1.8-6.4	
Thereafter	7-18			2.5-6.4	
Uric acid		mg/dL	×59.48		μmol/L
1-5 years	1.7-5.8			100-350	
6-11 years	2.2-6.6			130-390	
12-19 years					
Male	3.0-7.7			180-460	
Female	2.7-5.7			160-340	

On Call Formulary

Commonly Prescribed Medications

The On Call Formulary is designed as a quick reference for information on medications commonly prescribed by the pediatrician when on call. This list is abbreviated and therefore not all-inclusive. All medications are listed by generic names, with some common trade names also listed in parentheses after the generic name. Steroid preparations are included in a separate table. Doses listed are for children and/or infants with normal renal and hepatic function.

ACETAMINOPHEN (Tylenol)   *Analgesic/Antipyretic*

Indications:	Pain, fever
Actions:	Raises the pain threshold; acts directly on the hypothalamic heat regulation center
Side effects:	Uncommon: rash, drug fever, mucosal ulcerations, leukopenia, pancytopenia; overdose can lead to hepatic necrosis
Comments:	Unlike aspirin, acetaminophen has no anti-inflammatory action, does not irritate the stomach, does not affect platelet aggregation, and does not interact with oral anticoagulants. Overdoses, usually as suicide gestures, are serious, with onset of severe hepatotoxicity after about 36 to 48 hours
Dose:	10-15 mg/kg q4-6h PO or PR PRN for pain or fever; maximum for children >12 yr old, 650 mg q4-6h and 5 doses/ 24 hr

ACYCLOVIR (Zovirax)   *Antiviral*

Indications:	Herpes simplex infection in a neonate or immunosuppressed patient, varicella-zoster in the immunosuppressed; prophylaxis in bone marrow transplant recipient
Actions:	Selective inhibition of viral DNA synthesis

Side effects:	GI symptoms, headache, malaise, bone marrow suppression
Comments:	Dosage must be adjusted if renal function is not normal
Dose:	Neonatal herpes: 20 mg/kg/dose IV q8h × 14-21 days
	Immunocompromised patients with suspected HSV or varicella: 7.5-10 mg/kg/dose IV q8h

ADENOSINE (Adenocard) — *Antiarrhythmic*

Indications:	Supraventricular tachycardia
Actions:	Briefly (half-life of 6-10 sec) blocks atrioventricular node conduction, breaking a reentrant circuit
Side effects:	Chest pain, bradycardia, hypotension, SOB (bronchoconstriction), facial flushing
Comments:	Must be given as a rapid IV push because of short half-life; preferable to have an IV above the diaphragm
Dose:	0.01 mg/kg IV push with an immediate flush; if no response, double the dose and administer q2min to a maximum one-time dose of 12 mg

ALBUTEROL (Ventolin, Proventil) — *Bronchodilator*

Indications:	Bronchospasm
Actions:	β_2-Adrenergic receptor agonist with preferential effect on β_2-receptors of bronchial smooth muscle
Side effects:	Tachycardia, jitteriness, nausea, palpitations, hypokalemia
Comments:	May be used as continuous nebulization therapy for status asthmaticus
Dose:	Neonates: 0.1-0.5 mg/kg/dose via nebulizer q2-6h
	Children: 1.25-2.5 mg via nebulizer q2-6h

ALUMINUM HYDROXIDE (Amphojel) — *Antacid*

Indications:	Pain from peptic ulcer disease, reflux esophagitis; reduction of urinary phosphate in patients with phosphate-containing urinary calculi
Actions:	Buffers gastric acidity, binds phosphate in the intestine
Comments:	May bind and reduce intestinal absorption of medications such as tetracyclines and thyroxine
Dose:	For peptic ulcer disease: 5-15 mL/dose q3-6h or 1 and 3 hr after meals and at bedtime

For prophylaxis of GI bleeding: infants, 2-5 mL q1-2h NG; children, 5-15 mL q1-2h NG

For hyperphosphatemia: 50-150 mg/kg/day divided q4-6h

Note: Maalox is aluminum hydroxide with magnesium hydroxide and has laxative properties in addition to its antacid effect

AMIODARONE (Cordarone)   *Class III Antiarrhythmic*

Indications: Hemodynamically significant dysrhythmia, especially junctional ectopic tachycardia, ventricular tachycardia, ventricular fibrillation

Action: Prolongs the action potential and therefore prolongs PR, QRS, and QT intervals, as well as the effective refractory period. It inhibits inactivated sodium channels, noncompetitively binds α- and β-adrenergic receptors, and is a calcium antagonist

Side effects: Hypotension, bradycardia as a result of inhibition of both the SA and AV nodes, pulmonary fibrosis, hypothyroidism, fatigue, nausea, rash, hepatotoxicity; prolongs the prothrombin time

Comments. Amiodarone interacts with other medications through inhibition of cytochrome P-450 enzymes and may be proarrhythmic; contraindicated in patients with bradycardia and AV block; slow onset with very long half-life

Dose: Acute pulseless VT/VF "code" situation: 5-mg/kg IV rapid bolus

Recurrent VT: 5-mg/kg IV infusion over 20-60 min; may be repeated to a maximum of 15 mg/kg with a single-dose maximum of 300 mg

Oral: <1 year, 600-800 mg/1.73 m^2/day divided q12-24h for 4-10 days to "load," then reduce to 5 mg/kg/day divided q12-24h; >1 year, 10-20 mg/kg/24 hr divided q12h for 10 days, then 5-10 mg/kg/24 hr; adolescents and adults, 800 mg/day divided q12h

Note: Long-term follow-up of thyroid hormone and TSH levels; periodic ECG, pulmonary function test, and chest radiograph

AMOXICILLIN
(Amoxil and Others)

Indications:

Actions:
Side effects:
Comments:
Dose:

Oral Antibiotic

Bacterial upper respiratory infection, otitis media, sinusitis, pharyngitis, urinary tract infection, skin infections, bacterial endocarditis prophylaxis
Inhibits bacterial cell wall formation
Rashes, urticaria, diarrhea
Inactivated by β-lactamase
20-50 mg/kg/day divided q8-12h; for otitis media, 80-90 mg/kg/day; for SBE prophylaxis, give 50 mg/kg 60 min before the procedure and 25 mg/kg 6 hr after

AMOXICILLIN WITH CLAVULANIC ACID
(Augmentin)

Indications:

Actions:

Side effects:
Comments:

Dose:

Oral Antibiotic

Same as for amoxicillin; may also be useful in infections not responding to amoxicillin because of β-lactamase–producing organisms
Contains a β-lactamase inhibitor (clavulanic acid)
Diarrhea, rash, urticaria
Side effects generally caused by clavulanic acid
Same as for amoxicillin

AMPHOTERICIN B LIPID COMPLEX
(Abelcet, AmBisome)

Indications:
Actions:
Side effects:

Comments:

Dose:

Antifungal

Systemic fungal infections
Disrupts fungal cell membranes
Fever, chills, hypotension, nausea, vomiting, diarrhea, nephrotoxicity, hepatotoxicity, hypercalciuria, hypokalemia, phlebitis
Premedication with acetaminophen and meperidine may reduce side effects of fever, chills, nausea. Hydrocortisone added to bottle may also reduce side effects
2.5-5 mg/kg IV over 1-2 hr q24h. If tolerated, may increase to 7.5-10 mg/kg/24 hr

AMPICILLIN

Indications:

Actions:
Side effects:
Comments:

Antibiotic

Septicemia, meningitis, urinary tract infection, bacterial endocarditis prophylaxis
Inhibits bacterial cell wall synthesis
Diarrhea, rash, urticaria
Inactivated by β-lactamase

Dose:	Varies by age and size

Neonates ≤7 days:
- ≤2000 g: 50-100 mg/kg/day IM or IV divided q12h
- >2000 g: 75-150 mg/kg/day IM or IV divided q8h

Neonates >7 days:
- ≤1200 g: 50-100 mg/kg/day IM or IV divided q12h
- 1200-2000 g: 75-150 mg/kg/day IM or IV divided q8h
- >2000 g: 100-200 mg/kg/day IM or IV divided q6h

Children: 100-200 mg/kg/day IM or IV divided q6h; for severe infections (meningitis): 200-400 mg/kg/day IM or IV divided q4-6h

Adults: 250-500 mg IM or IV q4-8h

AMPICILLIN/SULBACTAM (Unasyn)

IV Antibiotic

Indications:
Septicemia, meningitis, urinary tract infection, sinusitis

Actions:
Inhibits bacterial cell wall synthesis, contains a β-lactamase inhibitor

Side effects:
Diarrhea, rash, urticaria, pseudomembranous colitis, hypersensitivity reactions, including anaphylaxis

Comments:
β-Lactamase–resistant combination with same spectrum and side effects as for ampicillin

Dose:
100-200 mg/kg/day IV or IM divided q4-6h

ASPIRIN

Analgesic, Antipyretic, Anti-inflammatory

Indications:
Pain from inflammation, fever (nonviral diseases only), antiplatelet use in selected cardiac patients

Actions:
Acts peripherally by interfering with prostaglandin synthesis, thus reducing pain and inflammation; acts centrally to reduce pain perception and reduce temperature by increasing heat loss

Side effects:
Gastritis, gastric erosion and ulceration, tinnitus, fever, thirst, diaphoresis, allergic reactions, bronchospasm in those with asthma, hepatitis

Comments:
Must not be used for fever control in children with viral syndromes because of the risk for Reye's syndrome

Dose:
10-15 mg/kg/dose q4-6h PRN
High-dose regimen for juvenile rheumatoid arthritis, Kawasaki disease: 80-100 mg/kg/day divided q6h

BISACODYL (Dulcolax)   *Laxative*

Indications: Constipation
Actions: Stimulates peristalsis
Side effects: Abdominal cramping, rectal bleeding
Comments: Onset PO, 6-10 hr; onset PR, 15-60 min
Dose: <2 yr: 5-mg rectal suppository
                        2-6 yr: 10-mg rectal suppository
                        >6 yr: 5-10 mg PO at bedtime or
                            before breakfast

BUMETANIDE (Bumex)   *Diuretic*

Indications: Fluid overload, renal failure
Actions: Inhibits sodium and chloride
                            reabsorption in the ascending loop
                            of Henle, interferes with concentration
                            of urine
Side effects: Hyponatremia, hypochloremia,
                            dehydration, hypotension
Comments: 1.0 mg is equivalent to 40 mg
                            furosemide
Dose: Neonates: 0.01-0.05 mg/kg/dose
                            q24-48h PO, IV, or IM
                        Infants and children: 0.015-0.1 mg/kg/
                            dose q6-24h PO, IV, or IM
                            (maximum dose, 10 mg/24 hr)

CALCIUM   *Essential Mineral*

	mg of Calcium/g	mEq/g of Calcium
Calcium carbonate	400	20
Calcium chloride	270	13.5
Calcium gluconate	90	4.5

Indications: Hypocalcemia manifested by tetany,
                            seizures, myocardial dysfunction,
                            hypoparathyroidism
Actions: Restores serum as well as intracellular
                            calcium concentration, restores
                            cardiac automaticity, increases
                            cardiac resting potential
Side effects: Dysrhythmia, especially in patients
                            receiving digoxin; should avoid
                            peripheral IV administration because
                            of risk for burns
Comments: 10% IV solution = 100 mg/mL
Dose: Calcium carbonate (Tums, Os-Cal)
                        Neonatal hypocalcemia: 50-150 mg/
                            kg/day divided q4-6h (maximum,
                            1 g/day)
                        Children: 20-60 mg/kg/day PO
                            divided qid
                        Calcium chloride: used in acute
                            resuscitation, 20 mg/kg/dose
                            (0.2 mL/kg/dose) IV

Calcium gluconate
Infant hypocalcemia: IV, 200-500 mg/kg/
day divided q6h; PO, 400-800 mg/
kg/day divided q6h
Children: 200-500 mg/kg/day IV or
PO divided q6h

CEFADROXIL (Duricef)

Oral Cephalosporin (1st Generation)

Indications: Minor respiratory and skin infections
Actions: Bactericidal, inhibits bacterial cell wall
synthesis
Side effects: Rash, diarrhea
Comments: Expensive; long half-life allows bid dosing
Dose: 15 mg/kg/dose q12h PO (maximum,
2 g/dose)

CEFAZOLIN (Ancef, Kefzol)

IV Cephalosporin (1st Generation)

Indications: Gram-positive bacterial infection,
some gram-negatives
Actions: Bactericidal, inhibits bacterial cell wall
synthesis
Side effects: Rash, diarrhea
Dose: 50-100 mg/kg/day IV divided q6-8h
Neonates:
≤7 days: 40 mg/kg/day IV
divided q12h
>7 days: 40-60 mg/kg/day IV
divided q8h

CEFDINIR (Omnicef)

Oral Cephalosporin (3rd Generation)

Indications: Bacterial infections, gram positive and
negative
Actions: Bactericidal, inhibits bacterial cell wall
synthesis
Side effects: Rash, diarrhea
Comments: Reduce dose if renal insufficiency
Dose: 14 mg/kg/24 hr in 1 or 2 doses
(maximum, 600 mg/24 hr)

CEFEPIME

IV Cephalosporin (4th Generation)

Indications: Broad-spectrum antibacterial
Actions: Bactericidal, inhibits bacterial cell
wall synthesis
Side effects: Nausea, diarrhea
Dose: 100-150 mg/kg/24 hr divided q8-12h
IV or IM

CEFOTAXIME (Claforan)

IV Cephalosporin (3rd Generation)

Indications: Septicemia, meningitis
Actions: Bactericidal, inhibits bacterial cell wall
synthesis

Side effects:	Rash, diarrhea, acute hypersensitivity in penicillin-allergic patients
Comments:	Not effective against *Pseudomonas*, very good penetration into cerebrospinal fluid
Dose:	Neonates:

≤7 days: 50 mg/kg/dose IV q12h
>7 days, <1200 g: 50 mg/kg/dose IV q12h
>7 days, >1200 g: 50 mg/kg/dose IV q8h

Infants and children: 50 mg/kg/dose IV q8h (For meningitis: 50 mg/kg/dose IV q6h)

CEFOXITIN (Mefoxin)   *IV Cephalosporin (2nd Generation)*

Indications:	Pelvic inflammatory disease, urinary tract infection
Actions:	Bactericidal, inhibits bacterial cell wall synthesis
Side effects:	Rash, diarrhea
Dose:	Infants ≥3 mo and children: 80-160 mg/kg/day IV divided q6-8h

CEFTAZIDIME (Fortaz)   *IV Cephalosporin (3rd Generation)*

Indications:	*Pseudomonas* infection
Actions:	Bactericidal, inhibits bacterial cell wall synthesis
Side effects:	Rash, diarrhea
Comments:	Should be combined with an aminoglycoside for treating *Pseudomonas* infections
Dose:	Neonates:

≤7 days: 50 mg/kg/dose IV q12h
>7 days, ≤1200 g: 50 mg/kg/dose IV q12h
>7 days, >1200 g: 50 mg/kg/dose IV q8h

Infants and children: 50 mg/kg/dose IV q8h

CEFTRIAXONE (Rocephin)   *IV Cephalosporin (3rd Generation)*

Indications:	Respiratory infections, meningitis
Actions:	Bactericidal, inhibits bacterial cell wall synthesis
Side effects:	Rash, diarrhea, biliary sludging
Comments:	q24h dosing IM or IV
Dose:	Neonates: 50-75 mg/kg/day IV or IM divided q24h

Children: 50-75 mg/kg/day IV or IM divided q12-24h
For meningitis: 75 mg/kg for first dose, then 80-100 mg/kg/day IV or IM divided q12-24h (maximum, 4 g/day)

CEFUROXIME (Zinacef, Ceftin)   *Cephalosporin (2nd Generation)*

Indications: Respiratory infections, otitis, sinusitis
Actions: Bactericidal, inhibits bacterial cell wall synthesis
Side effects: Rash, diarrhea
Dose: Infants: 40-100 mg/kg/24 hr IV divided q12h IV or IM
Children: 200-240 mg/kg/24 hr divided q8h IV or IM
Note: Cefuroxime axetil (Ceftin) is an oral preparation generally given for otitis or sinusitis. Dose: 20-30 mg/kg/day PO divided q8h

CEPHALEXIN (Keflex)   *Cephalosporin (2nd Generation)*

Indications: Skin infections
Actions: Bactericidal, inhibits bacterial cell wall synthesis
Side effects: Rash, diarrhea
Comments: Does not cross blood-brain barrier
Dose: 25-100 mg/kg/day PO divided q6-8h (maximum dose, 4 g/24 hr)

CHARCOAL, ACTIVATED   *Adsorptive Agent*

Indications: Certain toxic ingestions
Actions: Adsorbs toxins and prevents absorption in gut
Side effects: Vomiting, constipation, black stool, hypernatremia
Comments: Will adsorb many but not all toxins (ineffective with hydrocarbons, iron, alcohols); will adsorb acetylcysteine and therefore cannot be given simultaneously to treat acetaminophen ingestion
Dose: 1-2 g/kg q2-6h PO or NG

CHLORAL HYDRATE   *Sedative, Hypnotic*

Indications: Conscious sedation for procedures, for sleep
Actions: Hypnotic
Side effects: Gastric irritation, rash
Comments: Not advised in liver or renal disease
Dose: Neonates: 25 mg/kg/dose PO q6-8h
Infants and children: 25-100 mg/kg/dose PO q6-8h

CHLORPROMAZINE (Thorazine)   *Antipsychotic Phenothiazine*

Indications: Acute psychosis, agitation and delirium, nausea

Actions:	Dopamine, histamine, muscarinic, and α-adrenergic antagonist
Side effects:	Jaundice, extrapyramidal effects (dystonia), CNS depression, hypotension, dysrhythmias
Comments:	In an acutely agitated patient, haloperidol may cause less blood pressure instability
Dose:	Children >6 mo:
	IV or IM: 0.5-1 mg/kg/dose q6-8h PRN
	PO: 0.5-1 mg/kg/dose q4-6h
	PR: 1 mg/kg/dose q6-8h
	Adolescents:
	IV or IM: 25 mg initial dose; increase dose by 25-50 mg/dose q1-4h; maximum single dose, 400 mg q4-6h
	PO: 10-25 mg/dose q4-6h

CIMETIDINE (Tagamet) — *Histamine-Blocking Agent*

Indications:	Peptic ulcer disease, gastroesophageal reflux
Actions:	Inhibits histamine-mediated release of acid in the stomach
Side effects:	Gynecomastia, impotence, confusion, lethargy, diarrhea, leukopenia, thrombocytopenia
Comments:	Reduces microsomal enzyme metabolism of drugs, including oral anticoagulants
Dose:	Neonates: 5-10 mg/kg/24 hr IV, PO, or IM divided q8-12h
	Infants: 10-20 mg/kg/24 hr divided q6-12h
	Children: 20-40 mg/kg/24 hr divided q6h

CIPROFLOXACIN — *Fluoroquinolone Antibiotic*

Indications:	*Pseudomonas* and other enteric pathogens, some gram positives
Actions:	Inhibits action of bacterial DNA gyrase (topoisomerase 2)
Side effects:	Photosensitivity, tendonitis, confusion, dizziness
Comments:	Use is discouraged before adolescence
Dose:	15-30 mg/kg/24 hr divided q12h PO or IV; dose should be adjusted in patients with creatinine clearance <20 mL/min

CLINDAMYCIN (Cleocin) — *Antibiotic*

Indications:	Gram-positive bacterial infections, anaerobic coverage

Actions:	Suppresses bacterial protein synthesis at the ribosome
Comments:	Used especially if anaerobic pathogens are suspected, as in puncture wounds and abscesses
Dose:	Neonates:

≤7 days, ≤2000 g: 10 mg/kg/24 hr divided q12h IV or IM

≤7 days, >2000 g: 15 mg/kg/24 hr divided q8h IV or IM

>7 days, <1200 g: 10 mg/kg/24 hr divided q12h IV or IM

>7 days, 1200-2000 g: 15 mg/kg/24 hr divided q8h IV or IM

>7 days, >2000 g: 20mg/kg/day divided q8h IV or IM

Older infants and children: 20-40 mg/kg/24 hr divided q6-8h IV, IM, or PO

CLOTRIMAZOLE

Topical Antifungal

Indications:	Skin and mucous membrane fungal infections
Actions:	Disrupts fungal cell membranes
Side Effects:	Erythema, blistering, urticaria
Comments:	Available as topical cream, oral troche, or vaginal tablet
Dose:	Skin: apply twice daily

Thrush: dissolve 1 troche in mouth 5 times each day

Vaginal candidiasis: 100-200 mg/day for 7-14 days

CODEINE

Narcotic Analgesic, Antitussive

Indications:	Pain, unrelenting cough
Actions:	Decreases pain threshold as well as cough threshold
Side effects:	Constipation, respiratory depression
Dose:	Antitussive: 1-1.5 mg/kg/24 hr PO divided q4-6h

Pain: 0.5-1 mg/kg/dose PO divided q4-6h PRN (maximum dose, 60 mg)

CO-TRIMOXAZOLE
(Bactrim, Septra)

Combination Antibiotic

Indications:	Urinary tract infection, shigellosis, salmonellosis, recurrent otitis media
Actions:	Interferes with synthesis of tetrahydrofolic acid in sensitive bacteria, including *Pneumocystis carinii*
Side effects:	Bone marrow suppression, rash
Comments:	Combination of trimethoprim (TMP) and sulfamethoxazole (SMX)

Dose:	Children: 6-20 mg/kg/24 hr TMP PO or IV divided q12h *Pneumocystis carinii* pneumonia: 15-20 mg/kg/24 hr TMP PO or IV divided q12h *Pneumocystis carinii* prophylaxis: 5 mg/kg/24 hr TMP 3 times/wk PO

DESMOPRESSIN (DDAVP) *Hormone Analogue*

Indications: Diabetes insipidus, nocturnal enuresis, certain hemophilias

Actions: Vasopressin analogue acting on the kidney to encourage water retention

Side effects: Excessive fluid retention, headache, crampy abdominal pain

Dose: Diabetes insipidus: 0.05 mg PO twice a day
Hemophilia: 0.3 µg/kg IV 30 min before procedures
Nocturnal enuresis: 20 µg at bedtime

DIAZEPAM (Valium) *Benzodiazepine Hypnotic, Anticonvulsant*

Indications: Seizure disorders, anxiety, sedation

Actions: Benzodiazepine sedative-hypnotic with antianxiety and anticonvulsant properties

Side effects: Sedation, respiratory depression, paradoxical agitation

Comments: Also used as a muscle relaxant in cerebral palsy

Dose: Status epilepticus: 0.05-0.3 mg/kg/dose IV by slow infusion, may be repeated every 30 min to maximum total dose of 10 mg; rectal: 0.5 mg/kg, then 0.25 mg/kg in 10 min PRN
Sedation, anxiety, or muscle relaxation: 0.1-0.3 mg/kg/dose PO q4-8h; 0.04-0.3 mg/kg IV or IM

DIGOXIN (Lanoxin) *Cardiac Glycoside*

Indications: Congestive heart failure, supraventricular tachycardias, including atrial flutter/fibrillation, reentrant SVT (non-WPW)

Actions: Slows AV nodal conduction and increases force of contraction by inhibiting sodium-potassium ATPase

Side effects: Dysrhythmias, nausea, vomiting, neuropsychiatric disturbances

Comments:	80% of drug renally excreted; adjust dose for renal insufficiency; avoid hypokalemia, which can precipitate digoxin-mediated dysrhythmias (AV block, ventricular dysrhythmias). Serum levels should be monitored but may be unreliable in infants and children because of serum digoxin-like immune substances
Dose:	Neonates: 10-30 µg/kg IV load, then 5-10 µg/kg/24 hr <2 yr: 30 µg/kg IV load, then 10-15 µg/kg/24 hr 2-10 yr: 30 µg/kg IV load, then 5-10 µg/kg/24 hr >10 yr: 10 µg/kg IV load, then 2-5 µg/kg/24 hr

DIPHENHYDRAMINE (Benadryl) — *Antihistamine*

Indications:	Allergic reaction, sedation, antiemetic
Actions:	Antihistamine and anticholinergic
Side effects:	Drowsiness, dizziness, dry mouth, urinary retention
Comments:	Anticholinergic effect is additive with that of other drugs, such as tricyclic antidepressants
Dose:	Children: 5 mg/kg/24 hr PO or IV divided q6h PRN Adolescents: 10-50 mg/dose PO or IV q4h PRN

DOCUSATE (Colace) — *Stool Softener*

Indications:	Constipation
Actions:	Stool softener, emulsifier
Side effects:	Diarrhea
Comments:	Onset of action 48-72 hr after 1st dose
Dose:	<3 yr: 10-40 mg/24 hr PO divided in 1-4 doses 3-6 yr: 20-60 mg/24 hr PO divided in 1-4 doses 6-12 yr: 40-150 mg/24 hr PO divided in 1-4 doses Adolescents: 50-400 mg/24 hr divided in 1-4 doses

EMLA (Eutectic Mixture of Local Anesthetics) — *Topical Anesthetic*

Indications:	Premedication for venipuncture, IV line placement, lumbar puncture, bone marrow aspiration

Actions:	Short-acting topical cutaneous anesthetic agent
Side effects:	Can cause localized systemic vasospasm; contraindicated in children at risk for methemoglobinemia
Comments:	Emulsion of 2.5% lidocaine and 2.5% prilocaine applied to intact skin, *not wounds*, under an occlusive dressing for 30-60 min before procedures
Dose:	Apply an opaque layer of EMLA to the procedure site, and cover with an occlusive dressing

EPINEPHRINE, RACEMIC
  (Vaponefrin)

Catecholamine

Indications:	Croup (parainfluenza, laryngotracheobronchitis)
Actions:	Dilates airways
Side effects:	Rare: headache, tachyarrhythmias, nausea, palpitations
Comments:	Symptoms of croup may worsen after initial benefit
Dose:	0.25-0.5 mL of 2.25% solution diluted to 3 mL with saline solution and given with nebulizer over 15 min; should not be given more often than q2h

ERYTHROMYCIN
  (EryPed, Pediazole)

Macrolide Antibiotic

Indications:	Upper airway infections, *Mycoplasma* infections, pertussis, *Legionella* and *Chlamydia* infections
Actions:	Bacteriostatic and occasionally bactericidal; inhibits messenger RNA translation
Side effects:	Common: nausea, abdominal pain, vomiting
Comments:	Avoid IM administration; should be used cautiously in those with liver disease; may interfere with hepatic metabolism of other drugs (astemizole, carbamazepine, terfenadine, theophylline) and result in toxicity; available as ethyl succinate, lactobionate, and estolate preparations; for pertussis, use of estolate salt may reduce relapse rate Pediazole is a combination of erythromycin ethyl succinate and sulfisoxazole in oral suspension

Dose:

Neonates:
  ≤7 days: 20 mg/kg/24 hr PO
    divided q12h
  >7 days, ≤1200 g: 20 mg/kg/24 hr PO
    divided q12h
  >7 days, >1200 g: 30 mg/kg/24 hr
    PO divided q8h
Children: 20-50 mg/kg/24 hr IV or
  PO divided q6-8h

FOSPHENYTOIN

Anticonvulsant

Indications:
Actions:

Side effects:

Dose:

Acute seizures
Reduces sodium transport across
  neuronal membranes
Lethargy, nystagmus, Stevens-Johnson
  syndrome, hypotension
Each 1.5 mg fosphenytoin = 1 mg
  phenytoin dosing equivalent. Loading
  dose is 15-20 mg/kg IV phenytoin
  dosing equivalents (maximum,
  150 mg/min). Maintenance dose is
  5-10 mg/kg/24 hr PO, IV divided
  q12-24 hr.

FUROSEMIDE (Lasix)

Loop Diuretic

Indications:

Actions:

Side effects:

Comments:

Dose:

Fluid overload, congestive heart failure,
  hypertension
Inhibits reabsorption of sodium and
  chloride in ascending limb of the
  loop of Henle
Electrolyte depletion, hyperuricemia,
  hyperglycemia, ototoxicity
Loop diuretics well absorbed PO, with
  a prompt onset of action; duration
  of action approximately 2 hr after
  IV administration
Premature infants: 0.5-2 mg/kg IV or
  1-4 mg/kg PO q12-48h
Infants and children: 1-2 mg/kg IV or
  1-4 mg/kg PO q6-24h
Adolescents: 10-600 mg/24 hr PO divided
  in 1-4 doses or 20-80 mg IV/dose

GENTAMICIN (Garamycin)

Aminoglycoside Antibiotic

Indications:
Actions:

Side effects:
Comments:

Gram-negative bacterial infections
Bactericidal; binds to 30S ribosomal
  subunit and inhibits mRNA binding
Ototoxicity, nephrotoxicity
Serum levels should be monitored;
  therapeutic peak levels, 6-12 mg/L;
  trough, <2 mg/L; eliminated more
  quickly in patients with burns or
  cystic fibrosis, so dosage and interval
  adjustment may be necessary

Dose: Neonates:
                                   ≤7 days, 1200-2000 g: 2.5 mg/kg/
                                       dose IV/IM q12-18h
                                   ≤7 days, >2000 g: 2.5 mg/kg/dose IV/
                                       IM q12h
                                   >7 days, 1200-2000g: 2.5 mg/kg/dose
                                       IV/IM q8-12h
                                   >7 days, >2000 g: 2.5 mg/kg/dose
                                       IV/IM q8h
                               Children: 6-7.5 mg/kg/24 hr divided q8h
                               Note: Monitor peak and trough levels
                                   closely. Adjust interval for renal
                                   impairment and prematurity

HALOPERIDOL (Haldol)   *Antipsychotic*

Indications: Psychotic disorders, acute agitation,
                                   chorea
Actions: Antipsychotic neuroleptic butyrophenone
                                   that blocks dopamine receptors in
                                   the mesolimbic system
Side effects: Extrapyramidal reactions, postural
                                   hypotension, sedation, jaundice,
                                   blurred vision, neuroleptic malignant
                                   syndrome, bronchospasm
Comments: Extrapyramidal and acute oculogyric
                                   effects can be reversed with
                                   benztropine or diphenhydramine
Dose: 3-12 yr: 0.25-0.5 mg/24 hr PO divided
                                   in 2-3 doses; increase weekly by
                                   0.25-0.5 mg PRN (maximum,
                                   0.15 mg/kg/24 hr)
                               6-12 yr: 1-3 mg/dose IM q4-8h
                               >12 yr: 0.5-5 mg PO 2-3 times each
                                   day; 2-5 mg/dose IM q4-8h

HEPARIN   *Anticoagulant*

Indications: Used for anticoagulation in a wide
                                   variety of settings, most commonly
                                   in patients who have had a stroke,
                                   deep venous thrombosis, or central
                                   line thrombosis and for clot
                                   prophylaxis during hemodialysis,
                                   cardiopulmonary bypass, plasma-
                                   pheresis, or exchange transfusion
Actions: Binds to antithrombin III and inhibits
                                   the coagulation cascade by increasing
                                   the breakdown of thrombin, as well
                                   as factors Xa, IXa, and XIa
Side effects: Bleeding is the most common side
                                   effect. Heparin allergy has been
                                   reported, as has heparin-induced
                                   thrombocytopenia

Comments:	Heparin is usually given as a bolus followed by a continuous infusion
	Heparin may be reversed by protamine sulfate, 1 mg/100 U heparin given in the preceding 4 hr
Dose:	Infants and small children: 50 U/kg IV followed by a continuous infusion of 10-35 U/kg/hr, with a target PTT of 1.5-2 times the control value (best checked 4-6 hr after initiation). Intermittent dosing may be used with 50-100 U/kg/dose q4h
	Older children and adolescents: initial bolus of 50-100 U/kg followed by a maintenance infusion of 15-25 U/kg/hr; for intermittent dosing, 75-125 U/kg/dose every 4 hr
	Central lines and arterial lines: used with a final concentration of 0.5-1 U/mL; heparin flush solution usually standardized for peripheral IV at 10 U/mL, 1-2 mL per flush; for central lines, a 100-U/mL concentration used with 2- to 3-mL flush volume
	SC: 5000 U q8-12h for prophylaxis

HYDRALAZINE (Apresoline)   *Arteriolar Vasodilator*

Indications:	Hypertension, hypertensive crisis
Actions:	Relaxes arteriolar smooth muscle, causing vasodilation
Side effects:	Tachycardia, headache, nausea, vomiting, SLE-like reaction in high doses
Comments:	Limited effect on veins; therefore, little postural hypotension
Dose:	Emergency hypertension: 0.1-0.2 mg/kg/dose IM or IV q4-6h; maximum, 3.5 mg/kg/24 hr
	Chronic hypertension: 0.75-1 mg/kg/24 hr PO divided q6-12h; maximum, 200 mg/24 hr **or** 7.5 mg/kg/24 hr

HYDROXYZINE   *Histamine Receptor Blocker*
(Atarax, Vistaril)

Indications:	Sedation, pruritus
Actions:	Blocks H_1 receptors
Side effects:	Dry mouth, drowsiness, tremor, convulsions, blurred vision
Dose:	Children: 0.6 mg/kg/dose PO or IM q6h
	Adolescents: 10-100 mg/dose PO or IM q6-8h

IBUPROFEN (Motrin, Advil)

	Nonsteroidal Anti-inflammatory
Indications:	Pain, fever
Actions:	Inhibits prostaglandin synthesis
Side effects:	Nausea, abdominal pain, gastritis, ulcers, acute tubular necrosis
Comments:	May prolong bleeding time because of antiplatelet effects; use with caution in those with renal or hepatic disease
Dose:	Antipyretic, mild analgesia: 10-15 mg/kg/dose PO q6-8h
	Anti-inflammatory: 30-70 mg/kg/24 hr PO divided q6h

IMIPENEM-CILASTATIN

	Antibiotic
Indications:	Broad spectrum against gram-positive and gram-negative bacteria, including *Pseudomonas*
Actions:	Inhibits bacterial cell wall synthesis
Side effects:	Rash, nausea, seizures
Dose:	Neonates:
	≤7 days, ≤1200 g: 20 mg/kg IV or IM q18-24h
	≤7 days, >1200 g: 20 mg/kg IV or IM q12h
	>7 days: 1200-2000 g: 40 mg/kg IV or IM q12h
	>7 days, >2000 g: 60 mg/kg IV or IM q8h
	Children: 60-100 mg/kg/24 hr IV or IM divided q6-8h

INSULIN

	Hypoglycemic
Indications:	Diabetes mellitus, hyperkalemia
Actions:	Enhances hepatic glycogen storage, enhances entry of glucose and potassium into cells, inhibits breakdown of protein and fat
Side effects:	Hypoglycemia
Comments:	Less immunogenicity seen with human insulin preparations
Dose:	Variable for management of diabetes mellitus
	DKA: 0.1 U regular insulin/kg/hr IV initially, with adjustment based on glucose monitoring
	Hyperkalemia: give IV (with 50% dextrose, 0.5-1 mL/kg) as 1 U regular insulin per 4 g glucose

IPRATROPIUM BROMIDE (Atrovent)

	Bronchodilator
Indications:	Status asthmaticus
Actions:	Anticholinergic, bronchodilator

Side effects:	Dry mouth, urinary retention, dizziness, headache
Comments:	Use with caution in those with bladder obstruction, glaucoma; use 100 µg/dose in neonates
Dose:	125-500 µg nebulized every 20 min for 3 doses, then q4-8h

IVIG (intravenous immunoglobulin) *Immunoglobulin*

Indications:	Used in Kawasaki disease, idiopathic thrombocytopenic purpura (ITP), and as replacement therapy for immunodeficiency and/or HIV-mediated humoral deficiency
Actions:	Replenishes immunoglobulins in immunodeficiency states, non-specifically competitively binds antiplatelet antibodies in ITP, action in Kawasaki disease unknown
Side effects:	May cause fever, vasodilation, hypotension, chills, headache; anaphylaxis has been reported, especially in IGA-deficient patients
Comments:	IVIG is a pooled human plasma product and should be described to the family as such. Use in patients who are Jehovah's Witness followers must be done with adequate informed consent
Dose:	Varies by indication
	Kawasaki disease: 2 g/kg IV generally administered over 10-12 hr
	ITP: 1 g/kg/IV over 4-6 hr with repeat doses as needed
	Antibody replacement therapy: 300-400 mg/kg/mo IV, with the frequency determined by monitoring serum immunoglobulin levels

KETOROLAC (Toradol) *Anti-inflammatory*

Indications:	Pain
Actions:	Inhibits prostaglandin synthesis
Side effects:	Dyspepsia, nausea, abdominal pain, dizziness, headache, renal failure
Dose:	Children 2-16 yr: 0.4-1 mg/kg/dose IV, PO, or IM q6h
	Adolescents: 60 mg IM or 30 mg IV q6h

LABETALOL *Antihypertensive*

Indications:	Moderate to severe hypertension
Actions:	Blocks α- and β-adrenergic receptors
Side effects:	Hypotension, bradycardia, fatigue, headache, bronchospasm

Comments:	Contraindicated in asthma; onset of action within minutes when given IV
Dose:	PO: begin at 4 mg/kg/24 hr divided in 2 doses and increase as needed to maximum of 40 mg/kg/24 hr IV infusion: 0.4-1.0 mg/kg/hr (maximum, 3 mg/kg/hr)

LANSOPRAZOLE (Prevacid)   *Proton Pump Inhibitor*

Indications:	Gastritis, peptic ulcer
Actions:	Inhibits gastric acid secretion
Side effects:	Diarrhea
Dose:	15-30 mg once a day

LIDOCAINE (Xylocaine)   *Antiarrhythmic*

Indications:	Prophylaxis and treatment of ventricular tachycardia
Actions:	Lengthens the effective refractory period in ventricular conducting system; decreases ventricular automaticity
Side effects:	Nausea, vomiting, hypotension, seizures, perioral paresthesias
Comments:	Those with impaired renal function may accumulate seizure-inducing metabolite
Dose:	1-mg/kg IV loading dose; repeat every 5-10 min until total dose of 3 mg/kg; maintenance therapy given by continuous infusion of 20-50 µg/kg/min (maximum, 4 mg/min)

LORAZEPAM (Ativan)   *Anticonvulsant, Sedative*

Indications:	Seizures, sedation
Actions:	Benzodiazepine; potentiates neuroinhibitory effect of GABA
Side effects:	Tachycardia, drowsiness, confusion, respiratory depression
Comments:	Longer duration of action than diazepam
Dose:	Status epilepticus: Neonates: 0.05-0.2 mg/kg/dose IV over 2-5 min; may repeat q10-15min Adolescents: 0.07 mg/kg/dose IV over 2-5 min; may repeat q10-15min Sedation: 0.05-0.1 mg/kg/dose IV q4-8h

MAGNESIUM HYDROXIDE/ ALUMINUM HYDROXIDE (Maalox)   *Antacid*

Indications:	Pain from reflux esophagitis, gastritis, peptic ulcer
Actions:	Buffers gastric acid

Side effects:	Diarrhea, hypermagnesemia in renal failure
Comments:	Aluminum salts cause constipation; magnesium salts cause diarrhea
	May bind and reduce absorption of thyroxine, tetracycline; use with caution in renal failure
Dose:	5-15 mL PO q3-6h or 1 and 3 hr PC and HS

MANNITOL — *Osmotic Diuretic*

Indications:	Cerebral edema
Actions:	Osmotic effect results in intravascular shift of water
Side effects:	Volume overload, hyperosmolality, hyponatremia
Comments:	Contraindicated in renal failure; often given with furosemide
Dose:	0.5-1.0 g/kg/dose IV push, then 0.25-0.5 g/kg IV q4-6h; targeting for serum osmolality of 310-320 mOsm/L

MEPERIDINE (Demerol) — *Narcotic Analgesic*

Indications:	Moderate to severe pain
Actions:	Narcotic analgesic, binds opiate receptors in CNS
Side effects:	Respiratory depression, hypotension, nausea, vomiting, constipation, agitation, rash, seizures
Comments:	Addictive; contraindicated in cardiac arrhythmias, asthma, increased ICP; use with caution in renal failure (seizures may occur secondary to accumulation of metabolite normeperidine); naloxone is antidote
Dose:	1.0-1.5 mg/kg/dose PO, IM, IV, or SC q3-4h

METOCLOPRAMIDE (Reglan) — *GI Motility Stimulant*

Indications:	Gastroesophageal reflux disease or GI dysmotility
Actions:	Stimulates motility of the upper GI tract without increasing gastric, pancreatic, or biliary secretions; also used as an antiemetic
Side effects:	Motor restlessness, drowsiness, rare dystonic reactions and even tardive dyskinesia reported
Dose:	Infants and small children: 0.03-0.1 mg/kg/dose PO, IV, or IM q8h
	Older children and adolescents: 10-15 mg/dose PO before meals and qhs

METRONIDAZOLE (Flagyl)   *Antibiotic*
Indications: Anaerobic infections
Actions: Bactericidal via production of
                               intracellular free radicals
Side effects: Dizziness, seizures, nausea
Dose: Neonates:
  ≤7 days, <1200 g: 7.5 mg/kg IV or
    PO q18h
  ≤7 days, 1200-2000 g: 7.5 mg/kg IV
    or PO q24h
  ≤7 days, >2000 g: 7.5 mg/kg IV or
    PO q12h
  >7 days, 1200-2000 g: 7.5 mg/kg IV
    or PO q12h
  >7 days, >2000 g: 15 mg/kg IV or
    PO q12h
  Children: 30 mg/kg/24 hr IV or PO
    divided q6-8h (maximum, 4 g/24 hr)

MIDAZOLAM (Versed)   *Sedative*
Indications: Sedation
Actions: Benzodiazepine; potentiates
                               neuroinhibitory effect of GABA
Side effects: Tachycardia, drowsiness, confusion,
                               respiratory depression
Comments: Generally used as sedative, less
                               commonly as anticonvulsant
Dose: Neonates: 0.15-0.5 μg/kg/min IV by
                               continuous infusion
                             Infants and children: 0.05-0.2 mg/kg IV,
                               may be repeated in 1-2 hr or 2.5 mg
                               intranasally in each naris

MORPHINE SULFATE   *Narcotic Analgesic*
Indications: Moderate to severe pain
Actions: Narcotic analgesic
Side effects: Respiratory depression, hypotension,
                               nausea, vomiting, constipation,
                               increased ICP, biliary spasm
Comments: Addictive; naloxone is antidote; 10 mg
                               morphine IM or SC = 100 mg
                               meperidine IM or SC
Dose: Neonates: 0.05-0.2 mg/kg/dose IM, IV,
                               or SC q4h
                             Children: 0.1-0.2 mg/kg/dose IM, IV,
                               or SC q2-4h

NAFCILLIN   *Penicillinase-Resistant
                               Penicillin*
Indications: Bacterial infections with sensitive
                               organisms
Actions: Inhibits bacterial cell wall synthesis

Side effects:	Phlebitis, allergic reactions, rash
Comments:	Poorly absorbed orally; allergic cross-reactivity with other penicillins
Dose:	Neonates:
	≤7 days, 1200-2000 g: 50 mg/kg/24 hr IV or IM divided q12h
	≤7 days, ?2000 g: 75 mg/kg/24 hr IV or IM divided q8h
	>7 days, 1200-2000 g: 75 mg/kg/24 hr IV or IM q8h
	>7 days, >2000 g: 100 mg/kg/24 hr IV or IM divided q6-8h (meningitis: 200 mg/kg/24 hr IV divided q6h)
	Infants and children: 100-200 mg/kg/24 hr IV or IM divided q4-6h (maximum, 12 g/24 hr)

NALOXONE (Narcan)　　*Narcotic Antagonist*

Indications:	Narcotic antidote
Actions:	Competitive antagonism of opiate receptors
Side effects:	Nausea, vomiting; may precipitate withdrawal in narcotic addicts
Comments:	Multiple doses may be necessary because effect is shorter in duration than that of many narcotics
Dose:	0.1 mg/kg/dose IM, IV, or SC (maximum, 2 mg/dose); repeat every 2-3 min as needed

NIFEDIPINE (Adalat, Procardia)　　*Calcium Channel Blocker*

Indications:	Hypertension, hypertrophic cardiomyopathy
Actions:	Arterial vasodilator
Side effects:	Hypotension, headache, dizziness, peripheral edema, syncope, flushing, tachycardia
Comments:	For sublingual use, capsule contents must be aspirated and placed into mouth with syringe (each 0.175 mL = approx 5 mg)
Dose:	Hypertension: 0.25-0.5 mg/kg/dose PO or SL q4-6h
	Cardiomyopathy: 0.2-0.3 mg/kg/dose PO divided q8h

NYSTATIN (Mycostatin)　　*Antifungal*

Indications:	Oral and esophageal candidiasis
Actions:	Disrupts fungal cell membranes
Side effects:	Nausea, vomiting, diarrhea
Comments:	Poorly absorbed orally

Dose:

Preterm infants: 0.5 mL (50,000 U)
  spread to each side of mouth qid
Neonates: 1 mL (100,000 U) as above
Infants: 2 mL (200,000 U) as above
Children: 4-6 mL (400,000-600,000 U),
  swish and swallow qid

ONDANSETRON (Zofran)   *Antiemetic*

Indications:

Nausea and vomiting, especially
  associated with cancer chemotherapy;
  also useful after anesthesia and with
  drug toxicity

Actions:

Competitive antagonist of the
  serotonin-3 receptor

Side effects:

Bronchospasm, tachycardia,
  hypokalemia, lightheadedness,
  headache, seizures, transient
  transaminase elevation

Comments:

Works especially well when given before
  emetogenic chemotherapy

Dose:

0.15 mg/kg/dose IV q8h; 4-8 mg
  PO q8-12h

PENICILLIN G   *Antibiotic*

Indications: Infections with susceptible bacteria
Actions: Inhibits bacterial cell wall synthesis
Side effects: Anaphylaxis, rash, interstitial nephritis,
  hemolytic anemia

Comments:

In meningitis, higher doses at shorter
  intervals should be used
Concurrent use of probenecid will
  prolong half-life

Dose: Neonates:

≤7 days, 1200-2000 g: 50,000 U/kg/
  24 hr IV/IM q12h (meningitis:
  100,000 U/kg/24 hr divided q12h)
≤7 days, >2000 g: 75,000 U/kg/24 hr
  IV/IM divided q8h (meningitis:
  150,000 U/kg/24 hr divided q8h)
>7 days, ≤1200 g: 50,000 U/kg/24 hr
  IV/IM divided q12h (meningitis:
  100,000 U/kg/24 hr divided q12h)
>7 days, 1200-2000 g: 75,000 U/kg/
  24 hr IV/IM divided q8h
  (meningitis: 225,000 U/kg/24 hr
  divided q8h)
>7 days, >2000 g: 100,000 U/kg/24 hr
  IV/IM divided q6h (meningitis:
  200,000 U/kg/24 hr divided q6h)
Children: 100,000-400,000 U/kg/24 hr
  IV/IM divided q4-6h (maximum,
  24 million U/day)

PENICILLIN V POTASSIUM | *Antibiotic*
(Pen-Vee K)

Indications:	Less serious infections with susceptible bacteria
Actions:	Inhibits bacterial cell wall synthesis
Side effects:	As with penicillin G
Comments:	Oral absorption better than with penicillin G; should be taken 1 hr before or 2 hr after meals
Dose:	25-50 mg/kg/24 hr PO divided q4-8h (maximum, 3 g/day)

PHENOBARBITAL | *Barbiturate*

Indications:	Seizures, sedation
Actions:	CNS depressant
Side effects:	Respiratory depression, hypotension, hyperactivity, irritability
Comments:	Contraindicated in hepatic or renal disease; long duration of action; may decrease blood levels of other drugs because of hepatic metabolism induction; therapeutic levels, 15-40 mg/L
Dose:	Sedation: 6 mg/kg/24 hr PO divided tid
	Seizures: 15-20 mg/kg IV as loading dose followed by maintenance dose as follows:
	Neonates: 3-4 mg/kg/24 hr PO or IV divided q12-24h
	Infants and children: 5-6 mg/kg/24 hr PO or IV divided q12-24h
	>12 yr: 1-3 mg/kg/24 hr PO or IV divided q12-24h

PHENYTOIN (Dilantin) | *Anticonvulsant*

Indications:	Seizures
Actions:	Reduces sodium transport across cerebral membranes
Side effects:	Cardiac dysrhythmias, hypotension, ataxia, nystagmus, SLE-like reaction, Stevens-Johnson syndrome, hepatotoxicity, gingival hyperplasia, hirsutism, megaloblastic anemia, lymphadenopathy
Comments:	IV push should not exceed 0.5 mg/kg/min; hepatic metabolism may affect serum levels of many other drugs. Drug is metabolized in fixed amount per unit time; therefore, small changes in dose may cause significant changes in serum concentration. Therapeutic levels, 10-20 mg/L

Dose:
15-20 mg/kg IV as loading dose, followed by maintenance dose as follows: Start at 5 mg/kg/24 hr and adjust based on serum levels
Neonates: 5-8 mg/kg/24 hr PO or IV divided q12-24h
Infants and children: 5-10 mg/kg/24 hr PO or IV divided q12-24h
Note: Oral suspension is unreliable in concentration unless thoroughly mixed or shaken

PIPERACILLIN (Pipracil)
Broad-Spectrum Penicillin

Indications: Infections with susceptible bacteria
Actions: Inhibits bacterial cell wall synthesis
Side effects: As with penicillin G
Comments: Only available parenterally; extends penicillin coverage to include most *Pseudomonas aeruginosa* infections
Dose: Neonates:
≤7 days: 150 mg/kg/24 hr IV divided q8-12h
>7 days: 200 mg/kg/24 hr IV divided q6-8h
Infants and children: 200-300 mg/kg/24 hr IV/IM divided q4-6h (maximum, 24g/24 hr)
In cystic fibrosis: 300-500 mg/kg/24 hr IV/IM divided q4-6h

PREDNISONE (See Systemic Corticosteroids)

PROPRANOLOL (Inderal)
Nonspecific β-Blocker

Indications: Hypertension, migraine, SVT, tetralogy of Fallot "spells"
Actions: Nonspecific (β_1 and β_2) β-adrenergic blockade
Side effects: Hypotension, bradycardia, bronchospasm, congestive heart failure, nausea, vomiting, fatigue, nightmares
Comments: Effect may be diminished if indomethacin, rifampin, or barbiturates are used concurrently; effect may be enhanced by chlorpromazine, hydralazine, verapamil, or cimetidine
Dose: Arrhythmias: 0.01-0.1 mg/kg/dose IV given slowly q6-8h (maximum, 1 mg/dose in infants; 3 mg/dose in children)

Hypertension: 0.5-1.0 mg/kg/24 hr
  PO q6-8h; dose can be gradually
  increased over 3-5 days to maximum
  of 5 mg/kg/24 hr
Migraine prophylaxis: 0.6-2 mg/kg/
  24 hr PO divided q6-8h
Tetralogy "spells": 0.15-0.25 mg/kg/
  dose IV; may repeat in 15 min

RANITIDINE (Zantac)   *Histamine Receptor Blocker*

Indications: Gastroesophageal reflux, gastritis,
                          peptic ulcer
Actions: Inhibits histamine-induced gastric
                          acid secretions
Side effects: Headache, leukopenia, gynecomastia,
                          jaundice
Comments: May cause increased levels of
                          warfarin
Dose: Neonates: 1.5-2 mg/kg/24 hr IV or
                          PO divided q12h
                        Infants and children: 1-5 mg/kg/24 hr
                          IV or PO divided q6-8h
                        Adolescents: 150 mg/dose PO q12h
                          or 300 mg/dose q24h; 50-100 mg/
                          dose IV q6-8h

SODIUM POLYSTYRENE   *Cation Exchange Resin*
  SULFONATE (Kayexalate)

Indications: Hyperkalemia
Actions: Nonabsorbable cation exchange resin
Side effects: Nausea, vomiting, gastric irritation,
                          sodium retention
Dose: Children: 4 g/kg/24 hr PO divided
                          q4-8h; 4-12 g/kg/24 hr PR divided
                          q2-6h
                        Adolescents: 15 g/dose PO q6-12h

SUCRALFATE (Carafate)   *Aluminum Salt*

Indications: Gastritis
Actions: Adheres to mucosal surface
Side effects: Abdominal cramping, constipation,
                          headache
Dose: 40-80 mg/kg/24 hr PO divided q6-8h

TETRACYCLINE   *Antibiotic*

Indications: Infections with susceptible organisms
Actions: Binds to 30S ribosomal subunit,
                          inhibiting transfer RNA attachment
Side effects: Nausea, abdominal pain, hepatotoxicity,
                          stomatitis, photosensitivity, rash,
                          pseudotumor cerebri

Comments: SHOULD NOT BE USED IN
CHILDREN <8 YR or in pregnant
women because of effects on teeth
(staining) and bone growth.
Should be given 1 hr before or
2 hr after meals

Dose: 25-50 mg/kg/day PO divided q6h
(maximum, 2 g/day)

TICARCILLIN (Ticar) *Broad-Spectrum Penicillin*

Indications: Infections with susceptible organisms
Actions: Inhibits bacterial cell wall synthesis
Side effects: Decreased platelet function, rash,
hypocalcemia, hypernatremia
Comments: As with piperacillin, extends penicillin
coverage to include *Pseudomonas*
Dose: Neonates:
≤7 days, ≤1200 g: 150 mg/kg/24 hr
IV divided q8-12h
≤7 days, >1200 g: 225 mg/kg/24 hr
IV divided q8h
>7 days, <1200 g: 150 mg/kg/24 hr
IV divided q12h
>7 days, 1200-2000 g: 225 mg/kg/
24 hr IV divided q8h
>7 days, >2000 g: 300 mg/kg/24 hr
IV divided q6-8h
Children: 200-400 mg/kg/24 hr IV/IM
divided q4-6h (maximum, 24 g/24 hr)

TOBRAMYCIN (Nebcin) *Aminoglycoside*

Indications: Infections with susceptible organisms
Actions: Binds to 30S ribosomal subunit, inhibiting attachment of messenger RNA
Side effects: Ototoxicity, renal toxicity, marrow
suppression
Comments: Therapeutic levels: peak, 6-10 mg/L;
trough, <2 mg/L
Dose: Neonates: 2.5 mg/dose IV, with dosing
interval as follows:
≤7 days, 1200-2000 g: q12-18h
≤7 days, >2000 g: q12h
>7 days, 1200-2000 g: q8-12h
>7 days, >2000 g: q8h
Children: 6-7.5 mg/kg/24 hr IV divided
q8-12h

VANCOMYCIN (Vancocin) *Antibiotic*

Indications: Infections with susceptible organisms
Actions: Inhibits bacterial cell wall synthesis
Side effects: Ototoxicity, renal toxicity, "red man
syndrome"
Comments: Diphenhydramine may be used to treat
"red man syndrome"

Dose:

Neonates:

≤7 days, ≤1200 g: 15 mg/kg/24 hr IV divided q24h

≤7 days, 1200-2000 g: 15 mg/kg/24 hr IV divided q12-18h

≤7 days, >2000 g: 30 mg/kg/24 hr IV divided q12h

>7 days, <1200 g: 15 mg/kg/24 hr IV divided q24h

>7 days, 1200-2000 g: 15 mg/kg/24 hr IV divided q8-12h

>7 days, >2000 g: 45 mg/kg/24 hr IV divided q8h

Infants and children: 45-60 mg/kg/24 hr IV divided q8-12h (meningitis: 15 mg/kg/dose)

For *Clostridium difficile* colitis: 40-50 mg/kg/24 hr PO divided q6h (maximum, 500 mg/day)

WARFARIN (Coumadin)	*Anticoagulant*
Indications:	Hypercoagulable state
Actions:	Antagonizes vitamin K synthesis, depleting vitamin K–dependent clotting factors (II, VII, IX, X)
Side effects:	Bleeding
Comments:	Avoid green leafy vegetables in diet because of high vitamin K content; be aware of multiple drug interactions
Dose:	0.2 mg/kg PO once each day, then titrate to desired INR

Systemic Corticosteroids

I. RELATIVE POTENCY

Equivalent effects are seen with the doses listed.

Drug	Glucocorticoid Effect	Mineralocorticoid Effect
Cortisone	5 mg	5 mg
Hydrocortisone	4 mg	4 mg
Prednisone	1 mg	5 mg
Prednisolone	1 mg	5 gm
Methylprednisolone	0.8 mg	None
Dexamethasone	0.15 mg	None

II. INDICATIONS AND DOSES

Anti-inflammatory and/or immunosuppressive

Preparation and dose: Prednisone, 0.05-2 mg/kg/day PO divided qd-qid

Methylprednisolone, 0.05-2 mg/kg/day divided qd-qid

Prednisolone, 0.05-2 mg/kg/day PO divided qd-qid

"Pulse" methylprednisolone = 30 mg/kg IV qd for 1-3 days (maximum, 1 g/day)

Cerebral edema
Preparation and dose: Dexamethasone, 0.5-1.5 mg/kg/dose IV initially, then 0.2-0.5 mg/kg/day IV divided q6h (adults: 10 mg initially, then 4 mg q6h)

Airway edema
Preparation and dose: Dexamethasone, 0.25-0.5 mg/kg/dose IV or IM q6h

Meningitis
Preparation and dose: Dexamethasone, 0.15 mg/kg/dose IV q6h for 4 days

Reactive airway disease
Preparation and dose: Prednisone, 1-2 mg/kg/day PO divided qd-bid for 3-5 days
Prednisolone, 1-2 mg/kg/day PO divided qd-bid for 3-5 days
Methylprednisolone, 2 mg/kg IV initially, then 0.5 mg/kg/dose IV q6h

Adrenal crisis
Preparation and dose: Hydrocortisone, 1-2 mg/kg IV initially, then 25-250 mg/day IV divided bid-tid

Stress (e.g., surgery in those taking steroids long-term)
Preparation and dose: Cortisone, 50-62.5 mg/m^2/day IV

Physiologic replacement
Preparation and dose: Cortisone, 0.5-0.75 mg/kg/day PO divided q8h, **or**
Cortisone, 0.25-0.35 mg/kg IM qd
Hydrocortisone, 0.5-0.75 mg/kg/day PO divided q8h, **or**
Hydrocortisone, 0.25-0.35 mg/kg IM qd

Index

Note: Page numbers followed by the letter f refer to figures and those followed by t refer to tables.